2022

ADVANCES IN
SMALL ANIMAL CARE

EDITOR-IN-CHIEF
Philip H. Kass

SECTION EDITORS
Chiara Mariti
Angela J. Marolf
Silke Salavati Schmitz
Vanessa R. Barrs
Jonathan Stockman

ELSEVIER

Publishing Director, Medical Reference: Dolores Meloni
Editor: Stacy Eastman
Developmental Editor: Jessica Cañaberal

Reprints: For copies of 100 or more of articles in this publication, please contact the Commercial Reprints Department, Elsevier Inc., 360 Park Avenue South, New York, NY 10010-1710. Tel: 212-633-3874; Fax: 212-633-3820; E-mail: reprints@elsevier.com.

Editorial Office:
Elsevier, Inc.
1600 John F. Kennedy Blvd,
Suite 1800
Philadelphia, PA 19103-2899

International Standard Serial Number: 2666-450X
International Standard Book Number: 978-0-323-84977-7

ADVANCES IN SMALL ANIMAL CARE

EDITOR-IN-CHIEF

PHILIP H. KASS, BS, DVM, MPVM, MS, PhD,
Diplomate ACVPM (Specialty in Epidemiology)
Office of Academic Affairs
School of Veterinary Medicine
School of Medicine
University of California, Davis One Shields Avenue
Davis, CA 95616, USA
phkass@ucdavis.edu

SECTION EDITORS

CHIARA MARITI, DVM, PhD
European Veterinary Specialist in Animal Welfare
Science Ethics and Law
Associate Professor at Dep. Veterinary Sciences,
Università di Pisa (viale delle Piagge 2 Pisa, Italy)
ETOVET lab
chiara.mariti@unipi.it

ANGELA J. MAROLF, DVM, DACVR
Professor, Environmental and Radiological Health
Sciences
College of Veterinary Medicine and Biomedical
Sciences
Colorado State University
Fort Collins, Colorado, USA
angela.marolf@colostate.edu

SILKE SALAVATI SCHMITZ, DR.MED.VET., PhD,
DIPL.ECVIM-CA, FHEA, MRCVS
Senior lecturer in Small Animal Internal Medicine
University of Edinburgh Royal (Dick) School of
Veterinary Studies and The Roslin Institute Hospital
for Small Animals
Easter Bush, Midlothian, UK
Silke.Salavati@ed.ac.uk

VANESSA R. BARRS, BVSc(Hons), PhD,
MVetClinStud, FANZCVS (Feline Medicine)
BOHK Endowed Chair Professor of Veterinary
Medicine
Jockey Club College of Veterinary Medicine and Life
Sciences
Hong Kong, SAR China
vanessa.barrs@cityu.edu.hk

JONATHAN STOCKMAN, DVM, DACVN
Assistant Professor, Department of Veterinary Clinical
Sciences
College of Veterinary Medicine
Long Island University
Old Brookville, New York, USA
jonathan.stockman@liu.edu

CONTRIBUTORS

EDITOR

PHILIP H. KASS, BS, DVM, MPVM, MS, PhD
Diplomate, American College of Veterinary Preventive Medicine (Specialty in Epidemiology); Office of Academic Affairs, University of California, Davis, Davis, California, USA

AUTHORS

MARIANGELA ALBERTINI, DVM, PhD
Professor, Department of Veterinary Medicine and Animal Sciences, University of Milan, Lodi, Italy

ELEONORA AMADEI, DVM, MVSc
Independent Researcher, Carpi, Modena, Italy

PAWEŁ M. BĘCZKOWSKI, DVM, PhD, MRCVS
Diplomate, European College of Veterinary Internal Medicine–Companion Animals; Department of Veterinary Clinical Sciences, Jockey Club College of Veterinary Medicine and Life Sciences, City University of Hong Kong, Kowloon, Hong Kong

JULIA A. BEATTY, BSc(hons), BVetMed, PhD, FANZCVS (Feline med), GradCertEd (Higher Ed), FRCVS, GAICD
Department of Veterinary Clinical Sciences, Jockey Club College of Veterinary Medicine and Life Sciences, City University of Hong Kong, Kowloon, Hong Kong

KATHRIN BUSCH, DVM, Dr med vet
Diplomate, European College of Veterinary Internal Medicine–Companion Animals; Clinic of Small Animal Medicine, Centre for Clinical Veterinary Medicine, Ludwig Maximilians University, Munich, Germany

DANIEL L. CHAN, DVM
Diplomate, American College of Veterinary Emergency Critical Care; Diplomate, European College of Veterinary Emergency and Critical Care; Diplomate, American College of Veterinary Internal Medicine (Nutrition); Section of Emergency and Critical Care, Department of Clinical Science and Services, The Royal Veterinary College, Hertfordshire, United Kingdom

JENNIFER C. CHAN, DVM
William R. Pritchard Veterinary Medical Teaching Hospital, University of California, Davis, Davis, California, USA

JULIEN DANDRIEUX, BSc, Dr med vet, PhD
Diplomate, American College of Veterinary Internal Medicine (Small Animal Internal Medicine), U-Vet, Faculty of Veterinary and Agricultural Sciences, University of Melbourne, Werribee, Victoria, Australia

VALERIE FREICHE, Dr med vet, PhD, DESV-IM
Ecole Nationale Vétérinaire d'Alfort, CHUVA, Unité de Médecine Interne, Maisons-Alfort, France

CHRISTINE GRIEBSCH, Dr med vet, GradCertEdStud (HigherEd), FHEA, PhD Candidate
Diplomate, European College of Veterinary Internal Medicine–Companion Animals; Sydney School of Veterinary Science, University of Sydney, New South Wales, Australia

SARAH HEATH, BVSc, PgCertVE DipECAWBM(BM), CCAB, FHEA, FRCVS
RCVS Veterinary Specialist in Behavioural Medicine, EBVS European Veterinary Specialist in Behavioural Medicine, Visiting Lecturer in Small Animal Behavioural Medicine, University of Liverpool School of Veterinary Science, Behavioural Referrals Veterinary Practice, Chester, United Kingdom

SILKE HECHT, Dr med vet
Diplomate, American College of Veterinary Radiology; Diplomate, European College of Veterinary Diagnostic Imaging; Department of Small Animal Clinical Sciences, University of Tennessee College of Veterinary Medicine, Veterinary Medical Center, Knoxville, Tennessee, USA

SEAN E. HULSEBOSCH, DVM
Diplomate, American College of Veterinary Internal
Medicine; Department of Veterinary Medicine and
Epidemiology, University of California, Davis, Davis,
California, USA

LYNELLE R. JOHNSON, DVM, MS, PhD
Diplomate, American College of Veterinary Internal
Medicine; Department of Veterinary Medicine and
Epidemiology, University of California, Davis, Davis,
California, USA

AARTI KATHRANI, BVetMed (Hons), PhD, FHEA,
MRCVS
Royal Veterinary College, Hatfield, Hertfordshire,
United Kingdom

ANGELA J. MAROLF, DVM
Diplomate, American College of Veterinary
Radiology; Department of Environmental and
Radiological Health Sciences, Colorado State
University Veterinary Teaching Hospital, College of
Veterinary Medicine and Biomedical Sciences,
Colorado State University, Fort Collins, Colorado,
USA

JACQUELINE M. NORRIS, BVSc, MVS, PhD,
FASM, RCVS (Microbiology),
GradCertEdStud(HigherEd)
Sydney School of Veterinary Science, University of
Sydney, New South Wales, Australia

LUDOVICA PIERANTONI, DVM
Diplomate, European College of Animal Welfare and
Behavioural Medicine–Behavioural Medicine; CAN
(Comportamento Animale Napoli) s.s.d.r.l., Naples,
Naples, Italy

PATRIZIA PIOTTI, Dr, DVM, MSc, PhD
Department of Veterinary Medicine and Animal
Sciences, University of Milan, Lodi, Italy

FEDERICA PIRRONE, DVM, PhD
Professor, Department of Veterinary Medicine and
Animal Sciences, University of Milan, Lodi, Lodi, Italy

SILKE SALAVATI SCHMITZ, Dr med vet, FHEA,
PhD, FRCVS
Diplomate, European College of Veterinary Internal
Medicine–Companion Animals; Hospital for Small
Animals, Royal (Dick) School of Veterinary Studies,
College of Medicine and Veterinary Medicine,
University of Edinburgh, Easter Bush, Midlothian,
United Kingdom

BRIAN A. SCANSEN, DVM, MS
Diplomate, American College of Veterinary Internal
Medicine (Cardiology); Professor and Service Head,
Cardiology and Cardiac Surgery, Department of
Clinical Sciences, Colorado State University, Fort
Collins, Colorado, USA

LAUREN VON STADE, DVM
Department of Environmental and Radiological
Health Sciences, Colorado State University Veterinary
Teaching Hospital, College of Veterinary Medicine
and Biomedical Sciences, Colorado State University,
Fort Collins, Colorado, USA

JONATHAN STOCKMAN, DVM
Diplomate, American College of Veterinary Internal
Medicine (Nutrition); Long Island University,
Greenvale, New York, USA

CAMILLE TORRES, DVM
Diplomate, American Board of Veterinary
Practitioners; Diplomate, American College of
Veterinary Internal Medicine (Nutrition); Camille
Torres - Associate Professor Colorado State University
Jonathan Stockman, Assistant Professor Long Island
University, Affiliate Faculty Colorado State University

STEFAN UNTERER, DVM, Dr med vet, Dr habil
Diplomate, European College of Veterinary Internal
Medicine–Companion Animals; Clinic for Small
Animal Internal Medicine, Vetsuisse Faculty,
University of Zurich, Zurich, Switzerland

MICHAEL P. WARD, BVSc(Hons), MSc, MPVM,
PhD, DVSc, FANZCVS
Sydney School of Veterinary Science, University of
Sydney, New South Wales, Australia

CONTENTS

VOLUME 3 • 2022

achieve recognition within the profession. One of the most important developments in the field of feline behavior is an increasing understanding of the fact that emotional and cognitive health are important components of overall health and are of equal significance to physical health, which has been the traditional focus of the veterinary profession. In order for behavioral medicine to become a more mainstream feature of veterinary practice, it is helpful to emphasize the fact that it is another form of internal medicine and requires a very similar approach in terms of diagnosis and selection of management and treatment approaches for specific reported behavioral concerns. In addition, taking a behavioral medicine approach to veterinary practice enhances the diagnosis and treatment of physical disease in patients with feline.

Peripheral Concentration of Amyloid-β, TAU Protein, and Neurofilament Light Chain as Markers of Cognitive Dysfunction Syndrome in Senior Dogs: A Meta-analysis, 23

Patrizia Piotti, Mariangela Albertini, and Federica Pirrone

Canine cognitive dysfunction syndrome (CCDS) is an age-related neurodegenerative disease. The authors reviewed and performed a meta-analysis of the literature covering in vivo peripheral markers for CCDS. The quantitative analysis focused on 6 papers on amyloid-β 40 and 42 in the serum or plasma. Fixed effect models indicated a significant difference between dogs with CCDS and healthy senior controls in the pooled effect for Aβ42, but not Aβ42, showing moderate heterogeneity. Overall, the evidence for clinical use of Aβ as a peripheral marker of CCDS is not sufficient, but the current findings suggest that it is worthy of further research.

SECTION II: DIAGNOSTIC IMAGING

Cardiac Computed Tomography Imaging, 39

Brian A. Scansen

The heart is a 3-dimensional structure, yet nearly all cardiac imaging performed in animals relies on 2-dimensional imaging techniques such as radiography, fluoroscopy, and ultrasonography. Cross-sectional imaging of the heart using cardiac computed tomography (cCT) allows visualization and reconstruction of cardiac anatomy in unique and useful ways and is particularly useful for planning surgical or catheter-based interventions. This review provides an overview of the technical aspects required for cCT as well as methods to optimize imaging protocols, with particular focus on aspects relevant to imaging small animals.

Advanced Imaging of the Pancreas, 57
Lauren von Stade and Angela J. Marolf

Disorders of the pancreas in dogs and cats are often difficult to diagnose with radiographic and conventional ultrasonographic methods. The increased availability and research advancement in imaging technologies including contrast-enhanced ultrasonography, computed tomography, and magnetic resonance imaging are improving clinician options for the detection of diseases such as acute pancreatitis and pancreatic neoplasia, including insulinoma and adenocarcinoma. Advantages of these modalities include detailed assessment of full anatomy, decreased operator dependence, improved patient comfort, and evaluation of organ perfusion. Advanced imaging is now considered the gold standard for the detection and evaluation of pancreatic disease and associated sequelae.

Update on Magnetic Resonance Imaging of the Brain and Spine, 73
Silke Hecht

Compared to radiography, ultrasound, and computed tomography (CT), magnetic resonance imaging (MRI) is considered a "newcomer" in the world of diagnostic imaging. The first MR imaging-related articles were published in the late 1970s and early 1980s. Reports on the use of MRI in animals were largely limited to animal models at that point. Over the following decades and with increasing recognition of the superb imaging capabilities of MRI in combination with the apparent low risk to patients, MRI research and clinical use especially in the area of neurology rapidly grew in both human and veterinary medicine. Today, with few exceptions, MRI is generally recognized as the gold standard for the evaluation of the central nervous system in people and animals. MRI advances over time included improvement of available hardware (eg, type of magnet) and development/improvement of imaging techniques (eg, specialized MRI sequences). This article provides a brief comparison between low and high field MRI systems, gives an overview of recent advances in imaging technology as it pertains to small animal neuroimaging, provides recommendations for MRI protocols for the imaging of the canine and feline brain and spine, and discusses possible limitations of MRI in the evaluation for certain neurologic diseases in dogs and cats.

SECTION III: GASTROENTEROLOGY

Modifying the Gut Microbiota – An Update on the Evidence for Dietary Interventions, Probiotics, and Fecal Microbiota Transplantation in Chronic Gastrointestinal Diseases of Dogs and Cats, *95*
Silke Salavati Schmitz

Modifications of the intestinal microbiota can be achieved by dietary manipulations, introduction of probiotics, and fecal microbiota transplantation (FMT). Most dietary changes have a moderate impact on microbiota composition and diversity. For individual macro- and micronutrients such as dietary fiber and other prebiotics, changes in "gut health" parameters have been observed in healthy animals, but the effect on gastrointestinal disease is less clear. For probiotics, results are mixed, likely due to the use of different probiotic strains, dosages, durations, and the assessment of different outcomes. While FMT is a promising new treatment modality, information on its optimal use in small animals is currently too scarce to make recommendations.

Nutrition in Canine and Feline Gastrointestinal Disease, *109*
Aarti Kathrani

This comprehensive review focuses first on the principles of nutritional management of canine and feline gastrointestinal diseases by detailing the process of nutritional assessment of the patient, the current diet, feeding management, environment, and reassessment and monitoring once the chosen dietary strategy has been implemented. Then a detailed review of the relevant nutritional strategies for the management of acute gastroenteritis, adverse reaction to food, chronic inflammatory enteropathy, intestinal lymphangiectasia, and feline constipation is provided.

Challenges in Differentiating Chronic Enteropathy from Low-Grade Gastrointestinal T-cell Lymphoma in Cats, *121*
Julien Dandrieux and Valérie Freiche

Chronic enteropathies (CEs) are common diseases, particularly in elderly cats. The differentiation between CE and low-grade gastrointestinal T-cell lymphoma (LGITL) remains challenging. The end diagnosis is reached by combining clinical signs with gastrointestinal tract sampling for histology, immunohistochemistry, and molecular testing. There is currently a lack of international guidelines on molecular testing, with variable results depending on the laboratory used. The clinician needs to keep this in mind when requesting and interpreting a test. Although LGITL is neoplastic, the progression is slow, and most cats can be stabilized for 2 years or more with a combination of prednisolone and chlorambucil.

Update on Acute Hemorrhagic Diarrhea Syndrome in Dogs, 133

Kathrin Busch and Stefan Unterer

Clostridial overgrowth and associated release of their toxins is responsible for the pathogenesis of acute hemorrhagic diarrhea syndrome. Diagnosis is based on exclusion of other causes for acute hemorrhagic diarrhea, because only invasive tests, such as small intestinal biopsies identifying clostridial colonization on the surface of a necrotic intestinal mucosa, support a diagnosis. These are not usually performed in unstable, hypovolemic patients with an acute disease. In the absence of complications, most dogs rapidly improve with intensive fluid replacement and symptomatic therapy. The short-term prognosis is good, but one-third of dogs develop signs of chronic gastrointestinal disease later in life.

SECTION IV: INFECTIOUS DISEASE

Feline Immunodeficiency Virus: Current Knowledge and Future Directions, 145

Paweł M. Bęczkowski and Julia A. Beatty

Based on clinical observations and the increasing number of published reports, it is evident that many feline immunodeficiency virus (FIV)-positive cats display mild or inapparent clinical signs and frequently achieve normal life spans. Although the clinical manifestation of infection is determined by unknown viral, host, and environmental factors, the relative intrahost genetic stability of FIV may play an important role in the apparent clinical stability observed in many naturally infected cats. Performance of the commercial Fel-O-Vax FIV vaccine documented in recent field studies is suboptimal, reminding us that the fully efficacious lentiviral vaccine remains elusive.

SECTION V: NUTRITION

Nutritional Management of Acute Pancreatitis, 221
Daniel L. Chan

Medical management of acute pancreatitis has shifted from the concept of "pancreatic rest" to early reinitiation of enteral feeding as soon as it is feasible. This shift is due to improved understanding of the pathophysiology of acute pancreatitis and growing evidence of the benefits of enteral feeding in this disease. Nutritional planning for patients with acute pancreatitis centers on nutritional assessment, selecting the most appropriate approach of nutritional support, and initiating enteral feeding as soon as it is feasible. Monitoring for tolerance of enteral feeding and adjusting the nutritional plan as appropriate is key in the management of these patients.

Creating a Weight Loss Plan with Owner Engagement, 229
Camille Torres and Jonathan Stockman

The obesity epidemic affects more than half of dogs and cats in westernized countries. This disease has several negative implications on the quality of life, risk of concurrent disease, and longevity. Many pet owners may not recognize their pet is obese or realize the implications of obesity. Weight loss is a lengthy process that requires the owner's commitment and diligence. There are multiple hurdles that can impede a successful outcome; however, there are steps that the veterinary team can take to mitigate some of the challenges during the pet's weight loss and increase the chances for success.

Preface

Year Three of This Journal: Bringing Future Developments in Veterinary Medicine Closer to Reality

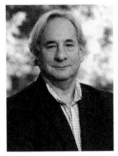

Philip H. Kass, BS, DVM, MPVM, MS, PhD
Editor

As any astute editor will tell you, there are often vast chasms between the transmission of discovery and the perturbation of empirical practice and standard of care. Auspicious developments in research may fail the test of time, and those with the most promise may still be years away from entering medical curricula, much less becoming available for widespread use.

The philosophy of this journal is to bring the future closer to reality and create a sense of anticipation among readers about not only what soon lies ahead, but also what is sufficiently ready to alter our standards of practice and questions the dogma of our engrained knowledge and belief. Scarcely an easy feat, it is accomplished by receiving exciting, new contributions solicited from a distinguished cadre of scientific experts from all over the world. The time between receipt of

the initial drafts of these articles and the publication date is less than one year, guaranteeing that this new knowledge is truly cutting-edge veterinary medicine. And far from being opinion pieces, these review articles are extensively documented to ensure that they adhere to the highest scientific standards.

This issue's Section I begins with a topic that has particular relevance during the COVID-19 pandemic: cat and dog behavior. A consequence of sheltering in place and remote work is that it not only profoundly affected the relationship between worker and workplace, but also has redefined the human-animal bond in an unexpected way. As people began to develop home or hybrid work environments, they sought pet companions, which in some regions led to a shortfall of adoptable pets from traditional sources, such as animal shelters. As the pandemic inevitably evolves into a

https://doi.org/10.1016/j.yasa.2022.08.001
2666-450X/22/ © 2022 Published by Elsevier Inc.

state of endemicity, it remains to be seen if these relationships similarly endure. Understanding behavior, and the challenges it can bring, may become even more vitally important than in past times if we are to avoid a relinquishment backlash as people begin to return to more traditional workplaces.

Section II provides three articles on new advances on the imaging of the heart, pancreas, brain, and spine. What once were diagnostic tools restricted to only the most advanced tertiary care facilities are now becoming far more accessible and affordable, meaningfully raising the standards of veterinary medical practice as they already have in human health.

Section III returns to a familiar yet urgently important topic to every veterinarian: gastroenterology. Understanding the relationships between gut microflora, food, and systemic health is still in the early stages, but the two articles examining these topics bring such understanding far closer. Diagnostic gastroenterology is a long-standing area for growth, whether differentiating between chronic inflammation and neoplasia, or between the different causes of hemorrhagic gastroenteritis and diarrhea, and the two new articles bring readers up-to-date on these ubiquitous medical challenges.

Section IV of this issue introduces readers to emerging knowledge about two important small animal infectious diseases: feline immunodeficiency virus infection, as well as the widespread zoonotic disease leptospirosis. It also provides an important roadmap for the diagnosis of infectious diseases of the respiratory tract, allowing more precise medical interventions than the broad-spectrum approaches of earlier times.

Finally, the issue ends in Section V with two articles that will be of interest and vital importance to any small animal practitioner: nutritional management of acute pancreatitis, and developing a functional weight loss program that owners will adhere to and achieve success with.

As this journal continues to flourish, it remains essential that we provide the most up-to-date and topical resources for practitioners that bridge the gap between peer-reviewed scientific journals, publishing the discovery of new knowledge, and the textbooks that can be years in the making. I value your feedback about the contents of this issue and welcome suggestions for future issues if the topics can fortuitously fall into this exciting opportunistic publication niche.

Philip H. Kass, BS, DVM, MPVM, MS, PhD
Office of Academic Affairs
University of California, Davis
One Shields Avenue
Davis, CA 95616, USA

E-mail address: phkass@ucdavis.edu

SECTION I: BEHAVIOR

Advances in Small Animal Care 3 (2022) 1–11

ADVANCES IN SMALL ANIMAL CARE

Factors to Consider when Selecting Puppies and Preventing Later Behavioral Problems

Ludovica Pierantoni, DVM, Dipl ECAWBM-BM[a],*, Eleonora Amadei, DVM, MVSc[b], Federica Pirrone, DVM, PhD[c]

[a]CAN (Comportamento Animale Napoli) s.s.d.r.l., Rione Sirignano, 9, Naples, NA, Italy; [b]Via E.Curiel, 14, 41012, Carpi, MO, Italy; [c]Department of Veterinary Medicine and Animal Science, University of Milan, Via dell'Università, 6, Lodi 26900, LO, Italy

---

KEYWORDS

- Behavior • Dog • Early experiences • Maternal care • Puppy development

KEY POINTS

- Appropriate handling of prenatal and early life aspects could help to improve human–pet bond and prevent the outcome of negative behavioral consequences, which may become long-lasting.
- Critical aspects in puppy behavioral development may be maternal environment and early life stress, attachment and maternal care, age of adoption and puppy origin, and early life experiences and socialization.
- Environment should provide an adequate level of stimulation customized by type and timing but the definition of "adequate" is still lacking.
- General and behavioral medicine veterinarians and professional dog trainers should play a key role in managing the delicate phases of the early life of a puppy.

INTRODUCTION

In 2020, the dog population in Europe was measured at approximately 89.82 million, registering an increase from around 87.5 million in the previous year. Dogs are today part of the human family, who provide for their needs and desires, and consider them as family members (93.3% according to Kubinyi and colleagues [1]), particularly like children (62% according to Pirrone and colleagues [2]).

The role of dogs as companions heavily depends on the development of a successful dog–owner relationship, and many dogs are known to be abandoned because they display behaviors that their owners find unacceptable [3]. A dog's maladaptive behaviors may compromise the benefits associated with dog ownership [4] as well as the overall welfare of the dog [3].

In a changing environment, genes interact with the environment and with past experiences, thus contributing to the modification of the behavioral phenotype [5]. Evidence supports a genetic component for psycho-behavioral traits in dogs such as anxiety/fear, noise phobia, human aversion, obsessive-compulsive disorder, predatory behavior, and at least 2 types of aggression: impulse/control and conspecific [6–9]. Moreover, the psycho-pathological outcome from early trauma may have, at least in part, a hereditary basis [10]. However, the observable behavior of an animal is due to the complex interaction of genetics, environment, and experiences [11] (Fig. 1). The combination

---

*Corresponding author, *E-mail address:* ludovica.pierantoni@gmail.com

https://doi.org/10.1016/j.yasa.2022.05.001
2666-450X/22/

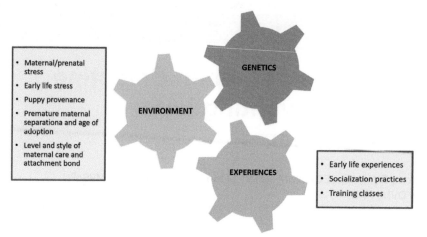

FIG. 1 Determining factors of the puppy behaviors.

of these factors may affect the physiology and behavior of puppies, having neuroendocrine, behavioral or epigenetic consequences that may persist throughout life [12]. With regards to factors related to environment and experience, it is generally accepted that early life experiences and socialization, attachment and maternal care [13], age of adoption [14], and the origin of the dog [12,15] have long-lasting consequences for the behavioral and physiologic development of an individual.

Here, the authors will go through the intertwining of these factors and discuss how to best manage them in order to avoid the development of negative behavioral consequences which may become long-lasting.

CRITICAL ASPECTS IN BEHAVIORAL DEVELOPMENT

Prenatal Experiences

Exposure of a pregnant female to environmental stressors may have long-lasting effects on the mental health and behavioral outcomes of the offspring later in life, mainly as a result of dysregulation of the HPA axis that, in turn, involves decreased feedback inhibition of corticotropin-releasing hormone and prolonged elevation of plasma corticosteroids [16,17].

Research on the effects of prenatal experiences has associated maternal stress with many adverse effects among the offspring. In species other than canids an impaired ability to cope with stress, maladaptive social behavior, increased fearfulness, decreased exploratory behavior, impaired adaptation to conditions of conflict, and diminished attention span have been demonstrated [16,18,19].

Sensitive Periods and Early Life Stress

Sensitive periods represent phases in development during which certain capacities are readily shaped or altered by experience. Six sensitive periods, including the prenatal period, neonatal period, transitional period, socialization period, juvenile period, and adult period, have been described in domestic canine development [18,19].

In mammals, it is well known that stress during the formative periods of neural development, from the prenatal stage through adolescence, has a huge and often lifelong effect on brain structure and function and, as a consequence, on ontogeny of behavior [15].

A list of possible behavioral effects related to stressful events during sensitive periods is presented in Table 1.

Canine studies on the long-term effects of early life stress are rare. Foyer and colleagues [10] have reported long-term behavioral effects in dogs who were exposed to stressful environments and experiences during their first 10 days of life. That period is when they were in their neonatal sensitive period and, therefore, were immature from a sensory point of view and totally dependent on the mother for nourishment, warmth, and elimination.

It has to be said that a certain amount of stress, as that produced by gentle manipulation, is desirable during this time because it may help an individual cope with stressors as adult [20,21]. In rodents, human handling of newborns causes increased maternal care, which is suggested to be responsible for making the separated rats less reactive and more emotionally stable compared with unhandled controls, presumably by decreasing the release of corticotropin-releasing factor [22].

TABLE 1	
Prenatal/early life stress and likely behavioral effects	
Timing and kind of stress	**Behavioral effects**
Stressful environment during prenatal period [16,18,19]	• Impaired ability to cope with stress • Maladaptive social behavior • Increased fearfulness • Decreased exploratory behavior • Impaired adaptation to conflict-related conditions • Decreased attention span
Stressful environment during neonatal period [10]	• Long-lasting effects on coping styles in a stressful test situation encountered as adult
Gentle manipulation during neonatal and transitional period [20–23]	• Better ability to cope with stressors as adult • Increased emotional stability and desire to explore compared with unstimulated dogs
Stressful event during socialization period [39,40]	• Marked effect on the development of behavior (increase in aggression, fear, and stress-related disorders)

Handling also seems to accelerate the maturation of nervous structures in some species.

Dog puppies exposed to gentle handling daily from the third day postpartum until the 21st, and then tested at the age of 8 weeks to assess their emotionality, were found to be more emotionally stable and willing to explore than unstimulated control dogs [23].

Of course, if stress becomes excessive in this stage of neurologic development, detrimental effects may occur that impair an individual's both mental and physical health.

The third week of life is defined as the "transitional period." Conventionally, it begins with the opening of the eyelids and ends when the startle response appears [24]. As a consequence of sensory development, exposure to stimuli during this period facilitates rapid behavioral changes and states, sensory abilities, and physiologic adaptations [25].

During this period, puppies start to explore their environment and interact with social and environmental stimuli. Consequently, the environment must provide stimulation in adequate amount, type, and timing. Animal-based research suggests that poor or little sensory exposure at this stage can result in reduced sensory capacity [26], and modifications of normal patterns of postnatal sensory experience can have significant effects on early brain growth and development [27,28]. The authors of another study [29] compared the average age and dynamics of sensory-motor development and behavior of dog puppies on postnatal days 10 to 21. The duration and frequency of puppy behaviors varied significantly with breed and season of

birth. Breed and gender differences in gross motor and sensory development were also observed.

From 4 to 16 weeks of age, dog puppies are in their socialization period, when they readily acquire behaviors that define their future abilities to form social partnerships with dogs, other animals, and humans. Adequate socialization is necessary for producing a well-balanced and well-adjusted dog [30]. As long as the pup interacts with its environment and learns about relevant stimuli, the connections between neural synapses become stronger and neural circuits more stable [31]. Afterward, only the synapses that have been stimulated will survive. The stabilization of the synapses, as well as efficiency of sensory systems' discriminatory capacities, depends on the environmental conditions and leads to an "individualization" of the structural and functional characteristics of the nervous system. Thus, exposure to stimuli and social experiences in this phase has a proportionately greater effect on the formation of neural structures, temperament, and behavior than events later in life [32].

In Tables 2 possible correlations between socialization practices and behavioral effects are summarized.

When later exposed to social stimuli, puppies that were totally socially isolated from people or dogs until 14 to 16 weeks of age showed fear-related behaviors and avoidance [33,34], highlighting very clear negative impacts of poor socialization.

Puppies that have not had the opportunity to experience a variety of stimuli reportedly present several problematic behaviors later in life, including neophobic responses, hyperactivity, impaired social behavior and

TABLE 2
Socialization practices and likely behavioral effects

Socialization practices	Behavioral effects
Totally socially isolated from people or dogs until 14–16 wk [33,34]	• Fear-related behaviors and avoidance
Puppy isolated from other dogs [72]	• Possibility to recover social behaviors with later integration into the group
Poor or little sensory exposure during transitional period [26]	• Reduced sensory capacity
Poor socialization [36,38]	• Neophobic responses • Impaired social behavior and relationships • Reduced learning ability • Aggressive behaviors
Early socialization [36]	• Developed a thriving dog–owner bond
Adequate socialization [30]	• Well-balanced and well-adjusted dogs
Extra socialization programs [41]	• Positive effects on the behavioral responses of puppies even after a year
Attended puppy class [60,63–66,68]	• Reduced risk of aggression toward unfamiliar people and dogs • Reduced odds of displaying family-dog aggression, nonsocial fear, and touch sensitivity and increased trainability. • Displayed fewer behavioral problems as adults • Not significantly improve puppies' behavior
Experienced thunder before than 4 mo of age [37]	• Fear of noises, such as thunders and fireworks

relationships, decreased exploratory behavior, diminished learning ability, and aggression [33–36]. Evidence of the importance of appropriate types of socialization comes from the study by Blackwell and colleagues [37], where it was shown that adult dogs with a fear of noises, such as thunder and fireworks, were more likely to have experienced thunder when they were younger than 4 months of age.

An Australian study used a retrospective questionnaire to quantify the amount and age of early social experiences of pet dogs with reported interdog aggression. Results showed that every week that an owner waited to begin public social exposure reduced the odds of their dog becoming aggressive to other dogs as an adult by 4.2%. There was no significant change in odds of dogs becoming aggressive to other dogs with increasing time spent with unfamiliar dogs or increasing numbers of dogs met per week in public areas during the first 8 weeks of public social exposure. It should be noted that, in this study, the quality of the interaction was not assessed, thus the results might be related to having lived negative experiences in unprotected environments rather than to the frequency of the experiences

themselves. However, one cannot exclude that negative experiences occurring to young puppies in public may predispose them to later aggression [38].

Overall, stressful events during the socialization period may have a particularly marked effect on the development of behavior [39,40].

The heightened sensitivity to positive environmental influences during the socialization period seems to be similarly sensitive to negative influences [33], leading to a deep impact of traumatic experiences on an animal's later responses.

Finally, extra socialization programs have positive effects on the behavioral responses of puppies even after a year [41].

Level of maternal care
Maternal care, expressed with physical contact with the pups, licking the pups (including anogenital licking) and nursing is crucial in the life of the offspring because it ensures neonatal survival and provides appropriate environmental and sensorial stimuli during the first period of life [42,43]. Furthermore, maternal care influences the expression of glucocorticoid receptors at the

hippocampus level and modulate behavioral responses to stress [44]. This is important to consider in altricial species, such as dogs, where offspring are unable to care for themselves at birth and effects of maternal care on stress-related behaviors may therefore be particularly marked.

High level of maternal care and responsiveness promote a less reactive stress response and an improvement in individual resiliency [45]. Low levels of maternal care may instead lead to increased activity of the HPA axis, thus impairing neural development and resulting in heightened stress response and higher risk of long-term disease in the adult animal [46].

A relatively novel concept in dogs is maternal care as a predisposing factor for dog anxiety. The correlation between maternal care in puppyhood and anxiety development in dogs has been identified by Tiira and Lohi [47]. In this study, in which more than 3000 dog owners were involved, dogs that had an owner-reported lowered maternal care score were significantly more likely to be at risk of anxiety.

Direct evidence for a link between maternal behavior and puppy anxiety later in life has also been recently documented [10]. Maternal and puppy behaviors of 22 German shepherd litters were observed and coded: at 18 months of age, puppy behaviors classified as physical and social engagement, as well as aggression were significantly affected by the level of maternal care received.

In contrast to these findings, however, the authors of an earlier study [48] found higher level of maternal care as positively associated with undesirable anxiety-related behaviors and performance in young adult dogs. Further studies are needed to unravel these issues.

Style of Maternal Care

Bitches are known to use 3 different postures to breast-feed: they may lie on their side (lateral nursing), stand or sit down (vertical nursing), or lie on their belly (ventral nursing). These different nursing styles can make the accessibility of the nipple more or less easy, having consequences on the pups.

In a study on guide dogs, the nursing style of the mother seemed to influence the success rate of guide dog training in the pups, with ventral nursing being associated with failure and vertical nursing with success [49].

Vertical nursing requires more effort than ventral nursing because it is harder for the pups to breastfeed. Puppies whose mothers chose the vertical style were subjected to small challenges in their early days and this gave them the opportunity to acquire a certain degree of independence, leading to a reduced incidence of anxiety-related behaviors. A higher chance of success in the training was described in these puppies.

Maternal Care–separation

Another critical aspect in behavioral development is the relationship between the mother and pup and the weaning process. In nature, weaning of mammalian young is usually a relatively slow process. Separation, especially if it occurs before the natural age of weaning, is itself stressful/traumatic [50] impairing the individual's ability to cope with additional stressors in the future [51]. Slabbert and Rosa [52] evaluated the expression of social behaviors toward humans as well as physical development in dogs separated from their mother early (6 weeks) and late (12 weeks). Puppies separated at 6 weeks of age showed more distress vocalizations, greater weight loss, illness, and mortality compared with puppies separated later. In another study, Pierantoni and colleagues [14] examined the prevalence of behaviors in dogs separated from the litter for adoption at different ages. The odds of displaying destructiveness, excessive barking, fearfulness on walks, reactivity to noises, toy possessiveness, food possessiveness, and attention-seeking were significantly greater for those that had been removed from the litter earlier in the socialization period (30–40 days old). In particular, dogs separated early were 15 times more likely to be fearful on walks, and 7 times more likely to display noise fear and attention seeking. These results confirm how early separation of a puppy from the litter is an experience that may increase the animal's chances of showing potentially problematic behaviors as an adult.

Maternal Care–attachment

To optimize the chances of survival, individuals need to explore the environment while maintaining a line of protection: this is achieved by behavioral strategies related to the attachment bond [51]. When an attachment bond is structured, the reference figure acts as a safe haven providing comfort in stressful situation, and as a secure base that gives confidence to explore the environment [B4 [53], B1 [54]]. Most studies on attachment bonds in dogs have investigated the human–dog relationship, whereas intraspecific attachment bond has received much less attention [55]. Prato-Previde and colleagues [56] suggested that an attachment behavioral system exists in the puppy–mother relationship: when exposed to a social or environmental stressor, puppies seek proximity with their mother, who act as a secure-base. In the study by Mariti and colleagues [57], a human stranger was found to have a stronger ameliorative effect than a cohabitant dog on the stress response to isolation in family dogs exposed to a modified version of the Ainsworth strange situation test.

However, dogs tested with their mother displayed both social and nonsocial behaviors in a very similar manner when in the company of the stranger or of the mother [58] demonstrating that adult dogs showed a stronger bond for their mother.

A puppy's provenance

It is a common thought among veterinarians and canine professionals that dogs obtained as puppies from pet shops have a higher prevalence of health and behavioral problems. However, studies reported inconsistent results [59,60] (Table 3). In a very small sample size of dogs (n = 20), Jagoe [60] found that those coming from a pet shop had a significantly higher prevalence of owner-directed (dominance-type) aggression and social fears (fear of strangers, children, and unfamiliar dogs) than did dogs from 5 other sources, namely breeders, animal shelters, friends or relatives, found or rescued off the streets, and home bred. In a convenience sample of 413 companion dogs, of which 47 were obtained from pet shops, Bennett and Rohlf [59] discovered that dogs purchased from pet shops or shelters were considered by their owners to be more unfriendly or aggressive than dogs purchased from breeders, and significantly more nervous than dogs bred by the owner. Casey and colleagues [61] found an increased risk of aggression toward family members in dogs obtained from sources such as pet shops, as compared with those obtained directly from breeders. According to authors, puppies acquired from pet shops may be less socialized or be subjected to less careful selections. Owners that adopt a puppy from this source may also be less

prone to dedicate time and effort to the training of the newly adopted puppy or less tolerant of the misbehavior of their dogs compared with people who adopt dogs from official breeders. The authors of [62] found that dogs acquired from pet shops showed a higher incidence of problematic behaviors related to aggression than those obtained from noncommercial breeders. In this study, however, demographic and background information that could influence the results were not included. In a subsequent study, Pirrone and colleagues [12] evaluated the effect of store provenance on the puppy's later behavior while controlling owner-related confounders. After adjusting for potential confounders, the odds of displaying owner-directed aggression were significantly greater for the dogs that had been purchased from a pet shop as puppies than those purchased from a breeder.

Many factors might account for this finding. First, assuming that genotype contributes to the development of adult behavioral phenotypes in dogs, one cannot consider that pet shops may obtain their puppies from so-called puppy mills or puppy factories, that are high-volume, substandard dog-breeding operations, which sell purebred or mixed-breed dogs where little attention is paid to the selection of dogs for breeding [https://www.sciencedirect.com/science/article/pii/S1558787817300102?via%3Dihub59]. Second, we know that if the mother undergoes stressful treatments, this may affect the later stress response in the offspring by inducing epigenetic effect on glucocorticoid receptors, which causes hyperreactivity in rodents and humans [63]. Third, pet shop dogs might be less adequately socialized as puppies and may be subjected to several stressors including those related to transport of puppy from their breeding facility, handling, confinement, acting as potential predisposing factors for problematic behaviors [62].

TABLE 3
Provenance and likely behavioral effects

From pet shop vs other origins	Behavioral effects
Pet shops/shelters vs bred by the owner [58]	• Considered by their owners to be significantly more nervous
Pet shops/shelters vs breeders [12,60,61]	• Considered by their owners to be more unfriendly or aggressive • Increased risk of aggression toward family members • Higher incidence of problematic behaviors related to aggression
Pet shop vs breeders/animal shelters/friends or relatives/found or Rescued off the streets/and home bred [59]	• Significantly higher prevalence of owner-directed (dominance-type) aggression and social fears (fear of strangers, children, and unfamiliar dogs)

Learning and Experiences

The early socialization of puppies is known to also exert an important role in developing a thriving dog–owner bond [36].

In puppy socialization and training classes, puppies are exposed to a variety of stimuli, which are presented in a nonthreatening way, and they have the opportunity to learn acceptable behaviors to better adapt to the society in which they live [63]. This contributes to the development of normal social relationships in adult dogs. Nevertheless, studies on the effects of puppy classes gave controversial results (see Table 2). Puppies that attended socialization classes were less likely to be surrendered to a shelter [64], presented a reduced risk of aggression toward unfamiliar people and dogs [61,65] and displayed fewer behavioral problems as adults [66]. However, many other factors were found to be related to these aspects, so that it seemed likely that puppy classes were only one of the potential factors that predicted those outcomes. Other studies suggested that puppy socialization programs did not significantly improve puppies' responses, if compared with nonattending puppies [67,68]. A possible explanation arises from the fact that puppies living in human families are already receiving a sufficient amount of stimuli, and therefore additional stimulation may not ensure a tangible result.

In contrast to the afore mentioned studies, using the standardized assessment tool C-BARQ to assess the effect of puppy class attendance on the behavior of participant dogs 1 year later, Gonzalez- Martinez A. and colleagues [69] found that puppy class attendance was significantly correlated to reduced odds of displaying family-dog aggression, nonsocial fear, and touch sensitivity and increased trainability.

One of the reasons why puppy classes do not always seem to be effective could relate to the ways in which some of the classes are run. Considering that many behavioral problems may potentially derive from a lack of owners' knowledge of canine behavior, studies aimed at assessing the effectiveness of advice provided to owners of newly adopted puppies were carried out which offered encouraging results.

Information given to the owners turned out as important in improving training and reducing confrontational methods, which can lead to conflict between owners and dogs and increased anxiety and uncertainty in the dog [3]. According to the author of ref. [70], counseling owners at the time of pet acquisition may have beneficial effects in the prevention of inappropriate behaviors. Similarly, dogs whose owners received advice by a veterinary behaviorist concerning puppy raising during the first visit displayed fewer undesirable behaviors than the control group in their later life [71].

DISCUSSION AND PRACTICAL IMPLICATIONS

In this review, we have summarized and analyzed the existing literature on socialization and sensitive periods, maternal care and attachment bond, provenance of the dogs, experiences, and training, providing evidence on the importance of all these aspects in the adult behavioral expression.

The applications of this review can be summarized in the following points:

- Correct age of adoption: the adoption of puppies aged between 30 and 40 days may have negative consequences on their behavior [14]. However, a recent study [72] also showed that puppies adopted between 13 and 17 weeks of life presented an increased risk of displaying behavior problems mainly related to social fear and aggression. Therefore, the correct time of rehoming of puppies may be a balance between the need for receiving enough maternal care and the need to have enough time to adapt to the new environment.
- A clear demonstration of a mechanistic link between a premature maternal separation and the development of behavior problems would reduce the prevalence of prematurely adopted dogs and allow intervention for those who have been adopted out too early.
- As in human newborns, the attachment bond between the puppies and the mother is likely to be affected by quality and quantity of maternal care, ultimately influencing the dog–human attachment bond as well. Information on the link between maternal care and attachment is lacking as well as information on the potential role of the mother's temperament and behavior, type of litter, and previous maternal experiences on the quality of the attachment bond [13]. Further investigations are therefore strongly needed.
- Although socialization occurs throughout the life of the dog for maintenance of social relationships and behaviors, the socialization period in dogs is considered to be the period from 4 to 16 weeks of age, during which a dog defines his abilities to form social relationship. Moreover, as for dogs, the term "socialization" should not be simply intended as the process by which an animal learn species recognition because it includes also habituation, by which they

get used to nonthreatening environmental stimuli, learning to ignore them. It is not surprising, in fact, that dogs grown up in a nondomestic environment and deprived of experience of urban environments between 3 and 6 months of age were found more likely to exhibit aggression toward unfamiliar people and avoidance behavior [73]. Moreover, dogs born at home where they will remain later had a reduced risk of displaying fearful behaviors as adults as compared with dogs purchased from breeder by a second owner [74]. This means that the more the environment where growth occurs is similar to the future life environment, the lower is the risk of developing behavioral problems later. Dog's population may be divided into different classes according to the level of relationship they have with humans. In southern Italy, there are many "stray dogs," abandoned by humans living in the city, suburbs, or rural communities, who live as free-ranging dogs but are still dependent on humans for nutrition. Otherwise, "feral dogs" are elusive and have a greater flight distance from humans, on whom they do not depend for food and protection. In southern Italy, there is a very particular situation: regional laws provide for the release of stray dogs after being neutered in the area they came from. In the authors' opinion, the release into freedom is not only correct both ethically and ethologically but it is also necessary: the shelters in fact are chronically overcrowded, which often prevents their normal functioning. Many shelter dogs have no chance of being adopted due to their suspicious nature of people, which would lead them to experience very strong discomfort in a domestic situation. For feral dogs, the shelter risks becoming a life sentence, whereas the choice to release them in extraurban areas guarantees respect for their need of freedom, dignity, and overall welfare. Based on previously addressed issues, for feral dogs, adaptation to an anthropic urban context is very challenging. Therefore, if they are housed and adopted, many of them are candidates to develop problematic behaviors, particularly those related to fear and aggression.

- Poor socialization can have detrimental effects on behavior. Although we know there must be a required minimum, we are still unable to estimate it. Some of the puppies isolated from other dogs in the experiments conducted by Fisher and colleagues [75] were able to subsequently recover social behaviors that allowed them to integrate into the group. Moreover, a study by Fuller [35] found that the negative behavioral effects of social isolation of puppies from humans could be prevented by as little as 20 minutes of exposure to humans twice per week from age 4 to 16 weeks. Furthermore, it is unknown whether a maximum amount of socialization is required, beyond which any extra socialization is useless or even harmful. For ethical reasons, studies on environmental hypostimulation that were carried out in the past cannot be replicated, and it is possible that current research actually compares normal stimulation levels with enriched stimulation levels. Retrospective studies with questionnaires cannot demonstrate a causal link; it is possible that the reduced exposure to social stimuli in problematic puppies is a consequence, and not a cause, of the problem itself.

- Puppy socialization practices are considered crucial in the development of social relationship and psychological health in adult dogs; however, evidence is less clear on the benefit of puppy classes, specifically [36]. Many puppy classes are conducted by first-level trainers. Unfortunately, there are no standards in Europe on dog training, so the quality of courses could significantly vary. During the socialization period, it is imperative that puppies have their experiences in a gradual and positive way. If a puppy class is not properly conducted, it may end up being a stressful event for the puppies involved and potentially result in behavioral problems during the puppy's development.

- Finally, the first veterinary visit should be considered an important opportunity to provide owners with information on responsible and competent pet ownership.

Studies on these topics are lacking and more research is strongly needed to gain more precise information that might also help to regulate the delicate steps that occur between the birth of the puppy and the entry into the new home ultimately increasing the chances of a happy and peaceful human–pet bond.

CLINICS CARE POINTS

- Limit exposure of a pregnant female and puppy to environmental stressors may help to prevent negative long-lasting effects on the mental health and behavioral outcomes of puppy.

- When scheduling timing for rehoming of puppies, it is imperative to look for a balance between the need for receiving enough maternal care and the need to have enough time to adapt to the new environment.

- During anamnesis process, it is important to pick information about level and style of maternal care and the provenance of the puppy because it could influence their behavior.

- Be aware that during the socialization period, puppies must have their experiences in a gradual and positive way.

ACKNOWLEDGMENT

The authors would like to thank Macarena Acuna Kitto, native English speaker, for language revision.

DISCLOSURE

The authors have nothing to disclose.

REFERENCES

[1] Kubinyi E, Turcsán B, A M. Dog and owner demographic characteristics and dog personality trait associations. Behav Process 2009;81:392–401.

[2] Pirrone F, Pierantoni L, Mazzola S, et al. Owner and animal factors predict the incidence of, and owner reaction toward, problematic behaviors in companion dogs. J Vet Behav 2015;10(4):295–301.

[3] Landsberg GM, Hunthausen W, Ackerman L. Canine aggression. In: Hunthausen W, editor. Handbook of behaviour problems of the dog and cat. 3th edition. London: Saunders; 2012. p. 129–50.

[4] Serpell J, Jagoe JA. Early experience and the development of behaviour. In: Serpell J, editor. The domestic dog: its evolution, behaviour, and interactions with people. Cambridge, UK: Cambridge University Press; 1995. p. 79–102.

[5] Mills DS. Using learning theory in animal behaviour. Therapy Practice. Vet Clin North Am Small Anim Pract 1997;27(3):617–35.

[6] Murphree OD, Dykman RA. Litter patterns in the offspring of nervous and stable dogs. I. Behavioral tests. J Nerv Ment Dis 1965;141(3):321–32.

[7] Overall KL, Dunham AE. Clinical features and outcome in dogs and cats with obsessive-compulsive disorder: 126 cases (1989-2000). J Am Vet Med Assoc 2002;221: 1445–52.

[8] Liinamo AE, van den Berg L, Leegwater PAJ, et al. Genetic variation in aggression-related traits in Golden Retriever dogs. Appl Anim Behav Sci 2007;104:95–106.

[9] Dodman NH, Karlsson EK, Moon Fanelli A, et al. A canine chromosome 7 locus confers compulsive disorder susceptibility. Mol Psychiatry 2010;15:8–10.

[10] Foyer P, Wilsson E, Wright DE, et al. Early experiences modulate stress coping in a population of German shepherd dogs. Appl Anim Behav Sci 2013;146:79–87.

[11] Plomin R, Asbury K. Nature and nurture: genetic and environmental influences on behavior. Ann Am Acad Polit Social Sci 2005;600:86.

[12] Pirrone F, Pierantoni L, Pastorino GQ, et al. Owner-reported aggressive behavior towards familiar people may be a more prominent occurrence in pet shop-traded dogs. J Vet Behav Clin Appl Res 2016;11:13–7.

[13] Dietz L, Arnold A-MK, Goerlich-Jansson VC, et al. The importance of early life experiences for the development of behavioural disorders in domestic dogs. Behaviour 2018;155:83.

[14] Pierantoni L, Albertini M, Pirrone F. Prevalence of owner-reported behaviours in dogs separated from the litter at two different ages. Vet Rec 2011;169:468–73.

[15] Mc Millan FD. Behavioral and psychological outcomes for dogs sold as puppies through pet stores and/or born in commercial breeding establishments: Current knowledge and putative causes. J Vet Behav 2017;19: 14–26.

[16] Beydoun H, Saftlas AF. Physical and mental health outcomes of prenatal maternal stress in human and animal studies: a review of recent evidence. Paediatr Perinat Epidemiol 2008;22(5):438–66.

[17] Huizink AC, MulderEJ, Buitelaar JK. Prenatal stress and risk for psychopathology: specific effects or induction of general susceptibility? Psychol Bull 2004;130:115–42.

[18] Overall KL. Canine behavior. Normal canine behavior and ontogeny: neurological and social development, signaling, and normal canine behaviors. In: Elsevier editor. Manual of clinical behavioral medicine for dogs and cats. St. Louis, Missouri: Elsevier Mosby; 2013. p. 123–8.

[19] Scott J, Fuller J. Genetics and the social behavior of the dog. Chicago (IL): University of Chicago Press; 1965.

[20] Selye H. History of the adaption syndrome (told in the form of informal, illustrated lectures). Montreal: Acta med. Publishers; 1952.

[21] Fox MV, Stelzner D. The effects of early experience on the development of inter and intraspecies social relationships in the dog. Anim Behav 1997;15(2–3):377–86.

[22] Liu D, Diorio J, Day J, et al. Maternal care, hippocampal synaptogenesis and cognitive development in rats. Nat Neurosci 2000;3:799–806.

[23] Gazzano A, Mariti C, Notari L, et al. Effects of early gentling and early environment on emotional development of puppies. Appl Anim Behav Sci 2008;110(2): 294–304.

[24] Case LP. Developmental behavior: puppy to adult. the dog: its behavior, nutrition, and health. 2nd edition. Ames, Iowa: Wiley-Blackwell publishing; 2005.

[25] Houpt K. Domestic animal behavior for veterinarians and animal scientists. 6th edition. Hoboken, New Jersey: John Wiley & Sons Inc.; 2018.

[26] Bateson P. How do sensitive periods arise and what are they for? Anim Behav 1979;27:470–86.

[27] King AJ, Carlile S. Changes induced in the representation of auditory space in the superior colliculus by rearing ferrets with binocular eyelid suture. Exp Brain Res 1993;94: 444–55.

[28] Wallace MT, Stein BE. Early experience determines how the senses will interact. J Neurophysiol 2007;97:921–6.

[29] Albertini M, Pirrone F, Pierantoni L, et al. Different dynamics of sensory-motor development and behavior during the transitional period in puppies: preliminary results. Mac Vet Rev 2018;41(2).153–61.

[30] Kutzler M. Puppy behavior, socialisation, and personality. Adv Small Anim Med Surg 2014;27(6):1–3.

[31] Knudsen EI. Sensitive periods in the development of the brain and behavior. J Cogn Neurosci 2004;16(8): 1412–25.

[32] Braastad BO. Effects of prenatal stress on behaviour of offspring of laboratory and farmed mammals. Appl Anim Behav Sci 1998;61:159–80.

[33] Weinstock M. The long-term behavioural consequences of prenatal stress. Neurosci Biobehav 2008;32:1073–86.

[34] Freedman DG, King JA, Elliot O. Critical period in the social development of dogs. Science 1961;133:1016–7.

[35] Fuller JL. Experiential deprivation and later behavior. Science 1967;158:1645–52.

[36] Howell TJ, King T, Bennett PC. Puppy parties and beyond: the role of early age socialisation practices on adult dog behaviour. Vet Med 2015;6:143–53.

[37] Blackwell EJ, Twells C, Seawright A, et al. The relationship between training methods and the occurrence of behavior problems, as reported by owners, in a population of domestic dogs. J Vet Behav 2008;3:207–17.

[38] Wormald D, Lawrence AJ, Carter G, et al. Analysis of correlations between early social exposure and reported aggression in the dog. J Vet Behav 2016;15:31–6.

[39] Sterlemann V, Ganea K, Liebl C, et al. Long-term behavioral and neuroendocrine alterations following chronic social stress in mice: Implications for stress-related disorders. Horm Behav 2008;53(2):386–94.

[40] Serpell JA, Duffy DL. Aspects of juvenile and adolescent environment predict aggression and fear in 12-month-old guide dogs. Front Vet Sci 2016;3:49.

[41] Vaterlaws-Whiteside H, Hartmann A. Improving puppy behavior using a new standardized socialisation program. Appl Anim Behav Sci 2017;197:55–61.

[42] Guardini G, Bowen J, Mariti C, et al. Influence of maternal care on behavioural development of domestic dogs (canis familiaris) living in a home environment. Animals 2017;7:93.

[43] Guardini G, Mariti C, Bowen J, et al. Influence of morning maternal care on the behavioural responses of 8-week-old Beagle puppies to new environmental and social stimuli. Appl Anim Behav Sci 2016;181:137–44.

[44] Weaver IC. Shaping adult phenotypes through early life environments. Birth Defects Res C Embryo Today 2009; 87:314–26.

[45] Gunnar M, Quevedo K. The neurobiology of stress and development. Annu Rev Psychol 2007;58:145–73.

[46] De Kloet ER, Joëls M, Holsboer F. Stress and the brain: from adaptation to disease. Nat Rev Neurosci 2005;6: 463–75.

[47] Tiira K, Lohi H. Early life experiences and exercise associate with canine anxieties. PLoS One 2015;10:11.

[48] Bray EE, Sammel MD, Cheney DL, et al. Characterizing early maternal style in a population of guide dogs. Front Psychol 2017;8:175.

[49] Bray EE, Sammel MD, Cheney DL, et al. Maternal style and guide dog success. Proc Natl Acad Sci 2017; 114(34):9128–33.

[50] Panksepp J. Affective Neuroscience: the foundations of human and animal emotions. New York: Oxford University Press; 1998. p. 166.

[51] Slabbert JM, Rasa O. Observational learning of an acquired maternal behaviour pattern by working dogs: An alternative training method? Appl Anim Behav Sci 1997;53:438–81.

[52] Cassidy J. The nature of child's ties. Handbook of Attachment: theory, research and clinical applications. Third ed. New York, New York: Guilford press; 2016. p. 3–24.

[53] Bowlby J. Attachment and loss: vol 1. Attachment. New York, New York: Basic Books; 1969.

[54] Ainsworth MDS, Blehar MC, Waters E, et al. Patterns of Attachment: a psychological study of the strange situation. Hillsdale, New Jersey: Lawrence Erlbaum Associates; 1978.

[55] Savalli C, Mariti C. Would the dog be a person's child or best friend? Revisiting the dog-tutor attachment. Front Psychol 2020;11:2649.

[56] Prato-Previde E, Ghirardelli G, Marshall-Pescini S, et al. Intraspecific attachment in domestic puppies (Canis familiaris). J Vet Behav 2009;4:89–90.

[57] Mariti C, Carlone B, Ricci E, et al. Intraspecific attachment in adult domestic dogs (Canis familiaris): preliminary results. Appl Anim Behav Sci 2014;152:64–72.

[58] Mariti C, Carlone B, Ricci E, et al. Intraspecific relationships in adult domestic dogs (Canis familiaris) living in the same household: A comparison of the relationship with the mother and an unrelated older female dog. Appl Anim Behav Sci 2017;194:62–6.

[59] Bennett PC, Rohlf VI. Owner-companion dog interactions: relation- ships between demographic variables, potentially problematic behaviours, training engagement and shared activities. Appl Anim Behav Sci 2007;102: 65–84.

[60] Jagoe JA. Behaviour problems in the domestic dog: a retrospective and prospective study to identify factors influencing their development. UK: Department of Clinical Veterinary Medicine and St Catharine's College, University of Cambridge; 1994 PhD thesis.

[61] Casey RA, Loftus B, Bolster C, et al. Human directed aggression in domestic dogs (Canis familiaris): occurrence in different contexts and risk factors. Appl Anim Behav Sci 2014;152:52–61.

[62] McMillan FD, Serpell JA, Duffy DL, et al. Differences in behavioral characteristics between dogs obtained as

puppies from pet stores and those obtained from noncommercial breeders. J Am Vet Med. Assoc 2013; 242:1359–63.

[63] Radtke KM, Ruf M, Gunter HM, et al. Transgenerational impact of intimate partner violence on methylation in the promoter of the glucocorticoid receptor. Transl Psychiatry 2011;1(7):e21.

[64] Duxbury M, Jackson J, Line S, et al. Evaluation of association between retention in the home and attendance at puppy socialisation classes. J Am Vet Med Assoc 2003; 223(1):61–6.

[65] Casey RA, Loftus B, Bolster C, et al. Inter-dog aggression in a UK owner survey: prevalence, co-occurrence in different contexts and risk factors. Vet Rec 2013;172:127.

[66] Ward MR. Behavioural therapy success and the effect of socialisation on subsequent behaviour in dogs. Palmerston North, New Zealand: Veterinary Science, Massey University; 2003.

[67] Seksel K, Mazurski E, Taylor A. Puppy socialisation programs: short and long term behavioural effects. J Appl Anim Welf Sci 1999;62:335–49.

[68] Batt L, Batt M, Baguley J, et al. The effects of structured sessions for juvenile training and socialisation on guide dog success and puppy-raiser participation. J Vet Behav 2008;3:199–206.

[69] González-Martínez A, Martínez MF, Rosado B, et al. Association between puppy classes and adulthood behavior of the dog. J Vet Behav 2019;32:36–41.

[70] Herron M, Lord L, Hill L, et al. Effects of preadoption counseling for owners on house-training success among dogs acquired from shelters. J Am Vet Med Assoc 2007; 231:558–62.

[71] Gazzano A, Mariti C, Alvares S, et al. The prevention of undesirable behaviors in dogs: effectiveness of veterinary behaviorists' advice given to puppy owners. J Vet Behav 2008;3(3):125–33.

[72] Jokinen O, Appleby D, Sandbacka-Saxen S, et al. Homing age influences the prevalence of aggressive and avoidance-related behaviour in adult dogs. Appl Anim Behav Sci 2017;195:87–92.

[73] Appleby DL, Bradshaw JWS, Casey RA. Relationship between aggressive and avoidance behaviour by dogs and their experience in the first six months of life. Vet Rec 2002;150:434–8.

[74] Blackwell EJ, Bradshaw JWS, Casey RA. Fear responses to noises in domestic dogs: Prevalence, risk factors and co-occurrence with other fear related behaviour. Appl Anim Behav Sci 2013;145(1–2):15–25.

[75] Fisher AE. The effects of differential early treatment on the social and exploratory behavior of puppies, . PhD dissertation. The Pennsylvania State University, University Park; 1955.

Advances in Small Animal Care 3 (2022) 13–22

ADVANCES IN SMALL ANIMAL CARE

Feline Behavioural Medicine – An Important Veterinary Discipline

Sarah Heath, BVSc, PgCertVE DipECAWBM(BM), CCAB, FHEA, FRCVS[a,b,*]

[a]Behavioural Referrals Veterinary Practice, 10 Rushton Drive, Upton, Chester CH2 1RE, United Kingdom; [b]University of Liverpool School of Veterinary Science

---

KEYWORDS

• Behavioural medicine • Cat • Emotional • Cognitive • Physical • Feline • Health • Mental well-being

KEY POINTS

- Provision of comprehensive and effective health care involves recognizing the three equally important parts of the health triad, namely emotional, cognitive and physical health.
- The three components of the health triad are inextricably linked and it is not appropriate to think in terms of presenting problems as being either medical or behavioral.
- A behavioral medicine approach to veterinary work will result in improved diagnosis and treatment of feline health issues in their broadest sense.
- Positive (engaging) and negative (protective) emotions are both beneficial in terms of survival and both have the potential to contribute to behaviors that are considered problematic.
- Emotional arousal, regardless of the motivations involved, can be a contributory factor to compromised emotional health which can impact on physical and cognitive well-being.

INTRODUCTION

Mental well-being can be defined as being that aspect of well-being that relates to the emotional and cognitive health of an individual. Within the context of veterinary behavioral medicine, the author has proposed that health care for non-human animals is a multidimensional process and that the health of veterinary species should be considered as a triad of equally important aspects that are inextricably linked to one another [1]. As this health triad is composed of physical, emotional, and cognitive health, comprehensive health care involves acknowledging and optimizing all three. The veterinary profession is charged with safeguarding the health of non-human species and traditionally the emphasis has been on striving to optimize physical health. Due to the complex interconnections between all 3 aspects of the health triad, this aim cannot be achieved unless emotional and cognitive health are also considered. Feline behavioral medicine is the veterinary discipline that considers all 3 aspects of feline health and the interplay between them.

TAKING AN INTERNAL MEDICINE APPROACH

One of the features of behavioral medicine is the aim to identify the underlying cause of any presenting signs. There is a recognition, as in other branches of internal medicine, that the signs identified by the caregiver at home, or the veterinary professional in the consultation room, may be the result of a range of different factors. Cats that vomit or have diarrhea can do so for a myriad of reasons and they require a diagnostic process that

---

*Behavioral Referrals Veterinary Practice, 10 Rushton Drive, Upton, Chester CH2 1RE, United Kingdom.
E-mail address: office@behaviouralproductions.co.uk

https://doi.org/10.1016/j.yasa.2022.07.001
2666-450X/22/

identifies the specific cause in order for treatment to be successful in the long term. Of course, symptomatic treatment may be indicated in the short term, while diagnostic procedures take place, and this is also true when the presenting sign is one of the altered behaviors. The institution of so-called "barrier methods," which prevent the consequence of a behavioral response, can be an important part of immediate management. Examples would include the physical segregation of cats in a multi-cat household when confrontational behaviors are being expressed toward one another. Identifying potential differential diagnoses involves the consideration of the potential emotional motivations for the behavior, the range of physical health changes which could be impacting the cat's responses and the involvement of cognitive factors, such as past learning experiences or age or physical disease-related compromises in cognitive function.

THE CONCEPT OF EMOTIONAL VALENCE

Traditionally there has been a lot of emphasis in behavioral work on the identification of the underlying emotional motivation. The Panksepp model [2] is widely used to explain the link between emotion and behavioral response and an understanding of the different motivational systems, and their function, is central to the discipline of behavioral medicine. It holds the key to preventing, managing, and treating reported behavioral problems in veterinary patients. It is also a major factor in ensuring positive welfare for non-human animals kept as companion animals, minimizing the negative impact of the veterinary visit on pets and their caregivers and optimizing detection, management, and treatment of physical diseases.

EMOTIONS NOT FEELINGS

There has been some resistance to the acceptance of emotional health as an important topic in the veterinary context. Some of that resistance stems from human perception of emotions in terms of feelings and the use of verbal reporting as a means of assessing them. It is important to clarify that, within the field of veterinary behavioral medicine, the emotions being described are motivational-emotional systems that are responsible for emotional arousal rather than feelings of emotion that may be more familiar to most of the people. Research studying "aggressive" behaviors in cats which seemed to be very similar in appearance found that the motivations and neural circuits responsible for the behaviors were in fact different [3].

MOTIVATIONAL-EMOTIONAL SYSTEMS

From an affective neuroscientific perspective, adapted and developed from Panksepp [2], the motivational-emotional systems can be classified into different systems. Panksepp groups these into positive and negative emotional motivations, which can be used to understand the normal behavioral responses of a species but also the ways in which those behaviors may become problematic. The use of this terminology is in keeping with other disciplines, such as learning theory, whereby positive and negative are used to describe the adding or the removing of something, rather than a concept of good and bad. However, in everyday language, there is a perception that something that is described as negative is detrimental, while something that is described as positive is inherently desirable. As a result, for many caregivers and for some veterinary professionals, these terms lead to a perception that the positive emotions will be good and the negative emotions will be bad. This is not the case. Negative emotions serve to protect the individual and they are very adaptive and beneficial in terms of ensuring survival. Healthy negative emotion is desirable and leads to appropriate behavioral responses. An aim to create an environment that is free of negative emotions, such as fear, is misguided and an alternative approach of recognizing such emotions and ensuring that the patient can respond to them appropriately and effectively, will be far more effective in safeguarding animal welfare as well as resolving unwanted behaviors. Positive emotions lead to interaction and engagement with others and with the environment and this can be beneficial to the individual. However, emotions that trigger engaging behavioral responses need to be context appropriate and when they are experienced in unsuitable situations or at problematic intensities they can be associated with unwanted behaviors. It can, therefore, be seen that both groups of emotion are essential for good emotional health, but both can become compromised and be involved in the expression of behaviors that are classed as being problematic. This problem with the misinterpretation of the terms positive and negative is addressed in the Heath Model of Emotional Health (developed by Dr Sarah Heath in 2010) by the use of the words engaging and protective to describe the valence of an emotion [4],[5]. Engaging emotions are the ones that lead to the individual engaging or interacting with someone or something and examples would include the systems of desire-seeking, social play, care, and lust. Protective emotions are responsible for behaviors that are designed to protect the individual from someone or something and these include fear-anxiety, pain frustration, and panic-grief. When emotions are triggered appropriately they are all beneficial to the individual and lead to behavioral responses which enhance their survival. This may be obvious when desire-seeking leads to predatory behavior which results in the acquisition of nutrition, but it is equally true when fear-anxiety motivation leads a cat to seek a high-up safety location and successfully avoid interaction with a potential predator. In cats, who are not obligately social, the role of the protective emotions is particularly important as they enable the individual to cope with potential challenges to their survival.

The emotional systems are listed below together with an overview of their function.

POSITIVE (ENGAGING) EMOTIONAL MOTIVATIONS
The Desire - Seeking System
This is a general-purpose neuronal system that motivates animals to move to places whereby they have more potential of finding and consuming resources needed for survival for example, food, water, and shelter [6]. In a clinical setting, the behavioral manifestations of this system include predatory behaviour, object play, engagement in social interaction and emotional drive to access survival resources such as food, water, and shelter. In cats, the fact that they are nonobligate in terms of social interaction in adulthood means that the desire-seeking motivational drive to acquire social interaction is very different from that demonstrated in socially obligate mammals such as dogs, horses, and humans. Learning though the delivery of appropriate reward is associated with the desire-seeking system [7] and it is, therefore, extremely important in the application of behavioral modification.

The Social Play System
This system gives information to individuals about their own social competence and potential in relation to others. As a social species, the domestic cat is motivated by this system in its interaction with other cats and young kittens have a high drive for social play [8]. In socially mature cats where social interaction is not an obligate requirement for survival the motivation for social play can be significantly diminished but there is considerable individual variation.

The Lust System
The "lust system" organizes the specific reproductive needs, ranging from the attraction or the selection of a partner through courtship to any potential bonding and on to the act of mating with a sexual partner. In

the UK and in a number of other countries, this system is the least likely to be relevant to the behavior of pet cats, since the vast majority of kittens are neutered prepubertally. For those individuals keeping cats for breeding and showing, the presence of entire cats in their households can be associated with behavioral responses which can cause a degree of inconvenience, and the cats may suffer from an inability to act on their lust motivation. In some situations housing to limit the negative effects of this motivation may place additional pressures on the cats by compromising their environmental needs and this must be taken into account if their welfare is to be protected. For example, if an entire male cat is urine spraying as a result of lust motivation this can lead to decisions to house the cat in an easily cleanable enclosure, which lacks the necessary environmental complexity to fulfill feline needs such as the ability to engage in play and predatory behavior. Using solitary pens away from the main housing areas to reduce scent communication with the entire females and reduce the risk of unpleasant olfactory working conditions for people can reduce the potential for the provision of consistent and predictable human social interaction [9].

The Care System
The "care system" is dedicated to maintaining the bond to individual offspring through recognizable parental care and is also involved in nurturing behavior toward others who are vulnerable. In socially obligate species such as horses, dogs, and people, the behavioral manifestation of the care system is seen in a variety of relationships and is not confined to the parent–offspring interaction. Cats are not obligate in their social behavior in adulthood and the motivation of care is often less significant once cats have become socially mature. However, there is considerable individual variation and many caregivers do report examples of care-motivated nurturing behaviors demonstrated by adult neutered pet cats toward other cats and sometimes other pet species within the household.

NEGATIVE (PROTECTIVE) EMOTIONAL MOTIVATIONS
The Fear-Anxiety System
This system relates to the preservation of comfort provided by predictable access to essential resources and the management of threats to personal or resource security. This "system" intrinsically helps animals to avoid dangers and it is more adaptive to feel anticipatory fear (anxiety) than to be attacked and harmed. The

behavioral responses to the emotion of fear-anxiety are designed to ensure survival and often result in an increase in space from the perceived challenge or a decrease in interaction with it. However, emotional systems are not mutually exclusive and in some situations, the coexistence of positive emotional motivation in the same context can lead to a desire to remain in the presence of the threat but adopt information gathering behavioral responses which aim to limit the potential for a negative outcome. As a result of their differing social behavior cats and dogs will often react differently to potentially fear inducing situations. However, for both species this emotional motivation leads to behavioral responses which are designed to limit potential for damage and increase the potential for survival. This is a very beneficial emotional motivation when triggered in an appropriate context but can be detrimental and potentially limiting for the individual when it is triggered inappropriately. Stimuli commonly encountered in a domestic environment can trigger fear-anxiety motivation and lead to reported behavioral concerns. Fear-anxiety motivation is often associated with feline responses within the veterinary clinic but understanding and recognizing the difference between frustration and fear-anxiety can be a particular challenge in a clinical context [10].

The Pain System

The "pain system" is related to the maintenance of body integrity and functioning and it is both a distinct sensation and a motivation [11]. The pain system is associated with the preservation of physical comfort and as such can also be considered to be part of the fear-anxiety system within the Panksepp model. In a veterinary clinical context, the importance of pain as a potential factor in behavioral presentations is significant [12] and consideration of pain as an emotional motivational system is beneficial. The most obvious contribution of pain to behavioral reactions may be the presence of acute pain, but the influence of chronic pain in behavioral cases is common and the potential for learned behavioral responses to persist following the experience of pain also needs to be considered.

The Panic-Grief System

This system is related to the safeguarding of the survival of young and vulnerable individuals, therefore, the protection of the genetic survival of the species. Before they are able to protect themselves young animals start to exhibit powerful emotional arousal indicating the desperate need for nurturing care. Kittens will "cry" when separated from their mother and this vocalization is designed to alert the queen to a need to seek, retrieve

and attend to her offspring. In the feline context, it is most commonly displayed by young kittens as they have a need for social interaction but is less strongly motivated in adult cats as a result of their solitary survivor social behavior. However, behavior that is motivated by the panic—grief system is reported in older cats and can be displayed in relation to the loss of a bonded feline such as a sibling. Some authors also suggest that separation from human caregivers can lead to a panic-grief motivated behavioral response in some individual cats. However, separation-related behaviors in cats have received far less research attention than corresponding behavioral presentations in dogs [13]; future studies on cats, including reviews of clinical behavioural cases, would be beneficial.

The Frustration System

The "frustration system" is triggered by a failure to meet expectations, obtain resources or retain control. This system intensifies and accelerates behavioral responses. It is associated with so-called "aggressive" behaviors when animals do not have control over a situation, when they are irritated or restrained. In a species which is non-obligate in terms of social interaction and is a solitary survivor, the need to be in control is a fundamental part of the feline behavioral repertoire. This increases the potential for cats to perceive a lack of control in a range of situations and to experience frustration as a result. This emotion is commonly associated with unwanted feline behavioral responses within the veterinary clinic [4,10]. Frustration is an important emotion to consider when investigating reported behavioural concerns from caregivers. It is triggered in association with any of the other systems when the cat perceives those emotions to be justified but is unable to respond to them successfully. Differences between human animals and non-human animals result in many discrepancies between the domestic environment and the optimal environment for cats and this can lead to the potential for frustration to be triggered. Frustration leads to increased intensity and speed of behavioral responses and is also associated with increased possibility of confrontational behavioral responses.

RECOGNIZING THE ROLE OF EMOTIONAL AROUSAL

Emotion is not only important in terms of its valence, whether it is negative (protective) or positive (engaging) in its function, but also in terms of arousal, which can be thought of as the amount of emotion that is present, regardless of its valence. The significance of arousal is related to the finite capacity of an individual for emotional input and the resulting need to be able to dissipate emotion that has served its purpose.

APPLICATION OF THE HEATH MODEL TO VETERINARY BEHAVIOURAL MEDICINE

As part of the Heath Model of Emotional Health [5], the author has developed a slightly different form of terminology for describing the potential behavioral responses to negative (protective) emotion and feels that these terms give a more accurate description of the behaviors that are exhibited in a clinical context. The use of this terminology helps to increase caregiver understanding and to increase awareness of the equal importance of each of the four behavioral options in a clinical context. There is a great deal of emphasis in the behavioral literature on behavioral responses which have previously been categorized as "fight" and this has led to frequent use of the word "aggression" to describe these responses. Confusion over the definition of the term "aggression" has increased misunderstanding about motivation and led to a concentration on so-called "aggression" as the behavioral response of most interest and significance in a domestic setting. In fact, the presence of any behavioral responses which indicate an underlying negative (protective) emotional motivation should be cause for concern both for pet caregivers and for members of the veterinary profession. Failure to place equal significance on the behavioral options available to domestic pets increases the potential for their welfare to be compromised. For this reason, the author proposes that the use of the terms flight, fight, freeze, and fiddle are not appropriate in a clinical behavioral medicine context [4].

When emotional motivations are triggered, the individual displays a range of behavioral responses. The aim of these behaviors is to fulfill the requirements of the emotional drive and return the individual to a state of emotional safety. For example, when desire-seeking motivation is triggered the individual responds by approaching and engaging with a resource, such as food, water, or shelter, and in doing so they increase their survival chances and achieve a state of satisfaction. Similarly, behavioural responses to the protective emotions lead to behavioral responses which protect the individual from harm. This protection is achieved in one of the two ways:

1. Increase distance from and decrease interaction with the trigger
2. Gather more information about the trigger

Within each of these categories of behavioral responses, there is a spectrum of behavior of increasing intensity which the individual can select from. Failure of a behavioral response to result in a perception of safety for the individual will increase the likelihood of selection of a response of greater intensity from the same category or selection of a response from a different category. In the Heath Model of Emotional Health these behavioural responses are referred to by using terms that assist us in understanding the purpose of the behaviour.

BEHAVIOURAL RESPONSES WHICH INCREASE DISTANCE FROM AND DECREASE INTERACTION WITH A TRIGGER FOR PROTECTIVE EMOTION

Repulsion describes those behaviours which increase distance and decrease interaction by repelling the potential threat. It is the response of the "threat" to the repulsion behaviour which determines whether or not the action is successful. The most commonly quoted examples of repulsion are intense and active responses such as swiping, chasing, and biting. These behaviors are often referred to as "aggressive" behaviors. In addition, repulsion can be achieved through lower intensity behaviors such as grumbling and intense staring, and these behaviors are often overlooked or misinterpreted. As with all of the behavioral options when triggered by protective emotion, repulsion is a spectrum of behaviors with the same aim. Fight is a description of one high-intensity version, but all forms of repulsion are significant and it is very important to be able to identify them. Cats are particularly associated with higher intensity forms of repulsion in the veterinary context, but this is explained by the perceived lack of success of other behavioral responses. If one of the other categories of behavioural responses has been attempted but, despite escalating to high intensity forms of those responses, they have been unsuccessful then the animal can change to the same intensity of an alternative response. Cats who have tried to use avoidance and inhibition without success can therefore change to a response of high intensity repulsion.

Avoidance describes behaviors with the same aim of increasing distance and decreasing interaction, but which achieve it directly through the action of the individual. There is a range of possible avoidance behaviours from the more passive eye aversion to a more active act of physically running away. The use of the term flight is, therefore, appropriate to describe one high-intensity version of the avoidance response but this response option is far more complex than that. Avoidance is often described as the preferred feline strategy, which makes perfect sense in terms of the social behavior of the domestic cat. As non-obligate social animals the protection of self is a primary aim and the increasing of distance and decreasing of interaction by taking action themselves, rather than inducing a reaction in others, is a more reliable way of maintaining control over the situation. However, the domestic environment is often limiting in relation to the selection of an avoidance response and the context of the veterinary practice is a good example of this. Cats are placed in cat carriers or restrained for examination and these interactions can limit the potential for an avoidance response to be successful in enabling the cat to reach a state of perceived safety. Well-meaning human caregivers may also try to encourage cats to interact with stimuli that are inducing fear-anxiety, in a misguided attempt to help the animal "overcome its fear." Such forced interactions can make avoidance responses unsuccessful and thereby increase the potential for one of the remaining three categories of protective behavioral response options to be used. For example, the cat that attempts to remain in its cat carrier in the consultation room is using an avoidance response to protect itself. If they are forced to leave the carrier and then held using forceful physical restraint, it is more likely that they will change their behavioural response to one of repulsion and swipe out in an attempt to resolve the threatening situation. If the cat is permitted to stay inside the carrier and the lid is removed and replaced with a towel, the cat remains "hidden" and avoidance is perceived to be successful. The towel can be moved to expose just the part of the cat's anatomy that is required to carry out the examination or procedure and the rest of the cat can remain "hidden" thus offering the cat a sensation of being protected. The perception that avoidance is being successful will make a change to a repulsion response less likely and this is the basis of a cat friendly approach to interactions during the veterinary visit [14].

BEHAVIOURAL RESPONSES WHICH INCREASE AVAILABILITY OF INFORMATION ABOUT A TRIGGER FOR PROTECTIVE EMOTION

Information can be gathered through a behavioral response that is referred to as inhibition in the Heath Model. This involves the passive collection of information about a trigger without becoming actively involved and can be achieved through auditory, olfactory and visual communication. Auditory inhibition behavior will involve passive listening, while visual inhibition involves passive looking or watching and olfactory inhibition

passive gathering of scent information. The cat may voluntarily remain at a distance from the trigger while engaging in these behaviors. In some situations the matter of proximity is out of the control of the individual and inhibition behavior can be seen when cats are in close proximity to a trigger, such as a veterinary surgeon during clinical examination or a caregiver during intended displays of affection. Cats will commonly select inhibition as it enables the individual to retain some control, but it may not be so readily recognized as a response to protective emotion which can result in it being overlooked or misinterpreted. The cat seems to be passive and doing nothing and this can be misinterpreted as them being "fine" and even "relaxed." This misinterpretation can lead to the inhibition behavioral response being unsuccessful in resolving the protective emotion and the individual selecting one of the other available behavioral responses (avoidance or repulsion) instead. A high-intensity form of inhibition may be referred to as freeze but there is a range of other possible inhibited behaviors through which an individual can passively take in information. The gathering of information can also be associated with engaging emotions such as desire-seeking and it is, therefore, important to interpret behaviors such as watching, listening, and sniffing with reference to the context in which they are displayed and to observe the accompanying body language of the individual which will give information about their emotional state.

The second form of behavior designed to increase information availability is referred to as appeasement and involves the gathering of information while also offering signs of non-hostility in return. While these responses are believed to be less common in cats, as a result of a decreased need to offer information to others when survival is a solitary responsibility, appeasement does occur in the feline world. It will involve the use of sensory communication which can take the form of auditory, visual, olfactory, or tactile communication and may be more readily utilized by kittens or individual more socially motivated adults. Tactile contact, such as rubbing and grooming, is usually reserved for individuals within the same social group, both feline and of other species, such as family dogs or people. Visual appeasement will involve the giving of information through body language signals while also collecting visual information from the trigger and vocal appeasement will involve vocalization as well as listening. Appeasement of an olfactory nature will involve active exchange of scent information between the cat and the trigger which obviously is difficult to achieve in the context of interspecific encounters. Appeasement is most likely to be displayed in situations of uncertainty involving familiar individuals whereby there is some benefit to the cat in reducing the protective emotions of the other party. It is less likely to be displayed in the veterinary practice context and more likely to be seen in interactions between socially compatible cats and between cats and their caregivers.

APPLICATION OF A BEHAVIORAL MEDICINE APPROACH TO THE VETERINARY VISIT EXPERIENCE

One of the reasons for the author developing new terminology, in relation to emotional motivations and behavioral responses, was a desire to make it easier for caregivers, veterinary professionals, and all individuals working with non-human animals, in whatever capacity, to determine the best way to respond to behaviors that an individual presents. This is just as applicable to interactions with wildlife as it is to the context of domestic pets. An understanding that protective emotions can be beneficial to the individual will increase the appreciation of the need to recognize them when they occur rather than simply seek to remove them from the emotional repertoire of the individual. The way in which humans respond to feline behavioral responses to protective emotion will be crucial in determining what happens next. In the context of the veterinary visit, identifying the style of behavioral response that a feline patient is selecting as a result of protective emotion can help professionals to find ways in which those responses can be perceived to be successful by the cat. This will reduce the risk of them escalating the intensity of that response or selecting an alternative [15]. For example, if a cat is attempting to use avoidance as a response to protective emotion by retreating to a perceived safe location within the veterinary consulting room, such as the high-sided feline weighing scales, it is possible to respond to this by allowing the cat to remain in its chosen location. By doing this the cat perceives that avoidance is successful in its aim of decreasing interaction with the trigger for their protective emotion (the veterinary environment and personnel) and there is no need for it to increase the intensity of the response by trying to physically flee or change the response to one of the repulsion and start to hiss and swipe. Failure to recognize the purpose of a behavioral response can result in the perception of failure for the cat and this can lead to the triggering of the emotion of frustration. This will increase the need for the patient to increase their perception of safety. Frustration is accompanied by

an increase in the intensity and speed of delivery of behavioral responses and it also increases the confrontational nature of those responses. Avoiding frustration through appropriate responses to protective behavioral responses is, therefore, important in the veterinary context. There is a lot of emphasis in the literature on the triggering of engaging emotions during a veterinary visit and this can be beneficial. However, the presence of engaging emotion does not remove the possibility of the presence of protective ones since both valences of emotion can be present at the same time. The provision of triggers for engaging emotion, such as food or toys, can increase the presence of engaging and interactive behavior but it is important to still monitor the patient for any body language or behavioral signs of protective emotion. The behaviour that an individual displays is the result of the predominant emotional motivation at that point in time. While using triggers to boost engaging emotion can be successful, there is a risk that unintentional escalation of protective emotional triggering can lead to the onset of behavioral responses, such as avoidance or repulsion, which are perceived by the human handler to be "out of the blue". Better understanding of feline behavioral medicine and emotional health, in particular, is key to achieving a truly cat-friendly experience.

CONSIDERING BEHAVIORAL MEDICINE IN FELINE PRACTICE

One important consequence of considering the behavioral responses of cats from a behavioral medicine perspective is an increased appreciation of the interplay between the underlying emotional and physiological factors involved in those behaviors and the physical health of the individual. Many years ago Professor Tony Buffington and colleagues made connections between the environments that domestic cats were living in and the physical disease state of feline interstitial cystitis (FIC) [16]. It was a very important moment in terms of our understanding of a connection between living in an environment that compromises natural feline behavior and expressing signs of physical disease. However, it was only the tip of the iceberg in terms of understanding the reality of the health triad and the need to consider veterinary health care in a much broader way than had traditionally been conducted. Other research groups have published papers emphasizing the need to consider emotional factors when dealing with a range of feline medicine cases [17–19] and understanding how emotional motivations, behavioral responses, and physiologic stress all impact physical health has certainly increased over recent years.

"PROBLEM" BEHAVIORS CAN RESULT FROM POSITIVE, ENGAGING, EMOTIONAL MOTIVATION

It is very important to remember that the definition of problem behavior, in the context of domestic pets, will usually be made by the humans involved, rather than the non-human animal. The "problem" usually relates to impact on caregivers, veterinary practices, or other people attempting to interact with the cat and not necessarily on the impact on the individual. It is also commonly assumed that problematic behavior is always motivated by negative (protective) emotion, but this is not necessarily the case. Triggering of positive (engaging) systems in unjustified or inappropriate contexts can also be linked to behavior that caregivers of domestic pets report as being problematic. For example, when cats are motivated to hunt via the desire-seeking system and their behavior is viewed by the caregiver or other members of society as being problematic [20]. Lust behaviors in entire domestic pets may also result in behaviors that the people caring for them find inconvenient and undesirable, although this is less frequently reported in domestic cats than in dogs.

DETERMINING THE SIGNIFICANCE OF EMOTIONAL MOTIVATION

Within the Heath Model approach to behavioral medicine the first step is to determine which of the emotional motivations are involved in triggering a given behavioral presentation, be that something reported by the caregiver or experienced by the practice staff. The model then asks three important questions to determine how to proceed in terms of adopting a treatment or management approach.
1. Is the emotional motivation(s) justified by the context?
2. Is the behavioral response justified by the emotion (s) ?
3. Is the behavioral response normal in terms of intensity and duration in relation to the context?

When "problematic" behaviors are motivated by emotional systems which are unjustified by the context and consist of behavioral responses which are out of proportion in terms of intensity and duration this indicates a compromised state of emotional health. It is important to remember that not all behavioral presentations in

domestic pets fit into the category of emotional disorder and that some behaviors which caregivers find unacceptable and undesirable are motivated by emotions that are entirely justified. The justification of the emotion needs to be considered from a species-specific and contextual perspective and also from an individual perspective. The latter will be influenced by prior learning and experiences and an in-depth chronologic history is, therefore, essential in every case.

BEHAVIOURAL PRESENTATIONS RELATED TO JUSTIFIED EMOTIONAL MOTIVATION AND "NORMAL" BUT UNWANTED BEHAVIORAL RESPONSES

All the emotional motivational systems are normal, adaptive, and beneficial. They are responsible for behavioral responses which ensure the survival of the individual and of the species. An understanding of normal feline behavior will increase the recognition of the different systems in behavioral responses of domestic cats. The most common engaging emotional systems involved in reported feline behavior problems related to justified emotional motivation are those involving desire-seeking and social play. If a cat is motivated to gain access to a resource or to engage in social play with a conspecific and is denied the opportunity to do so frustration will be triggered. This can lead to behaviors that are perceived to be "aggressive" in nature and yet the cat may be responding to perfectly justified emotion. The answer to this problem is to ensure that the pet can access necessary resources in an appropriate time scale and engage in suitably motivated social play. To this end, the environment that they live in must be optimal in relation to their species, age, and individual requirements. The topic of addressing feline environmental needs is outlined in the excellent AAPF and ISFM guidelines [9]. Determining whether frustration is involved in a behavioral presentation can be achieved through accurate history taking and comprehensive review of the physical and social environment from the cat's perspective.

The predominant protective emotional systems involved in reported feline behavior problems are fear-anxiety, pain, and frustration. In many cases, fear anxiety is a justified emotion in relation to the context but problematic behavior may also occur as a result of fear anxiety which results from a lack of appropriate emotional development. Pain can lead to unwanted behavioral responses, and the emphasis in dealing with these cases is to accurately diagnose and treat the underlying physical trigger for the pain, if one exists. This is clearly within the remit of the veterinary behaviorist or the general veterinary practitioner who has referred the case to a nonveterinary behavioral professional, which highlights the need for excellent levels of communication between veterinary and nonveterinary personnel involved with behavior cases. The relationship between pain and behavioral change can be complex [21] and a combination of history taking, direct observation, and assessment of remotely gathered information, for example, in video form, can be needed to identify it.

It has been shown that visual signaling is important in determining emotional motivation [22,23] and one study has looked specifically at the negative (protective) emotions of fear and frustration in relation to feline communication [24]. Studying visual communication has been shown to assist in the monitoring of acute pain in feline patients [25] and it is also important to consider the role of chronic pain and learned responses to pain when investigating behavioural presentations.

BEHAVIOURAL PRESENTATIONS RELATED TO UNJUSTIFIED EMOTIONAL MOTIVATION OR INVOLVING "ABNORMAL" BEHAVIORAL RESPONSES

Living in a domestic environment undoubtedly puts considerable pressure on domestic pets and optimizing their social and physical environment is a responsibility of anyone caring for or working with non-human animals. While suboptimal environments can often be involved in behavioral presentations this is not always the case and consideration of whether the emotional motivation of the patient is unjustified is necessary. Emotional motivation is always related to the perception of the individual and factors that can influence that perception will need to be investigated. These will include previous experiences or lack of them and chronological history taking is necessary to ensure that vital information is not missed. In the context of some domestic cats, such as those who have been rehomed, this past history may not be available and assessment of the justification of the emotional and behavioral response can only be made in relation to the context in which the behaviour is displayed.

RELEVANCE OF FELINE BEHAVIORAL MEDICINE TO GENERAL VETERINARY PRACTICE

Understanding of feline behavior in a clinical context has increased significantly over recent years. The application of learning theory to the explanation of how and why cats develop behavioral responses which cause difficulty for those around them has increased an awareness of the role of cognition. Substantial contributions from clinical behaviorists outside of the veterinary profession have improved the appreciation of the importance of understanding feline ethology and ensuring that species specific needs of cats are met within the domestic environment. More recently the role of the veterinary profession in the context of behavioral medicine has been explored. An understanding of the concept of the health triad has led to realization that to deliver comprehensive and effective health care to veterinary patients there must be consideration of emotional, cognitive, and physical health. The relationship between these three aspects of health is complex and it is no longer appropriate to think in terms of a clinical presentation being medical or behavioral. It is not a binary choice and appreciation that clinical cases result from an interplay between all aspects of health is essential to the delivery of high-quality veterinary care. Clinical feline behavior is traditionally thought about in terms of dealing with caregiver reporting of specific behavioral challenges in their pet but behavioral medicine has a far wider relevance to the veterinary profession. It is involved in developing preventative behavioral strategies to ensure that kittens, and young of other species, reach their emotional potential to the benefit of their physical health as well as their relationship with caregivers and others they interact with. Behavioural medicine also impacts on clinical veterinary practice in terms of improving diagnostic skills, enhancing the management and treatment of physical disease, informing clinical decisions, and making the veterinary experience as beneficial as possible for pets, caregivers, and practice staff.

SUMMARY

Feline behavioral medicine is a relatively new veterinary discipline and one that is central to the concept of cat-friendly veterinary practice. Traditionally veterinary education has focused exclusively on physical health but successful management and treatment of feline patients necessitates an appreciation of the impact of emotional and cognitive factors on their health. The veterinary profession is responsible for safeguarding the health and welfare of non-human animals and this responsibility can only be fulfilled by approaching health care in its broadest sense. Incorporating behavioral medicine into all veterinary undergraduate education programs is, therefore, something that should be considered a priority for the profession.

CLINICS CARE POINTS

- Taking a behavioral medicine approach to feline veterinary practice improves the diagnostic process and enables treatment approaches to be more comprehensive
- Recognizing protective behavioral responses during the veterinary visit gives the opportunity to ensure that they are perceived to be successful from the cat's perspective. This will reduce the risk of escalation of intensity of these behaviors and make clinical examination more successful and safer for patients and staff.
- Physiologic stress associated with persistent triggering of protective emotions can lead to physical disease
- A behavioral medicine approach can benefit the diagnosis and management of presented behavioral and physical signs of ill health and also improve the prevention of these conditions
- Considering emotional, physical, and cognitive health enables the veterinary profession to offer comprehensive health care to its patients

DISCLOSURE

No conflicts of interest to report.

REFERENCES

[1] Heath S. Environment and Feline Health: At Home and in the Clinic. Vet Clin North America - Small Anim Pract 2020;50(4):663–93. https://doi.org/10.1016/j.cvsm.2020.03.005.

[2] Panksepp J. Affective neuroscience: the foundations of human and animal emotions. Oxford University Press; 1998.

[3] Siegel A, Roeling TA, Gregg TR, et al. Neuropharmacology brain-stimulation-evoked aggression. Neurosci Biobehav Rev 1999;23:359–89.

[4] Heath S. Understanding feline emotions: … and their role in problem behaviours. J Feline Med Surg 2018; 20(5):437–44. Available at: https://journals.sagepub.com/doi/10.1177/1098612X18771205.

[5] Heath S, Dowgray N, Rodan I, et al. 10 years of Cat Friendly: a new model and terminology for understanding feline emotions. J Feline Med Surg 2022;24:934–5.

[6] Panksepp J, Moskal J. Dopamine and Seeking; subcortical "reward" systems and appetitive urges. In: Elliot A, editor. Handbook of approach and avoidance motivation New York. Taylor and Francis; 2008. p. 67–87.

[7] Wright JS, Panksepp J. An evolutionary framework to understand foraging, wanting and desire. Neuropsychol Seeking Syst Neuropsychoanalysis 2012;14:5–39.

[8] Kmecová NG, Peťková B, Kottferová J, et al. These Cats Playing? A Closer Look at Social Play in Cats and Proposal for a Psychobiological Approach and Standard Terminology. Front Vet Sci 2021;8. https://doi.org/10.3389/fvets.2021.712310.

[9] Ellis SL, Rodan I, Carney HC, et al. AAFP and ISFM Feline Environmental Needs Guidelines. J Feline Med Surg 2013;5:219–30.

[10] Ellis S. Recognising and assessing feline emotions during the consultation. J Feline Med Surg 2018;20:445–56.

[11] Craig AD. A new view of pain as a homeostatic emotion. Trends Neurosci 2003;26:303–7.

[12] Merola I, Mills DS. Behavioural Signs of Pain in Cats: An Expert Consensus. PLoS ONE 2016;11(2):e0150040.

[13] de Souza Machado D, Oliveira PMB, Machado JC, et al. Sant'Anna AC Identification of separation-related problems in domestic cats: A questionnaire survey. PLoS ONE 2020;15(4):e0230999.

[14] Rodan I, Dowgray N, et al. AAFP/ISFM Cat Friendly Veterinary Interactions Guidelines. 2022.

[15] Rodan I. Understanding Feline Behaviour and Application for Appropriate Handling and Management. Top Companion Anim Med 2010;25(4):178–88.

[16] Buffington CAT, Westropp JL, Chew DJ, et al. Clinical evaluation of multimodal environmental modification (MEMO) in the management of cats with idiopathic cystitis. J Feline Med Surg 2006;8(4):261–8.

[17] Horwitz DF, Rodan I. Behavioural awareness in the feline consultation: Understanding physical and emotional health. J Feline Med Surg 2018;20:423–36.

[18] Roberts C, Gruffydd-Jones T, Williams JL, et al. Influence of living in a multicat household on health and behaviour in a cohort of cats from the United Kingdom. Vet Rec 2020;187(1):27.

[19] Rusbridge C, Heath S, Gunn-Moore DA, et al. Feline orofacial pain syndrome (FOPS): A retrospective study of 113 cases. J Feline Med Surg 2010;12(6):498–508.

[20] Crowley SL, Cecchetti M, McDonald R. A Hunting behaviour in domestic cats: An exploratory study of risk and responsibility among cat owners. People Nat 2019;1(1):18–30.

[21] Mills DS, et al. Pain and Problem Behaviour in Cats and. Dogs Anim 2020;10(2):318.

[22] Bennett V, Gourkow N, Mills DS. Facial correlates of emotional behaviour in the domestic cat. Felis catus) Behav Process 2017;141(3):342–50. https://doi.org/10.1016/j.beproc.2017.03.011.

[23] Waller B, Caeiro C. The facial expressions of cats. Available at: http://www.feline-friends.org.uk/topics/the-facial-expressions-of-cats. Accessed June 19, 2022.

[24] Finka L, Ellis SLH, Wilkinson A, et al. The development of an emotional ethogram for Felis silvestris focused on Fear and Rage. J Vet Behav 2014;4(6):e5.

[25] Holden E, Calvo G, Collins M, et al. Evaluation of facial expression in acute pain in cats. J Small Anim Pract 2014; 55:615–21.

Advances in Small Animal Care 3 (2022) 23–38

ADVANCES IN SMALL ANIMAL CARE

Peripheral Concentration of Amyloid-β, TAU Protein, and Neurofilament Light Chain as Markers of Cognitive Dysfunction Syndrome in Senior Dogs

A Meta-analysis

Patrizia Piotti, Dr, DVM, MSc, PhD, Mariangela Albertini, DVM, PhD*, Federica Pirrone, DVM, PhD

Department of Veterinary Medicine and Animal Sciences, University of Milan, Via dell'Università; 6, 26900 Lodi, Italy

---

KEYWORDS

- Canine cognitive dysfunction • Biomarkers • Amyloid • Aβ42 • Aβ40 • Tau protein
- Neurofilament light chain • Meta-analysis

KEY POINTS

- A meta-analysis indicated that the difference between dogs with canine cognitive dysfunction syndrome (CCDS) and healthy senior controls did not have a significant a pooled effect for blood concentrations of Aβ40, while there was a significant difference for Aβ42.
- Overall, the evidence for the clinical use of Aβ as a peripheral marker of CCDS is not yet sufficient, but worthy of further research.
- There were insufficient studies to perform a quantitative analysis on peripheral concentrations of tau protein or neurofilament light chain.
- Methods such as proteomics and single molecule array assay have recently appeared particularly promising.
- The human literature also suggests that Aβ misfolding, rather than Aβ concentrations, might a better predictor for CCDS.

INTRODUCTION

In dogs, some behavioral and cognitive changes in cognition might be part of normal or healthy aging Supplementary Table 1 [1–3]. However, a small portion of the population is affected by pathological aging, which is characterized by a severe impairment in the function of the organism [4]. Canine cognitive dysfunction syndrome (CCDS) is a progressive, neurodegenerative disease associated with pathological aging in dogs [5]. Age is the main risk factor for CCDS, regardless of breed, size, or sex of the dog [6–8], with a reported prevalence of 8% to 14% in dogs aged 8 years and above, and up to 41% in dogs above the age of 14 years [6,9–12]. Overall, CCDS has a profound impact on the quality of life of the animal and the human-animal bond, leading to shortened life expectancy [7,13,14].

Clinical Signs of Canine Cognitive Dysfunction Syndrome

The clinical signs that are classically associated with CCDS can be described by the acronym DISHAA (Disorientation, altered Interactions, Sleep-wake cycle

---

*Corresponding author, *E-mail address:* mariangela.albertini@unimi.it

https://doi.org/10.1016/j.yasa.2022.07.002
2666-450X/22/ © 2022 Elsevier Inc. All rights reserved.

alterations, House soiling, altered Activity levels, Anxiety) [9,12,15–17] (Table 1):

Diagnostic Process
Authors have attempted to define various systems for staging of CCDS based on the clinical presentation of the condition, rather than the histopathological and instrumental findings, ranging from normal aging to severe cognitive decline [9,15]. Typically, 3 stages are recognized [8,15,17]:

- Normal aging: the dog's owners will not notice any changes in behavior, or these are mild and appear occasionally, affecting 0 to 2 domains
- Mild-to-moderate cognitive impairment: the dog's owners might not recognize the changes in the behavior or might notice the most undesirable changes, such as house-soiling or hyperactivity during the night; however, careful examination of the pet during the consultation and history taking can reveal further changes, such as altered social interactions and activity levels; typically, 2 to 4 domains are affected
- Severe cognitive impairment: the dog's owners clearly perceive the signs of the condition as detrimental to the pet and pervasive as they affect more

TABLE 1
Clinical presentation of canine cognitive dysfunction syndrome grouped based on the DISHAA domains

	Clinical presentation
Disorientation	The dog appears confused in the interaction with the environment: • Fails to recognize familiar people or pets • Gets stuck in corners, behind furniture or on the wrong side of doors • Gets lost in familiar environments • Responds more or less than usual to familiar stimuli and objects • Difficulty finding dropped food
Altered *I*nteractions, learning, and memory	Changes in the social interactions: • Avoids social interactions • Is clingy • Manifests aggressive behavior • Irritability • Inability to perform previously learned tasks (eg, sitting on command) • Inability to learn new tasks
Sleep-wake cycle alterations	Agitation beginning at dawn is often observed (sundown syndrome [21]), associated with increased sleeping during the day • Night restlessness, pacing, wandering at night • Vocalizations during the night • Decreased activity and increased sleeping time during the day
House-soiling	The dog eliminates in areas that were previously kept clean • House-soiling • Eliminating in the sleeping area • Fails to signal the need to eliminate • Alterations in the preferred soiling substrate/area • Eliminating indoors right after being outside
Altered *A*ctivity levels	Activity levels are increased or decreased • Increased pacing, circling, wandering aimlessly • Repetitive behavior (eg, tail chasing, fly biting) • Staring blankly at walls • Altered/reduced exploratory behavior • Reduced play
Anxiety	Increased anxiety and fear in response to changes in the environment, such as new stimuli or being left alone

Data from References [6,9,11,12,15,17–20].

than 4 domains; the dog's quality of life and, possibly, the human-animal bond are compromised

The symptoms associated with CCDS are common to several other medical and behavioral conditions [15,22–25]. It is therefore important that an accurate evaluation is performed in each case where CCDS is suspected. First, a veterinary behavior specialist should perform a thorough behavioral examination to identify all the signs potentially associated to CCDS and confirm whether they have had a late onset or have rather been present since a younger age. The initial assessment should be performed using a rating scale or scoring system (Supplementary Table 1). Some scales, such as the CCDR by Salvin and colleagues [19], are considered more appropriate for general screening and are designed completed by dog owners. Other scales, such as the CADES (CAnine DEmentia Scale) by Madari and colleagues [9], include the evaluation of the pet during consultation. In some cases, such as the CCAS scale by CAWEC, the scales have been associated with the cognitive evaluation of clinical patients [17]. Finally, some scales such as the RDR questionnaire by Rofina and colleagues [26] have demonstrated a positive relationship with histological and anatomical brain changes indicative of CCDS, although it was not possible to rule out medical causes for the symptoms when the questionnaire was developed, and the questionnaire's score does not provide staging of the condition. Ancillary examinations (eg, bloodwork, urinalysis, and imaging) may be prescribed based on the clinical case, in order to rule out medical differential diagnoses [15,22]. Overall, the diagnosis of CCDS is a diagnosis by exclusion; there are no pathognomonic clinical signs of CCDS, and a definitive diagnosis can only be reached post-mortem, considering the behavioral symptoms that occurred in vivo and histological changes in the brain [26]. For this reason, researchers have been focusing on the identification of peripheral biomarkers for the diagnosis of CCDS.

Histopathological Changes

At pathophysiological level, CCDS is considered analogous with the early stages of human Alzheimer Disease [27]. In fact, the main pathological brain changes linked to CCDS include brain atrophy, neuron loss, accumulation of Alzheimer disease-like neuropathology, vascular pathology, oxidative damage, and inflammation [15]. For example, cortical and hippocampal atrophy, as well as ventricular enlargement, have been observed in MRIs and confirmed by histological findings [28–30]. Furthermore, 2 hallmarks of human Alzheimer disease include the aggregation and deposition of amyloid-β (Aβ) as extracellular plaques and hyperphosphorylation of the microtubule-associated tau protein, which aggregates as intracellular neurofibrillary tangles (NFTs), which have also been associated with CCDS [20,26,31,32]. In addition, neurofilament light chain (NfL) is one of the subunits of neurofilament, which provides structural support to axons [33]. Low levels of NfL are constantly released from the axons; however, levels increase in the case of neurodegenerative and neuroinflammatory disease, trauma, and vascular disease [33]. Recent studies investigated the levels of Aβ amyloid, TAU filament, and NfL in dogs with various degrees of cognitive decline [34–38].

Amyloid plaques are extracellular depositions of the Aβ peptide, a 40 to 42 amino-acid-long by-product of a longer amyloid precursor protein [39]. There are 2 main isoforms of Aβ: the 42-residue Aβ42 and the 40-residue Aβ40, the only difference between Aβ42 and Aβ40 being that Aβ42 has 2 extra residues. Human research indicates that both Aβ42 and Aβ40 can aggregate in amyloid plaques in vitro, although in vivo there is a preferential deposition of Aβ42 at the extracellular space [40]. In dogs, Aβ accumulates in the brain cortex beginning in the prefrontal cortex and later in the temporal and occipital cortex [41]. There is evidence regarding the relationship between the extent of Aβ plaque deposition in the brain and the severity of cognitive deficits in dogs [26,42–44]. Some studies observed a positive relationship between brain Aβ deposits and canine cognitive decline measured in cognitive testing [43,44]. Colle and colleagues [42] found a moderate positive correlation ($r = 0.55$) between brain Aβ deposits and behavioral signs measured with the ARCAD scale [45], which is not specific for CCDS. A study by Borghys and colleagues [46] investigated the cognitive performance and the levels of Aβ42 in the CSF of laboratory beagle dogs aged 1.5 to 7 years. The authors compared 8 dogs with low mean Aβ42 levels in CSF (<600 pg/mL) and 10 dogs with high mean Aβ-42 levels (>600 pg/mL). The dogs with high Aβ42 levels showed significantly more errors in discriminative learning tasks, even in the absence of age effects [46]. The authors concluded that high Aβ42 levels in CSF early in life may be linked to decline in learning abilities in dogs, although confirmatory studies are necessary because of the difficulties in identifying dogs with consistent low and high CSF Aβ levels [46].

Similarly, Urfer and colleagues [47] found a linear relationship between the levels of Aβ42 deposits in 3 brain regions (prefrontal cortex, temporal cortex, hippocampus) and CCDR scale [48]. One study failed to identify a significant correlation between brain Aβ

deposition and signs of CCDS; however, only 16 dogs were analyzed, so it cannot be excluded [28].

Conversely, tau proteins are physiologically confined to neuronal axons. In Alzheimer disease, however, tau is hyperphosphorylated and mislocalized to somatodendritic areas, where it aggregates as NTFs [49]. Research on tau pathology in CCDS originally identified the accumulation of NTFs in less than 10% of dogs affected by CCDS, mostly localized at the hippocampal area [36,37]. However, recent studies have yielded more promising results. Abey and colleagues [50] investigated the presence of tau filaments in multiple brain regions of a small sample (n = 6) of dogs suspected to have CCDS following scoring with a scale by Salvin and colleagues [19], and compared them with healthy subjects (n = 6) [50]. The scale is designed for screening rather than diagnostic purposes [15]; however, the authors who developed it argued that high scores (>50) should be considered highly suspicious of CCDS [19]. Abey and colleagues [50] observed signs of p-tau accumulation in the thalamic and hippocampal areas of the Papez circuit [50]. In people, the Papez circuit comprises structures that are critically involved in episodic memory and contribute to cognitive impairment in Alzheimer disease [51]. The findings by Abey and colleagues [50] indicate that the hyperphosphorylated tau observed in brains of dogs affected by CCDS occurs in structures that are anatomically connected and functionally relevant to the clinical presentation of the condition. Similarly, Habiba and colleagues [52] have examined the brain of 37 dogs during routine necroscopies. Of these, n = 7 dogs had been previously assessed with the scale by Salvin and colleagues [19], and 5 had a score suspicious of CCDS (>50) [52]. The authors have identified signs of tau pathology in the hippocampus and frontal cortex region of the dog's brain, suggesting that newly refined immunostaining protocols for p-tau allow for better identification of the depositions [52].

Biomarkers of Canine Cognitive Dysfunction Syndrome

Interestingly, soluble Aβ can be measured in the cerebrospinal fluid (CSF) of dogs [46,53,54]. This led to the idea that Aβ levels in the CSF could be good markers for aging and cognitive decline [53] (Table 2).

One of the first investigations on the subjects was performed by Gonzales-Martinez and colleagues. [20], who measured the plasma concentration of Aβ40, Aβ42, detected with ELISA, and the Aβ42/40 ratio in dogs of various age groups, including 69 senior dogs aged at least 9 years. The senior dogs were classified as cognitively impaired (n = 31) and cognitively unimpaired (n = 38) following a clinical examination (physical and neurological examination, blood work, urinalysis, metabolic, mobility, and sensory deficits evaluation) and scoring with the RDR questionnaire by Rofina and colleagues [26] for CCDS [20]. The dogs in the cognitively impaired group had significantly higher levels of Aβ42 and Aβ42/40 ratio compared with the cognitively unimpaired dogs, while there were no statistical differences in the levels of Aβ40 [20]. In addition, the concentration of Aβ40 and Aβ42 was higher in young dogs (aged < 4 years, n = 9) compared to senior dogs, while the Aβ42/40 was lower. However, the authors reported significant overlap in the parameters' values between the 2 groups, thus compromising the discriminative capability of the test [20]. The overlap disappeared for the Aβ42 and the Aβ42/40, but not the Aβ40, when the authors compared the cognitively unimpaired dogs with a subgroup of mildly impaired dogs (n = 24, RDR score 2–5) [20].

Two more studies used the Salvin CCDR scale. Initially Schütt and colleagues [55] examined aged 8 years and more, free from medical conditions that could mimic CCDS, in a longitudinal study. They measured several biomarkers in the plasma using ELISA, including Aβ40 and Aβ42, and used the Salvin CCDR [19] and additional questions to create and compare 3 groups: cognitively unimpaired (n = 21), mild cognitive impairment (n = 16), and cognitively impaired CCDS (n = 12). As in the study by Gonzales-Martinez and colleagues. [20], Schütt and colleagues observed an overlapping in the biomarkers levels between the 3 groups [55]. However, Schütt and colleagues also found significantly higher levels of plasmatic Aβ42 in CCDS dogs compared with unimpaired and mildly impaired dogs [55]. They did not observe significant differences between groups in the levels of Aβ40 or Aβ42/40 [55]. More recently, Phochantachinda and colleagues [57] examined the plasma proteome of adult dogs (n = 4, age 1–7 years), normal aging dogs (n = 8, age > 7 years), and dogs suspected of CCDS (n = 10, age not reported) following the Salvin CCDR questionnaire [19], routine examination, and exclusion of dogs with potential neurological and metabolic conditions. In addition to proteomic analysis, they also used ELISA again to measure the plasmatic concentrations of Aβ42. Contrary to Gonzales-Martinez and colleagues. [20], Phochantachinda and colleagues [57] observed higher concentrations of Aβ42 in the normal aging dogs compared with the adult dogs. The discrepancy could be related to age differences, different cognitive status, or insufficient sample size. Phochantachinda and colleagues [57]

TABLE 2

Summary of the studies reporting comparisons in peripheral amyloid concentrations between senior dogs affected by canine cognitive dysfunction syndrome and healthy controls

		Gonzalez-Martinez [20] (2011)			Schütt [55] (2015)			Stylianaki [34] (2020)		Panek [56] (2021)			Phochantachinda [57] (2021)	Vikartovska [35] (2021)
		Aβ40	Aβ42	Aβ42/40	Aβ40	Aβ42	Aβ42/40	Aβ40	Aβ42	Aβ40	Aβ42	Aβ42/40	Aβ42	Aβ42
N	Controls	31	31	31	21	21	21	10	17	10	10	10	8	11
	Mild CCDS	21	21	21	17	17	17	4	10	4	4	4	-	13
	CCDS	17	17	17	13	13	13	5	20	5	5	5	10	-
Age (years)	Controls	12	12	12	12	12	12	11.9	13.5	11.9	11.9	11.9	>7	-
	Mild CCDS (years)	-	-	-	12.5	12.5	12.5	-	12.6	-	-	-	-	-
	CCDS	-	-	-	14	14	14	-	14.5	-	-	-	-	-
Concentration [ng/mL] Mean (SD)	Controls	64.7 (24.1)	23.3 (12)	0.35 (0.2)	0.2761 (0.063)	0.0749 (0.01)	0.28 (0.16)		10.42 (7.18)	0.19288 (0.14638)	0.01865 (0.01665)	0.1 (0.05)	0.17921 (0.1856)	0.0091 (0.0054)
	Mild CCDS	82.1 (38.8)	58.3 (65.5)	0.65 (0.37)	0.3148 (0.0894)	0.077 (0.0123)	0.26 (0.14)		23.03 (11.79)	0.19851 (0.09452)	0.01378 (0.0885)	0.08 (0.05)	-	0.0096 (0.0063)
	CCDS	75.3 (24.7)	31.1 (29.5)	0.37 (0.26)	0.3693 (0.1009)	0.0928 (0.024)	0.26 (0.24)		11.4 (12.98)	0.14326 (0.10776)	0.01087 (0.00578)	0.1 (0.05)	0.0754 (0.101)	-
Substrate		Plasma			Plasma			Plasma		Plasma			Plasma	Serum
Method		Enzyme-linked immunosorbent assay (ELISA)			ELISA			ELISA		Single molecule array assay (SIMOA)			ELISA	SIMOA
Balanced for sex:		Yes			Yes			No		No			Yes	?
Scale:		Rofina			Salvin + Rofina			CCAS		CADES			Salvin	CADES
Imaging:		No			No			No		No			No	No
Exclusion of neurological/ metabolic conditions:		Yes			Yes			Yes		Yes			No	Yes
Exclusion mobility conditions:		Yes			No			No		Yes			No	No
Exclusion sensory deficits:		Yes			Yes			Yes		Yes			No	No

also observed lower concentrations of Aβ42 in the CCDS dogs compared with the healthy controls, in accordance with the findings by Gonzales-Martinez and colleagues. [20]. Phochantachinda and colleagues [57] suggest that the decrease of Aβ42 may be caused by increased clearance and sequestration by Aβ sequester proteins. A study measured plasma Aβ40 and Aβ42 concentrations using ELISA.

Finally, 2 recent studies employed an innovative technology (SIMOA) that represents a highly sensitive platform that can detect thousands of single molecules simultaneously. Panek and colleagues [56] examined young dogs (n = 12, age 0.4–2 years), adult and mature dogs (n = 14, age 2.1–9 years), healthy senior dogs (n = 10, age 9.3–14.5 years), and dogs with suspected CCDS (n = 11, age 11–15.6 years), following scoring with the Madari CADES scale [9] and clinical examination to exclude other medical conditions. They found that plasma concentrations of Aβ40 and Aβ42 increased with age, while the Aβ42/Aβ40 ratio decreased [56]. They did not observe the decline in plasma amyloid in senior dogs observed in other studies. When they compared the dogs with suspected CCDS with the healthy senior dogs, however, they found significantly lower plasmatic levels of Aβ40 and Aβ42 in the CCDS group, but no differences in the Aβ42/Aβ40 ratio [56]. On the contrary, Vikartovska and colleagues [35] found different results. They measured the serum concentration of Aβ42, tau protein, and NfL in young dogs (n = 11, age < 3 years), 11 healthy senior dogs, and 13 dogs suspected of mild CCDS (dogs in both groups above the age of 8 years) following assessment with the Madari CADES scale and clinical evaluation [35], and found no statistical difference between the groups for Aβ42 and tau protein. On the contrary, they observed a sevenfold increase of serum NfL levels in normal aging compared with young dogs and a threefold increase in mild CCDS dogs compared with healthy aging dogs [35].

A few studies have focused on NfL as a potential biomarker for neurodegenerative disease. NfL is of interest as a biomarker for neurodegenerative disease due to ease of acquisition in blood samples. In humans, the use of NfL concentration has improved diagnostic accuracy of neurodegenerative disease and has been used as prognostic biomarker [58]. In dogs, it has been suggested that NfL can be a translational biomarker for aging and neurodegeneration [38]. One study by Panek and colleagues [38] has investigated the concentration of NfL in 36 healthy dogs of various age groups (n = 2 between 0.4 and 2 years, n = 14 between 2 and 9 years, n = 10 between 9 and 14.5 years), n = 11 senior dogs suspected diagnosis of CCDS (age

11–15.6 years), and n = 16 senior dogs affected with degenerative myelopathy (age 7.5–12.6 years). The diagnostic suspect of CCDS was corroborated by two scales, the CADES by Madari and colleagues [9] and the CCDR by Salvin and colleagues [19], in addition to physical, orthopedic, and neurological examinations; metabolic and neurological conditions, as well as sensory deficits and the use of medication that could affect the diagnosis were reasons of exclusion from the study [38]. The authors found that plasma NfL concentrations increased with age and in dogs suspected of CCDS according to CADES [38]. The positive relationship between plasma NfL concentrations and age in dogs was also confirmed in a study by Perino and colleagues [59], who examined 55 pure bred Labrador retrievers free from neuropathic and endocrine disease, chemotherapy, steroid administration, and any neurological symptom. In addition, the authors found a negative relationship between NfL concentration, the weight, and the height of the dog [59], supporting the idea that lifespan declines in dogs with increasing size [60].

Overall, the evidence on peripheral biomarkers for CCDS is unclear. The studies often have small sample size, which makes it difficult to interpret and weight their conclusions. In addition, the diagnostic methods and the scales vary between studies. For this reason, the authors briefly reviewed the literature covering in vivo peripheral markers for CCDS and performed a meta-analysis to systematically examine the articles published on this subject and strength of the evidence.

MATERIALS AND METHODS
The preferred reporting items for systematic reviews and meta-analysis (PRISMA) statement guidelines (Moher and colleagues, 2009) were followed when performing this study.

Search Strategy
The authors searched the PubMed, Web of Science (WOS), and Scopus databases for peer-reviewed studies reporting on serum or plasma amyloid-β 40 and 42, tau protein, and/or NfL markers in senior from 1995 to 2022 (ie, until February of 2022). The keyword terms were "(beta amyloid canine cognitive dysfunction) OR (beta amyloid cognitive dysfunction dog) OR (tau canine cognitive dysfunction) OR (tau cognitive dysfunction dog) OR (NfL canine cognitive dysfunction) OR (NfL dog cognitive dysfunction)." All searches were limited to original articles. Fig. 1 shows a flow diagram that summarizes all stages of the systematic

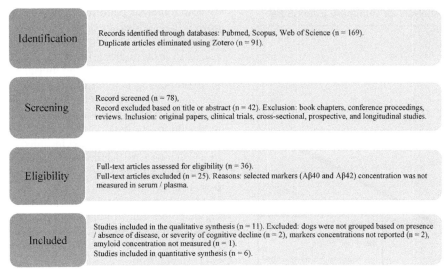

Identification
Records identified through databases: Pubmed, Scopus, Web of Science (n = 169).
Duplicate articles eliminated using Zotero (n = 91).

Screening
Record screened (n = 78),
Record excluded based on title or abstract (n = 42). Exclusion: book chapters, conference proceedings, reviews. Inclusion: original papers, clinical trials, cross-sectional, prospective, and longitudinal studies.

Eligibility
Full-text articles assessed for eligibility (n = 36).
Full-text articles excluded (n = 25). Reasons: selected markers (Aβ40 and Aβ42) concentration was not measured in serum / plasma.

Included
Studies included in the qualitative synthesis (n = 11). Excluded: dogs were not grouped based on presence / absence of disease, or severity of cognitive decline (n = 2), markers concentrations not reported (n = 2), amyloid concentration not measured (n = 1).
Studies included in quantitative synthesis (n = 6).

FIG. 1 Stages of the systematic review process.

review process, including the numbers of studies identified at each stage and any reasons for exclusion.

Inclusion Criteria

The retrieved studies were screened based on the titles, abstracts, and contents. Studies were identified as eligible for inclusion if they met the following criteria: (1) observational studies (case–control) or prospective studies, or (2) studies reporting circulating amyloid-β 40 and 42 concentrations in healthy senior dogs versus dogs affected by CCDS. Excluded studies are described in Supplementary Table 2. The exclusion criteria were absence of dogs affected by CCDS in the study and absence of reporting blood Aβ 40 and 42 measurements. Given the limited number of studies measuring tau protein (n = 4) and NfL (n = 2), these too have been excluded from further analysis, which has focused on Aβ markers. Studies using more than 1 experimental design or more than 1 assay method for blood Aβ 40 and 42 measurements determination were included. Some studies showed more than 2 groups for the comparative analysis of amyloid-β 40 and 42 (ie, normal aging, mild CCDS, and severe CCDS); however, the final analysis compared between normal aging and severe cases of CCDS.

Data Coding

Data extraction was performed for the studies found by a standardized Excel spreadsheet that was used to record all the relevant data and variables to be analyzed (see Table 2

and Supplementary Table 2). The data extracted were: title, first author, publication year, DOI, marker(s) measured, sample size, age of the dogs, study design, recruitment method, assay method used and brand, inclusion and exclusion criteria, and diagnostic scale for CCDS.

Risk of Bias and Quality Assessment

Given the heterogenicity of the studies retrieved from the literature, several sources of bias were assessed (Supplementary Table 3) based on the NHLBI study quality assessment tool [61]:

1. Identification of the research question: well defined in all studies
2. Definition of the research population: in some cases, the recruitment criteria or even the ages of the dogs were not clarified
3. Sample size justification: none of the studies reported a power analysis calculation
4. Time frame for recruitment: not reported
5. Inclusion and exclusion criteria: while the exclusion of comorbidities is usually reported, none of the studies provided details on the exact criteria and diagnostic examinations performed on each of the dogs
6. Clear definition between cases and controls: all studies but one [20] only reported in vivo diagnosis of CCDS
7. Justification for using less than 100% of eligible population: some of the studies analyzed the

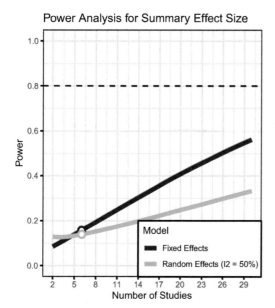

Power Analysis for Summary Effect Size

FIG. 2 Power analysis. The red line indicates the estimated power for fixed effect, and the blue line indicates the estimated power for random effects (power = 0.8 as reference reported as *dotted line*).

sample of a subgroup of dogs, but the selection of the dogs was not described

8. Use of concurrent controls (N/A)
9. Risk exposure (N/A)
10. Blinding method (N/A)
11. Control for confounding variables in the statistical analysis: while nearly all studies reported several confounding variables (sex, neutering status, weight, body condition score [BCS], weight), none adjusted the statistical analysis accordingly

RESULTS

All statistical analyses were performed with the statistical language R [62].

Power analysis performed using the package meta-poweR [63] yielded an estimated power of 0.16 with an expected effect size of d = 0.2 and an expected study size of 15 for 6 studies (Fig. 2).

The packages meta [64] and dmetar [65] were used to assess heterogeneity in the data and pool the effect sizes from the studies. Given the small number of studies, it was not possible to calculate a meta-regression for the data.

The first fixed-effect model included the concentrations on Aβ42 in healthy senior dogs versus CCDS (number of studies k = 5, number of observations o = 152, inverse variance method, Hedges' g calculated, bias corrected standardized mean difference using exact formula). Initial analysis indicated that the pooled effect according to the fixed-effects model (SMD) is g = 0.23, with the 95% confidence interval (CI) ranging from −0.1012 to 0.5711. The effect was not significant ($p = .170$). The restricted maximum likelihood method estimated a between-study heterogeneity variance of $\tau^2 = 0.269$. The confidence interval of τ^2 includes zero, meaning that the variance of true effect sizes is not significantly greater than zero ($I^2 = 60.8\%$; the heterogeneity H = 1.60 [ie, more than 50% of the variation in the data] is estimated to stem from true effect size differences [low heterogeneity, Table 3]).

No outliers were detected (ie, the CIs of the study do not overlap with the CIs of the pooled effect); however, influence analysis was used to identify if any given study had an extremely large effect on the results (Figs. 3–6).

Given that the study by Schütt and colleagues [55] consistently appeared to influence the data, it was decided to calculate again the fixed effect model without this study (number of studies k = 4, number of observations o = 118, inverse variance method, Hedges' g calculated, bias corrected standardized mean difference using exact formula). The analysis yielded a standardized mean difference of g = 0.02, which was

TABLE 3
Results of the meta-analysis

Analysis	g	95%CI	p	95%PI	I²	I² 95%CI
Aβ42: Healthy vs CCDS	0.23	−0.10–0.57	0.171	−1.76–2.04	61%	0% - 85%
Infl. Cases removed[a]	0.02	−0.35–0.40	0.901	−1.61–1.54	31%	0% - 75%
Aβ40: healthy vs CCDS	0.54	0.11–0.97	0.013	−7.87–8.84	61%	0% - 89%

[a] Removed an influential case: Schütt and colleagues, 2015.

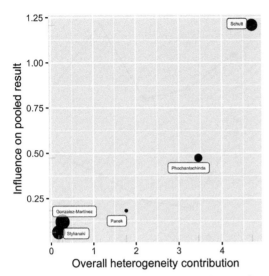

FIG. 3 Baujat plot. The plot shows the contribution of each study to the overall heterogeneity (measured by Cochran's Q) on the horizontal axis, and its influence on the pooled effect size on the vertical axis. The studies on the right side of the plot (Schütt, Phochantachinda) can be regarded as potentially relevant cases since they contribute heavily to the overall heterogeneity in the authors' meta-analysis. Studies in the upper right corner of the plot (Schütt) may be particularly influential, as they have a large impact on the estimated heterogeneity, and the pooled effect [66].

not significant (p=.926) and had a small heterogeneity of I^2 = 31% (see Table 3).

The second fixed effect model included the concentrations on Aβ40 in healthy senior dogs versus CCDS (number of studies k = 3, number of observations o = 97, inverse variance method, Hedges' g calculated, bias corrected standardized mean difference using exact formula). Initial analysis indicated that the pooled effect according to the fixed-effects model (SMD) is g = 0.54, p=.013, with the 95% CI ranging from 0.11 to 0.97. The restricted maximum likelihood method estimated a between-study heterogeneity variance of τ^2 = 0.28. The CI of τ^2 includes zero, meaning that the variance of true effect sizes is not significantly greater than zero (I^2 = 61.6%; the heterogeneity H = 1.61 [ie, more than 50% of the variation in the data] is estimated to stem from true effect size differences [low heterogeneity]). No outliers were detected. Given the limited number of studies, the authors did not calculate influential analysis. However, the authors inspected the data visually to better understand the observed heterogeneity; the graphs indicate a

marked separation between the study from Gonzales-Martinez and colleagues [20] and those from Panek and colleagues [56] and Schütt and colleagues [55] (Fig. 7).

DISCUSSION

The goal of this article was to review and perform a meta-analysis of the literature on peripheral biomarkers for CCDS. There were insufficient studies to address the findings on tau protein and NfL in dogs; therefore, the meta-analysis has focused on Aβ. In addition, the analysis has focused on the difference between dogs affected by CCDS and healthy controls of similar age. The main finding of this meta-analysis is that there is no compelling evidence that Aβ42 varies significantly between the 2 groups. However, the pooled effects on Aβ40 indicate that this marker varies significantly between dogs diagnosed with CCDS and healthy controls. Nevertheless, it should be noted that only 3 studies were available on Aβ40, which lead to a small size effect for both analyses.

Some of the studies examined in this meta-analysis analyzed the age effect on Aβ plasmatic concentrations and the relationship with CCDS. Gonzales-Martinez and colleagues [20] observed lower Aβ concentration in senior dogs compared with young and adults, then an increase in dogs affected by CCDS (especially mild presentations) compared with healthy senior controls. The authors suggested that the decreased concentration of Aβ in healthy senior dogs compared with young dogs might be caused by amyloid deposition or decreased production. In contrast, Aβ42 production might increase in dogs suffering from CCDS, thus reversing the pattern observed in successful aging [20]. In addition, according to the amyloid hypothesis, in human Alzheimer disease the condition begins when Aβ42 starts to aggregate and precipitate in the brain's interstitial space, slowly obstructing the ventricular system and reducing Aβ levels in the CSF and consequently in the bloodstream [67,68]. Similarly, the authors argued that, in dogs, the increase of Aβ might become apparent in the plasma in the early stages of the condition, when there is not yet extensive vascular damage, while the subsequent drop in Aβ42 could be related to the amyloid deposition around of capillaries, which might obstruct the brain-blood barrier [20].

Another potential issue with the study of CCDS biomarkers is that the diagnosis cannot be confirmed in vivo. Only one [20] of the studies included in the meta-analysis considered postmortem examination of

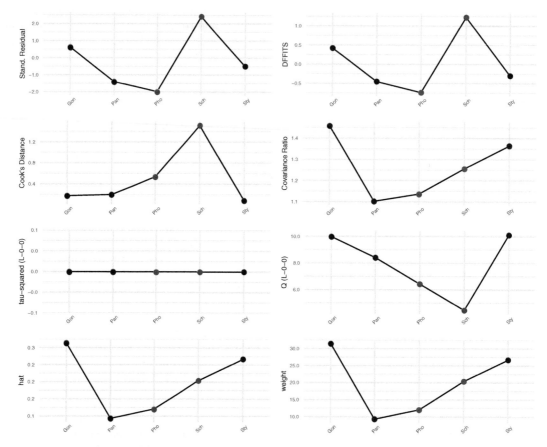

FIG. 4 Influence plots. Externally standardized residuals plot: these residuals are the deviation of each observed effect size from the pooled effect size. DFFITS value: indicates how (in standard deviations) the pooled effect changes when one or more studies are removed. Cook's distance: similar to the DFFITS value. Covariance ratio: calculated dividing the variance of the pooled effect (ie, its squared standard error) without each study by the variance of the initial average effect. Leave-One-Out $\tau 2$, Q Values, study weight and hat value of each study are calculated by the analysis but will not be considered. These metrics provide a visual indication of what studies might be influential cases and may negatively affect the robustness of the pooled result (displayed in red in the plot generated by the InfluenceAnalysis function [66]). Schütt and Phochantachinda are indicated as potentially influential.

the brains of the dogs, thus providing histological confirmation of the condition. Oftentimes the diagnosis relied on questionnaires, while details of the clinical examination were not provided on a case-by-case basis. The impact of co-occurring medical conditions on the symptoms of CCDS are largely understudied; however, the topic needs to be better understood, as, from a clinical point of view, it is often not possible to disentangle the two [22,23]. Recent research, however, is highlighting not only the behavioral manifestations of medical conditions in dogs [24], but also the indirect and not yet understood role of pain on

behavioral problems, including anxiety, and quality of life in dogs [69–71].

Some authors [46] argued that increased amyloid processing likely results in increased levels of amyloid, which might contribute to learning impairments. High levels of Aβ in the CSF, possibly caused by increased production and/or the anticipated subsequent increase in amyloid oligomers, may be predictive of significant learning impairments [46]. In turn, learning impairments likely precede cerebral amyloid deposition. Unsurprisingly, some recent studies have focused on the evaluation of the quality of life [13,72]

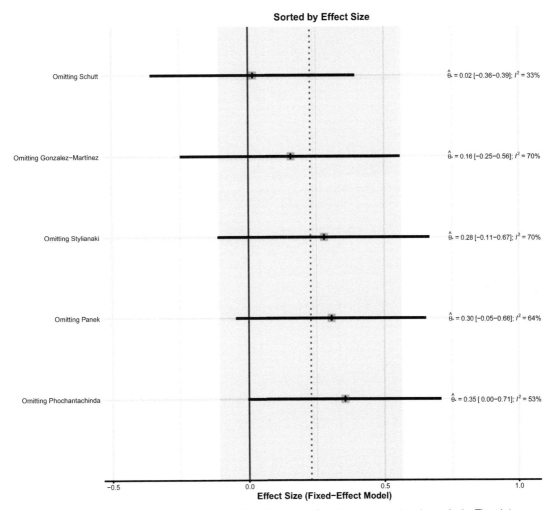

FIG. 5 Forest plot of effect sizes pooled by the effect size of the leave-one-out meta-analysis. The plot indicates effect size heterogeneity by calculating the effect size with 1 study omitted each time. The vertical dotted line and the green area represent the original pooled effect size and the 95% CIs.

and the cognitive decline occurring in apparently healthy aging dogs (ie, those dogs that are not specifically suspected of CCDS) [1–3,73]. Important age-related changes in memory, learning, and executive function can be measured through cognitive testing of the general pet dog population [1,2]. In accordance with this direction of research, the recently developed CCAS scale, by CAWEC, for the diagnosis of CCDS has triangulated clinical, behavioral, and cognitive data [17]. The most recent studies have focused on an integrated approach to assess the overall behavioral, cognitive, and health status of aging dogs [74,75]. Fleyshman and colleagues [75] proposed a multidimensional approach for the assessment of aging dogs,

focusing on the retired sled dog population. They proposed an assessment of the general health, physical fitness, immune system biomarkers, in vivo and questionnaire-based cognitive testing, and somatic cell genomic modification [75]. Similarly, Fefer and colleagues [74] examined the physical health, the cognitive status based on in vivo testing and questionnaires, and biomarkers. The authors concluded that a multidimensional approach using a combination of questionnaires, specific cognitive tests, and biomarkers concentration can be used to quantify cognitive decline in aging pet dogs [74].

Overall, the evidence for the clinical use of Aβ as peripheral markers of CCDS is not yet sufficient, but the

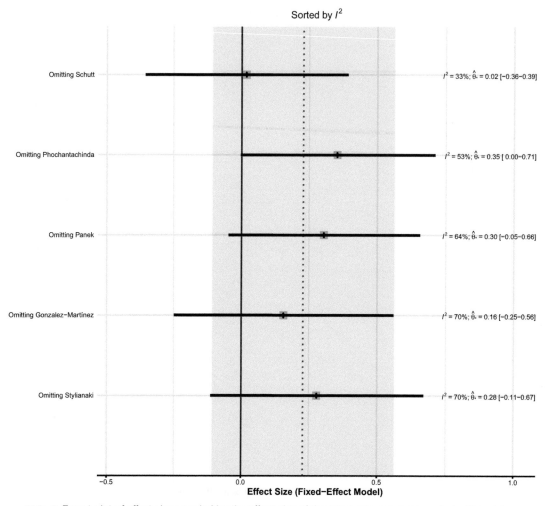

FIG. 6 Forest plot of effect sizes pooled by the effect size of the leave-one-out meta-analysis. The plot indicates effect size heterogeneity by calculating the effect size with 1 study omitted each time. The vertical dotted line and the green area represent the original pooled effect size and the 95% CIs.

current findings suggest that it is worthy of further research. Particularly, the most recent articles have adopted methodologies such as proteomics and SIMOA, which is a highly sensitive platform and can detect thousands of single molecules simultaneously, and immune-infrared measurements. In people, the methods have been recently adopted to investigate the predicting value of several biomarkers in plasma, such as Aβ misfolding, Aβ42/Aβ40 ratio, phosphorylated tau, NfL chain, and glial fibrillary acidic protein (GFAP) [76]. The authors found that Aβ misfolding showed the best discriminative performance, and a combination of Aβ misfolding and GFAP increased the value of the prediction accuracy of the incidence of Alzheimer disease [76]. SIMOA has been used in two of the studies examined in the current meta-analysis [35,56]; both looked at Aβ42 concentrations, though only 1 study also measured Aβ40 and other markers (eg, NfL) [56]. However, the findings in these 2 studies are contradictory as 1 study found a decrease in plasmatic Aβ in dogs diagnosed with CCDS compared with healthy senior controls [56], while the other did not find differences between the groups [35]. It is possible that, as suggested by the latest human literature, that Aβ misfolding, rather than Aβ concentrations, is a better predictor for the condition [76].

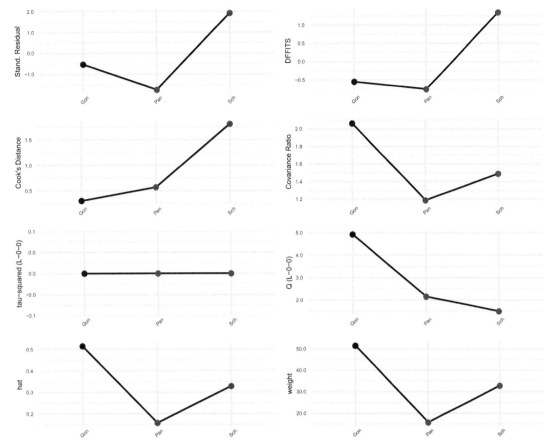

FIG. 7 Influence plots. Externally standardized residuals plot; DFFITS value; Cook's distance; covariance ratio. Leave-one-out τ2, Q values, study weight and hat value of each study are calculated by the analysis but will not be considered. The plots indicate a discrepancy between Gonzales-Martinez versus Schütt and Panek.

CLINICS CARE POINTS

- Canine Cognitive Dysfunction Syndrome (CCDS) is a diagnosis by exclusion when performed ante-mortem: the clinician should perform a clinical evaluation, including physical examination, behavioral consultation, cognitive assessment, and instrumental tests to exclude and/or identify comorbidities

- CCDS affects 6 domains following the acronym DIS-HAA: disorientation; altered interactions, learning, and memory; sleep-wake cycle alterations; house-soiling; altered activity levels; anxiety.

- Three stages of CCDS can be identified as part of the clinical assessment: 1) normal aging (0–2 domains mildly or occasionally affected, often not noticeable by owners); 2) moderate cognitive impairment (2–4 domains affected, usually the most undesirable changes are noticed, such as house-soiling or increased activity at night); severe cognitive impairment (more than 4 domains are affected).

- The CCDR scale from Salvin and colleagues can be used for routine screening aging dogs and the can be completed by dog owners.

- The CADES scale from Madari and colleagues or the CCAS scale by CAWEC could be used for diagnostic purposes.

- Diagnostic scales can be used to monitor the progression of the condition, but the same clinician should perform the consultation to ensure accuracy.

- Currently, there is no evidence that peripheral biomarkers could clinically confirm a diagnosis of CCDS.

SUPPLEMENTARY DATA

Supplementary data related to this article can be found online at https://doi.org/10.1016/j.yasa.2022.07.002.

REFERENCES

[1] Piotti P, Szabó D, Wallis L, et al. The effect of age on visuo-spatial short-term memory in family dogs. Pet Behav Sci 2017;(4):17. https://doi.org/10.21071/pbs.v0i4.10130.

[2] Piotti P, Szabó D, Bognár Z, et al. Effect of age on discrimination learning, reversal learning, and cognitive bias in family dogs. Learn Behav 2018;46(4):537–53.

[3] Szabó D, Gee NR, Miklósi A. Natural or pathologic? Discrepancies in the study of behavioral and cognitive signs in aging family dogs. J Vet Behav Clin Appl Res 2016;11:86–98.

[4] Hedden T, Gabrieli JDE. Insights into the ageing mind: a view from cognitive neuroscience. Nat Rev Neurosci 2004;5(2):87–96.

[5] Landsberg G, Araujo JA. Behavior problems in geriatric pets. Vet Clin North America - Small Anim Pract 2005;35(3):675–98.

[6] Azkona G, García-Belenguer S, Chacón G, et al. Prevalence and risk factors of behavioural changes associated with age-related cognitive impairment in geriatric dogs. J small Anim Pract 2009;50(2):87–91.

[7] Fast R, Schütt T, Toft N, et al. An observational study with long-term follow-up of canine cognitive dysfunction: clinical characteristics, survival, and risk factors. J Vet Intern Med 2013;27(4):822–9.

[8] Katina S, Farbakova J, Madari A, et al. Risk factors for canine cognitive dysfunction syndrome in Slovakia. Acta veterinaria Scand 2016;58(1):17.

[9] Madari A, Farbakova J, Katina S, et al. Assessment of severity and progression of canine cognitive dysfunction syndrome using the CAnine DEmentia Scale (CADES). Appl Anim Behav Sci 2015;(171):138–45.

[10] Neilson JC, Hart BL, Cliff KD, et al. Prevalence of behavioral changes associated with age-related cognitive impairment in dogs. J Am Vet Med Assoc 2001;218(11):1787–91.

[11] Osella MC, Re G, Odore R, et al. Canine cognitive dysfunction syndrome: prevalence, clinical signs and treatment with a neuroprotective nutraceutical. Appl Anim Behav Sci 2007;105(4):297–310.

[12] Salvin HE, McGreevy PD, Sachdev PS, et al. Under diagnosis of canine cognitive dysfunction: a cross-sectional survey of older companion dogs. Vet J 2010;184(3):277–81.

[13] Piotti P. Positive emotions and quality of life in dogs. Anim Sentience 2017;090:6.

[14] Manteca X. Nutrition and behavior in senior dogs. Top Companion Anim Med 2011;26(1):33–6.

[15] Landsberg G, Madari A, Žilka N, editors. Canine and feline dementia: molecular basis, diagnostics and therapy. 1st edition. Cham, Switzerland: Springer International Publishing; 2017.

[16] Landsberg G, Hunthausen W, Ackerman L. 3rd. Handbook of behavior problems of the dog and the cat. Missouri: Saunders; 2013.

[17] Le Brech S, Amat M, Temple D, Manteca X. Two feasible methods to detect cognitive impairment in aged dogs. Presented at: 3rd European Veterinary Congress of Behavioural Medicine and Animal Welfare; 2021; Online.

[18] Gunn-Moore D, Moffat K, Christie LA, et al. Cognitive dysfunction and the neurobiology of ageing in cats. J Small Anim Pract 2007;48(10):546–53.

[19] Salvin HE, McGreevy PD, Sachdev PS, et al. The canine cognitive dysfunction rating scale (CCDR): A data-driven and ecologically relevant assessment tool. Vet J 2011;188(3):331–6. https://doi.org/10.1016/j.tvjl.2010.05.014.

[20] González-Martínez Á, Rosado B, Pesini P, et al. Plasma β-amyloid peptides in canine aging and cognitive dysfunction as a model of Alzheimer's disease. Exp Gerontol 2011;46(7):590–6.

[21] Boronat AC, Ferreira-Maia AP, Wang YP. Sundown syndrome in older persons: a scoping review. J Am Med Directors Assoc 2019;20(6):664–71.e5.

[22] Bellows J, Colitz CMH, Daristotle L, et al. Defining healthy aging in older dogs and differentiating healthy aging from disease. J Am Vet Med Assoc 2015;246(1):77–89.

[23] Bellows J, Colitz CMH, Daristotle L, et al. Common physical and functional changes associated with aging in dogs. J Am Vet Med Assoc 2015;246(1):67–75.

24 Fatjó J, Bowen J. Medical and metabolic influences on behavioural disorders. In: Horwitz DF, Mills DS, editors. BSAVA Manual of Canine and Feline Behavioural Medicine. chapter 1. 2nd ed. Glouchester, UK: BSAVA; 2009. p. 1–9.

[25] Overall KL. Medical differentials with potential behavioral manifestations. Clin Tech small Anim Pract 2004;19(4):250–8.

[26] Rofina JE, Van Ederen AM, Toussaint MJM, et al. Cognitive disturbances in old dogs suffering from the canine counterpart of Alzheimer's disease. Brain Res 2006;1069(1):216–26.

[27] Andel IV, Ederen AMV, Papaioannou N, et al. Canine counterpart of senile dementia of the Alzheimer type : amyloid plaques near capillaries microglia and macrophages Canine counterpart of senile dementia of the Alzheimer type : amyloid plaques near capillaries but lack of spatial relationship with a. Amyloid 2009;(2017):6129. https://doi.org/10.3109/13506120309041730.

[28] Ozawa M, Chambers JK, Uchida K, et al. The relation between canine cognitive dysfunction and age-related brain lesions. J Vet Med Sci 2016. https://doi.org/10.1292/jvms.15-0624.

[29] Su M, Head E, Brooks WM, et al. Magnetic resonance imaging of anatomic and vascular characteristics in a canine

model of human aging. Neurobiol Aging 1998;19(5): 479–85.

[30] Tapp PD, Siwak CT, Estrada J, et al. Size and reversal learning in the beagle dog as a measure of executive function and inhibitory control in aging. Learn Mem 2003; 10(1):64–73.

[31] Ruehl WW, Bruyette DS, DePaoli A, et al. Canine cognitive dysfunction as a model for human age-related cognitive decline, dementia and Alzheimer's disease: clinical presentation, cognitive testing, pathology and response to 1-deprenyl therapy. Prog Brain Res 1995;106:217–25.

[32] Yu CH, Song GS, Yhee JY, et al. Histopathological and Immunohistochemical comparison of the brain of human patients with Alzheimer's disease and the brain of aged dogs with cognitive dysfunction. J Comp Pathol 2011;145(1):45–58.

[33] Gafson AR, Barthélemy NR, Bomont P, et al. Neurofilaments: neurobiological foundations for biomarker applications. Brain 2020;143(7):1975–98.

[34] Stylianaki I, Polizopoulou ZS, Theodoridis A, et al. Amyloid-beta plasma and cerebrospinal fluid biomarkers in aged dogs with cognitive dysfunction syndrome. J Vet Intern Med 2020;34(4):1532–40.

[35] Vikartovska Z, Farbakova J, Smolek T, et al. Novel diagnostic tools for identifying cognitive impairment in dogs: behavior, biomarkers, and pathology. Front Vet Sci 2020;7:551895.

[36] Schmidt F, Boltze J, Jäger C, et al. Detection and quantification of β-amyloid, pyroglutamyl Aβ, and tau in aged canines. J Neuropathol Exp Neurol 2015;74(9):912–23.

[37] Smolek T, Madari A, Farbakova J, et al. Tau hyperphosphorylation in synaptosomes and neuroinflammation are associated with canine cognitive impairment. J Comp Neurol 2016;524(4):874–95.

[38] Panek WK, Gruen ME, Murdoch DM, et al. Plasma neurofilament light chain as a translational biomarker of aging and neurodegeneration in dogs. Mol Neurobiol 2020;57(7):3143–9.

[39] Selkoe DJ. Normal and abnormal biology of the beta-amyloid precursor protein. Annu Rev Neurosci 1994; 17(1):489–517.

[40] Gu L, Guo Z. Alzheimer's Aβ42 and Aβ40 peptides form interlaced amyloid fibrils. J Neurochem 2013;126(3): 305–11.

[41] Head E, McCleary R, Hahn FF, et al. Region-specific age at onset of β-amyloid in dogs. Neurobiol Aging 2000; 21(1):89–96.

[42] Colle M, Hauw J, Crespeau F, et al. Vascular and parenchymal Aβ deposition in the aging dog. correlation. Behav 2000;21:695–704.

[43] Cummings BJ, Head E, Afagh AJ, et al. Beta-amyloid accumulation correlates with cognitive dysfunction in the aged canine. Neurobiol Learn Mem 1996;66(1): 11–23.

[44] Head E, Callahan H, Muggenburg BA, et al. Visual-discrimination learning ability and β-amyloid accumulation in the dog. Neurobiol Aging 1998;19(5):415–25.

[45] Pageat P. Pathologie du comportement du chien. 1st edition. France: Le Point Vétérinaire; 1995.

[46] Borghys H, Van Broeck B, Dhuyvetter D, et al. Young to middle-aged dogs with high amyloid-β levels in cerebrospinal fluid are impaired on learning in standard cognition tests. J Alzheimers Dis 2017;56(2):763–74.

[47] Urfer SR, Darvas M, Czeibert K, et al. Canine cognitive dysfunction (CCD) scores correlate with amyloid beta 42 levels in dog brain tissue. Geroscience 2021;43(5): 2379–86.

[48] Salvin HE, McGreevy PD, Sachdev PS, et al. Growing old gracefully-Behavioral changes associated with "successful aging" in the dog, Canis familiaris. J Vet Behav Clin Appl Res 2011;6(6):313–20.

[49] Wang JZ, Xia YY, Grundke-Iqbal I, et al. Abnormal hyperphosphorylation of tau: sites, regulation, and molecular mechanism of neurofibrillary degeneration. In: Perry G, Zhu X, Smith MA, et al, editors. JAD, 33 2012;. 2012. p. S123–39. https://doi.org/10.3233/-JAD-2012-129031, s1.

[50] Abey A, Davies D, Goldsbury C, et al. Distribution of tau hyperphosphorylation in canine dementia resembles early Alzheimer's disease and other tauopathies. Brain Pathol 2021;31(1):144–62.

[51] Aggleton JP, Pralus A, Nelson AJD, et al. Thalamic pathology and memory loss in early Alzheimer's disease: moving the focus from the medial temporal lobe to Papez circuit. Brain 2016;139(7):1877–90.

[52] Habiba U, Ozawa M, Chambers JK, et al. Neuronal deposition of amyloid-β oligomers and hyperphosphorylated tau is closely connected with cognitive dysfunction in aged dogs. J Alzheimers Dis Rep 2021; 5(1):749–60.

[53] Head E, Pop V, Sarsoza F, et al. Amyloid-β peptide and oligomers in the brain and cerebrospinal fluid of aged canines. JAD 2010;20(2):637–46.

[54] Sarasa L, Allué JA, Pesini P, et al. Identification of β-amyloid species in canine cerebrospinal fluid by mass spectrometry. Neurobiol Aging 2013;34(9):2125–32.

[55] Schutt T, Toft N, Berendt M. Cognitive function, progression of age-related behavioral changes, biomarkers, and survival in dogs more than 8 years old. J Vet Intern Med 2015;29(6):1569–77.

[56] Panek WK, Murdoch DM, Gruen ME, et al. Plasma amyloid beta concentrations in aged and cognitively impaired pet dogs. Mol Neurobiol 2021;58(2):483–9.

[57] Phochantachinda S, Chantong B, Reamtong O, et al. Change in the plasma proteome associated with canine cognitive dysfunction syndrome (CCDS) in Thailand. BMC Vet Res 2021;17(1):60.

[58] Olsson B, Portelius E, Cullen NC, et al. Association of cerebrospinal fluid neurofilament light protein levels with cognition in patients with dementia, motor neuron disease, and movement disorders. JAMA Neurol 2019; 76(3):318.

[59] Perino J, Patterson M, Momen M, et al. Neurofilament light plasma concentration positively associates with

age and negatively associates with weight and height in the dog. Neurosci Lett 2021;744:135593.

[60] Greer KA, Canterberry SC, Murphy KE. Statistical analysis regarding the effects of height and weight on life span of the domestic dog. Res Vet Sci 2007;82(2):208–14.

[61] NHLBI. Study. Quality assessment tool. 2013. https://www.nhlbi.nih.gov/health-topics/study-quality-assessment-tools. [Accessed 2 March 2022].

[62] Baayen RH. Analyzing linguistic data: a practical introduction to statistics using R. Processing 2008;2(3):353.

[63] Griffin J, Metapowe R. An R package for computing meta-analytic statistical power. 2020. Available at: https://CRAN.R-project.org/package=metapower.

[64] Balduzzi S, Rücker G, Schwarzer G. How to perform a meta-analysis with R: a practical tutorial. Evid Based Ment Health 2019;22(4):153–60.

[65] Harrer M, Cuijpers P, Furukawa T, et al. Dmetar: companion r package for the guide "doing meta-analysis in R. Available at: http://dmetar.protectlab.org/.

[66] Harrer M, Cuijpers P, Furukawa TA, et al. Doing meta-analysis with R: a hands-on guide. 1st. Oxon, UK: Chapman and Hall/CRC; 2021.

[67] Blennow K, Hampel H, Weiner M, et al. Cerebrospinal fluid and plasma biomarkers in Alzheimer disease. Nat Rev Neurol 2010;6(3):131–44.

[68] Kester MI, Verwey NA, van Elk EJ, et al. Evaluation of plasma Aβ40 and Aβ42 as predictors of conversion to Alzheimer's disease in patients with mild cognitive impairment. Neurobiol Aging 2010;31(4):539–40.

[69] Barcelos AM, Mills DS, Zulch H. Clinical indicators of occult musculoskeletal pain in aggressive dogs. Vet Rec 2015;176(18):465.

[70] Mills DS, Demontigny-Bédard I, Gruen M, et al. Pain and problem behavior in cats and dogs. Animals 2020;10(2):318.

[71] Piotti P, Albertini M, Lavesi E, et al. Physiotherapy improves dogs' quality of life measured with the Milan pet quality of life scale: is pain involved? Vet Sci 2022;9(7):335.

[72] Piotti P, Karagiannis C, Satchell LP, et al. Use of the Milan Pet Quality of Life instrument (MPQL) to measure pets' quality of life during COVID-19. Animals 2021;11:1336.

[73] Bognár Z, Piotti P, Szabó D, et al. A novel behavioural approach to assess responsiveness to auditory and visual stimuli before cognitive testing in family dogs. Appl Anim Behav Sci 2020;228:105016.

[74] Fefer G, Panek WK, Khan MZ, et al. Use of cognitive testing, questionnaires, and plasma biomarkers to quantify cognitive impairment in an aging pet dog population. JAD 2022;87(3):1367–78.

[75] Fleyshman DI, Wakshlag JJ, Huson HJ, et al. Development of infrastructure for a systemic multidisciplinary approach to study aging in retired sled dogs. Aging 2021;13(18):21814–37.

[76] Beyer L, Stocker H, Rujescu D, et al. Amyloid-beta misfolding and GFAP predict risk of clinical Alzheimer's disease diagnosis within 17 years. Alzheimer's & Dementia. Alzheimers Dement 2022. https://doi.org/10.1002/alz.12745.

SECTION II: DIAGNOSTIC IMAGING

Advances in Small Animal Care 3 (2022) 39–55

ADVANCES IN SMALL ANIMAL CARE

Cardiac Computed Tomography Imaging

Brian A. Scansen, DVM, MS, DACVIM (Cardiology)

Cardiology & Cardiac Surgery, Department of Clinical Sciences, Colorado State University, Campus Delivery 1678, Fort Collins, CO 80523, USA

KEYWORDS

- Dual-source computed tomography • Heart • Advanced imaging • Canine • Feline

KEY POINTS

- Cardiac computed tomography (CT) requires hardware and software that optimizes temporal resolution to freeze cardiac motion, that is gated to the cardiac cycle to allow reconstruction of different cardiac phases, and that offers sufficient spatial resolution to clarify important anatomy such as the coronary arteries.
- Cardiac CT in animals can be accomplished with a triphasic injection providing peak attenuation in the left heart, mixed attenuation in the right heart, and a saline flush, with variations on this protocol dependent on individual patient size, underlying disease, and heart rate.
- Dual-source CT scanners optimize temporal resolution, which may be advantageous for the rapid heart rates encountered in veterinary medicine.
- A regular heart rate is preferred for dual-source cardiac CT imaging, which may require administration of an anticholinergic agent due to the high prevalence and exaggerated variability of sinus arrhythmia in dogs.

INTRODUCTION

Cardiac computed tomography (cCT) has undergone rapid technological advancements in the last 2 decades and is now situated as an important imaging modality in human cardiovascular medicine. These advancements have positioned cCT as a screening tool for coronary artery disease [1], for the rapid evaluation of angina [2], and as a necessary tool for planning structural heart interventions [3,4].

Imaging the heart by CT, as compared with most other organs, is complicated by the rapid motion and complex internal architecture of this beating structure. The heart is in nearly constant motion, complicating our ability to freeze motion and clarify anatomy and pathology. For decades, CT technology was insufficient to obtain diagnostic images of the beating heart, although within 5 years of Hounsfield's first human CT scan

investigators evaluated the value of CT for cardiac imaging based on canine cadavers [5]. The advent of multidetector CT (MDCT) allowed for the temporal and spatial resolution necessary to make cardiac imaging feasible and the technology has evolved rapidly since.

In veterinary medicine, there are a few research publications [6–13] and case reports that describe the use of cCT [14–17]. Today, echocardiography remains the dominant imaging modality to understand and quantify cardiac structure and function in animals. However, ultrasound of the heart is limited by narrow acoustic windows and is predominately a 2-dimensional technique. Although 3-dimensional echocardiography is available and has been described in animals [18], it is limited by relatively poor spatial and temporal resolution. cCT overcomes these limitations, as it is not hindered by air or bone interfaces, and new scanners can

---

E-mail address: Brian.Scansen@colostate.edu

https://doi.org/10.1016/j.yasa.2022.05.002
2666-450X/22/

now achieve excellent spatial and temporal resolution even in small animals. This review highlights the author's experiences with use of cCT in animals, demonstrating the utility of this modality for understanding heart disease and describing the challenges to and potential solutions for high-quality cCT imaging in animals.

EVOLUTION OF COMPUTED TOMOGRAPHY TECHNOLOGY

- Early generation CT scanners lacked sufficient spatial and temporal resolution to characterize cardiac anatomy and freeze cardiac motion.
- The development of MDCT, also known as multi-slice CT, has improved both spatial and temporal resolution such that highly detailed visualization of cardiac and vascular structures is now clinically feasible.
- A detector is the portion of the scanner that receives the photons generated by the X rays passing through the patient. A single detector is composed of many elements along its circumference but is limited to a narrow width to allow it to resolve structures of interest.
- Multiple detectors allow the radiation effect to be collected along a broader slab width in the cranial-to-caudal direction known as the z-axis, which increases the thickness that can be scanned at one time.
- The first-generation MDCT scanners used 4 detectors to extend the z-axis thickness, with subsequent generations increasing to 8, 16, 64, 128, 320, and even 600 detectors. An MDCT with 320 detectors can typically cover the z-axis of a human heart, allowing the entire organ to be evaluated in one rotation of the CT gantry.
- The current top scanners from the major vendors that are optimized for and advertised as cardiac CT systems are listed with technical specifications in Table 1.

SPATIAL RESOLUTION

- Spatial resolution is defined as the ability to resolve structures that lie next to one another, specifically the smallest distance between structures that can accurately be resolved on the image.
- CT imaging can resolve a structure in all 3 anatomic axes. In CT parlance, these 3 axes are considered x (mediolateral), y (dorsoventral), and z (craniocaudal) when the dog sits on the CT table in sternal recumbency (Fig. 1).

- Spatial resolution in CT has been excellent for years in the x-y plane, but the z-axis (craniocaudal) resolution was historically challenging due to the available number, spacing, and width of detectors in the system.
- The width of the detector and the spacing between detectors largely determine the spatial resolution in the z-axis; a detector must be narrower than an object to resolve its border, and detectors must be sufficiently adjacent to resolve 2 objects that lie close to one another.
- A major advantage of CT compared with plain radiography or ultrasound is the ability to reconstruct the previously acquired dataset in any direction or plane and to generate a 3-dimensional volume. This multiplanar reconstruction requires isotropic resolution—meaning that the resolution of the imaging dataset is equivalent and adequate in all 3 directions (x, y, and z).
- Isotropic resolution at submillimeter resolution is now possible with MDCT scanners and is a requirement for cardiac imaging. Isotropic resolution of sufficient quality (eg, submillimeter) has greatly enhanced the visualization of small vascular structures and allows images to be reconstructed with excellent visualization in any plane even for small vessels such as the coronary arteries of dogs (Fig. 2).
- Spatial resolution is also improved by advancements in detector technology and reconstruction software. New high-definition scanners are available that can achieve spatial resolution down to 0.23 mm using novel detector material and advanced reconstruction algorithms.
- As dogs and cats are smaller in size than humans, adequate isotropic spatial resolution of small structures (eg, coronary vessels) remains a challenge in these species with all but the newest generations of scanners.

PITCH AND Z-AXIS COVERAGE

- For CT of a large moving organ such as the heart, the z-axis coverage is as important as the spatial resolution to allow reconstruction of the image in all planes without distortion.
- If the structure of interest cannot be completely imaged in one gantry rotation, multiple acquisitions will be required, as the patient moves through the scanner along the z-axis.
- Movement of the patient through the scanner is how CT has been performed since the advent of helical scanning. For an organ that does not move, stitching

TABLE 1
The Newest Generation Computed Tomography Systems from Major Vendors Are Listed with Technical Specifications

Manufacturer	Canon	GE	Philips	Siemens
Model	Aquilion One Genesis	Revolution Apex	Spectral CT 7500	Somatom Force
Number of x-ray sources	1	1	1	2
Detector rows	320	256 or 128	128	192 (2 × 96)
Slices per rotation	Up to 640	512 or 256	512	384 (2 × 192)
Voltage range	80–135 kVp	70–140 kVp	80–140 kVp	70–150 kVp
Amperage range	10–900 mA	10–1300 mA	10–1000 mA	20–1300 mA
Detector spacing	0.5 mm	0.625 mm	0.625 mm	0.4 mm
Z-axis coverage in one rotation	16 cm	16 cm or 8 cm	8 cm	5.76 cm
Fastest gantry rotation speed	0.275 s	0.28 s	0.27 s	0.25 s
Maximum acquisition speed	–	437 mm/s	–	737 mm/s
Novel features	Whole heart coverage; adaptive motion correction algorithm available to improve effective temporal resolution; arrhythmia detection software	Whole heart coverage; motion correction algorithm available to improve effective temporal resolution; arrhythmia detection software	Spectral detector allows for spectral imaging during all acquisitions; motion correction algorithm available to improve effective temporal resolution	True temporal resolution down to 66 ms; Turbo Flash mode allows single beat acquisition with steep pitch

These data were compiled by the author from publicly available information. As these systems undergo frequent revisions, this list is believed accurate at the time of publication but should be verified with each individual vendor.

these acquisitions together is relatively straightforward and unlikely to result in substantial artifact.

- In an organ such as the heart, however, constant motion complicates the ability to stitch sequential acquisitions together, and, for this reason, MDCT scanners with a high number of closely spaced detectors to capture as much of the heart as possible in one rotation are desired to optimize cCT imaging.

- Pitch is defined as the distance the table moves in a cranial-to-caudal direction per gantry rotation divided by the total thickness of the acquired slab (in the z-axis).

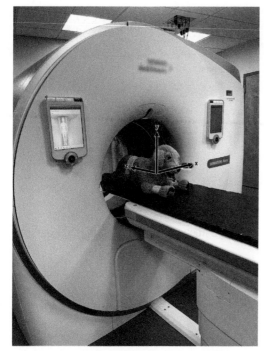

FIG. 1 A representative dog on a CT table with the anatomic axes represented as arrows demonstrating the x, y, and z axis imaging planes.

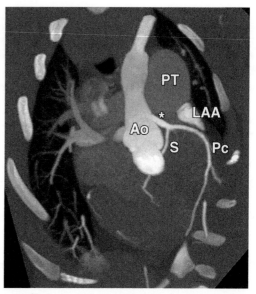

FIG. 2 Maximum intensity projection of the left coronary artery system in a 3-year-old 16.5-kg French bulldog with a heart rate of 74 beats per minute demonstrating submillimeter isotropic resolution and excellent visualization of small vessels. Ao, aorta; LAA, left auricular appendage; Pc, paraconal coronary artery; PT, pulmonary trunk; S, septal branch of the left coronary; *, left main coronary artery.

- A pitch greater than 1 implies gaps in the z-axis coverage, as the table moved faster than required for the scanner to image every slab in the field of view. Some degree of overlap in the z-axis is preferred to optimally reconstruct the full path of a blood vessel or the heart.
- Newer dual-source CT (DSCT) scanners can scan at a high pitch, as expected gaps will be covered by a second source and detector, allowing for more rapid acquisition of data and improving temporal resolution as discussed in the following section.

TEMPORAL RESOLUTION
- Temporal resolution describes the ability of the scanner to resolve a structure moving in time and is defined as the time required by the scanner to obtain the data necessary to reconstruct each image.
- A beating heart moves constantly and is only still for milliseconds of time throughout the cardiac cycle (typically in diastole or at end-systole). Fast scanners can image the organ of interest rapidly enough to effectively freeze motion and avoid artifacts of respiration, patient movement, and so forth.

- Temporal resolution depends on gantry rotation speed, mode of image acquisition, gating, and pitch.
- The fastest scanners currently on the market can perform a full gantry rotation in 250 msec (typically an optional feature). The CT software can generate an image from a half rotation of the gantry, as this is all that is required to capture photons from all angles through a body.
- Effective temporal resolution, or the minimal time required to obtain successive images, can therefore be thought of as half the gantry rotation time, which is approximately 125 msec with the fastest scanners available today.
- Adding an additional x-ray source and set of detectors placed 90° to the other is one strategy to minimize the time required to circumferentially rotate around the patient and can dramatically improve temporal resolution. These DSCT scanners are technically more complicated, given the extra hardware and heavier gantry (that must still rotate incredibly fast) but provide distinct advantages for cardiac imaging.
- Because DSCT scanners have 2 unique x-ray sources as well as 2 sets of detectors, sufficient data to

generate a complete image can be acquired with only a 90-degree rotation of the gantry. For a scanner with a gantry rotation speed of 250 msec, this results in an effective temporal resolution that is nearly one-fourth of the full rotation time or to a value of 66 msec for what is currently the fastest scanner on the market.

- DSCT scanners also have advantages for rapid acquisition at a greater pitch, as the 2 detectors can capture data twice as rapidly and need not overlap to the same proportion as a single source CT scanner. Very long z-axis coverage is therefore possible in a very short amount of time; current scanners can scan an entire thorax in one heart beat with a maximal pitch of 3.2 and a maximal table speed of 737 mm/s.

CONTRAST ADMINISTRATION

- All cCT studies require administration of iodinated contrast media. Only second- and third-generation, nonionic contrast media should be used. Meta-analyses of human studies suggest the third-generation agent, iodixanol, may pose a lesser risk for contrast-induced nephropathy, although most studies show no difference, and this has not been proved in animals [19].
- Relatively high concentrations of iodine are chosen for cCT imaging, typically 300 to 400 mg iodine/mL. As small animal patients have much smaller body size than humans, it may be feasible to use lower kVp settings and lower iodine concentrations in dogs and cats without loss of image quality, but this has not been investigated [20].
- Timing of contrast administration relative to scanning the structure of interest can be challenging but is paramount to obtaining a useful imaging study.
- cCT is achieved by delivering a bolus of contrast into a peripheral vein (typically cephalic in the dog or cat) and then initiating the scan when the contrast reaches the cardiac chamber of interest.
- Manual injection of contrast medium is generally unable to deliver the volume required fast enough to result in a tight bolus and full opacification of cardiac chambers in all but the smallest of patients. Power injectors made for CT that can control the rate, quantity, and pressure of contrast administration should be used for all cCT studies.
- Various protocols for contrast timing are available, with the 2 primary methods being a test scan or bolus tracking.
- A test scan involves monitoring a single slice that includes the structure of interest (typically the aortic arch) and then measuring the time it takes to reach peak opacification. The diagnostic scans are then planned based on these times so that the areas of interest are scanned when the contrast reaches the desired location or chamber.
- Automated bolus-tracking techniques use a machine-based monitoring scan that automatically initiates the full scan once an increase in attenuation (operator determined) is measured in the structure being monitored.
- Automated bolus tracking minimizes operator error in determining the optimal time for scan acquisition, although errors can still occur if the region of interest is not appropriately identified.
- Automated bolus tracking is often performed to initiate cCT, with the scan triggered when the contrast bolus reaches the pulmonary trunk or ascending aorta. The threshold, a predefined increase in the attenuation value of a particular region of interest, is set and then a single slice is repeatedly acquired at that region of interest to monitor change in attenuation over time (Fig. 3). Once threshold is reached, the scan is automatically initiated, although there is an inherent delay of 2 to 3 seconds before the scan commences both to position the scanner at the beginning scan position and to bring the gantry up to speed.
- The injection rate and concentration of contrast administration are also important considerations when imaging the heart.
- The rate of contrast injection is limited by the size (gauge) and length of the peripheral catheter, the concentration and temperature of the contrast medium, and the pressure limit of the power injector. Smaller gauge catheters, longer catheters, solutions of higher iodine concentration, and contrast at a colder temperature all cause greater resistance to flow. More resistance requires greater pressure to maintain a desired flow rate, which may not be possible with a given power injector or may not be tolerated by some peripheral catheters.
- A fast rate of contrast administration results in a tighter bolus as it moves through the vasculature; however, in small patients a rapid rate of injection can result in a very brief window for peak contrast opacification. As an example, consider a scenario where 2 mL/kg of iodinated contrast will be given for a cCT scan. If the patient weighs 3 kg and the contrast is delivered at 3 mL/s then the entire bolus will be injected in 2 sec (6 mL at 3 mL/s). The scan must be timed to acquire images of the heart within

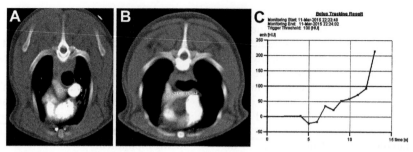

FIG. 3 Examples of automated bolus tracking. The region of interest may be placed on the aortic arch (**A**) for left heart studies or the pulmonary trunk (**B**) for right heart studies. Monitoring scans are performed through this region of interest until a threshold value above baseline is reached. In the enhancement curve in (**C**), the attenuation in Hounsfield units (HU) is shown on the y axis with time after injection on the x axis. The threshold in this example had been set at 100 HU, which was crossed on the final monitoring scan and the diagnostic cCT study then commenced.

this 2 sec window or contrast opacification will be suboptimal or nondiagnostic (eg, the bolus is "missed"). Conversely, if the injection rate is slowed to 1 mL/s then the window for image acquisition is increased to 6 sec and the operator has a better chance to obtain a diagnostic study.

- The downside to a slower rate of contrast administration is mixing in the vasculature and less attenuation in the chamber of interest.
- Flow rate limits are not always noted on peripheral catheters, but one study evaluated injection of iopromide, 370 mg iodine/mL, at an injection rate of 5 mL/s through various sizes of peripheral catheters [21]. Catheters from size 14 to 20 gauge did not reach the pressure limit of the power injector with this protocol and their injection was routine, but injection through the 22-gauge catheter at 5 mL/s did exceed the pressure limit, resulting in a reduced flow rate, and injection through a 24-gauge catheter was not possible at 5 mL/s [21].
- When choosing contrast injection rates in animals undergoing cCT, the author considers a maximum rate of 5 mL/s for an 18-gauge peripheral catheter, 4 mL/s for 20-gauge, 3 mL/s for 22-gauge, and 1 mL/s for 24-gauge to avoid complications. As noted earlier, the chosen injection rate may be lower than these limits based on the size of the animal, desired protocol, and total volume delivered.

GATING

- Gating refers to the timing of image acquisition relative to the cardiac cycle, usually based on a recording of the surface electrocardiogram.

- Timing the acquisition to the cardiac cycle enables reconstruction of systolic or diastolic datasets, as the image can be reconstructed at various time points.
- The animal's electrocardiogram (ECG) is linked to the time of image acquisition and used to reconstruct (retrospective) or trigger (prospective) the scan (Fig. 4).
- With retrospective gating, the entire cardiac cycle is scanned (usually several cardiac cycles depending on the size of the patient) and the desired image reconstructed from the raw dataset based on the simultaneous ECG; this allows for reconstruction of all phases of the cardiac cycle as desired and for dynamic analysis.
- Typically, phases are reconstructed as a percentage between consecutive R-R intervals such that at normal heart rates end-systole occurs at ∼30% and end-diastole at ∼100% (or 0%). Alternately, the phase may be reconstructed based on the absolute time in milliseconds from the peak of the R wave. End-systole in dogs is therefore around 220 ms (shorter for high heart rates, slightly longer for slow heart rates) and end-diastole is typically 0 to −10 ms.
- Retrospective gating increases radiation exposure to the patient, as the x-ray source is on throughout the cardiac cycle, rather than selectively turned on for a portion of the cardiac cycle as occurs with prospective gating.
- Retrospective gating allows for ECG editing, where premature beats or highly variable cycle lengths can be manually excluded to improve image quality (Fig. 5) [22]. ECG editing is generally not feasible with prospectively acquired data.

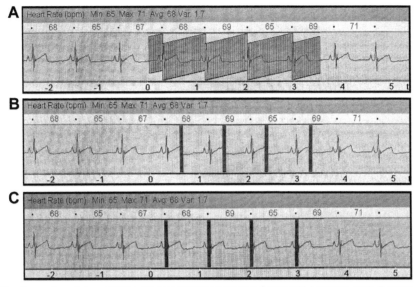

FIG. 4 Cardiac gating demonstrating 20 reconstructed phases (every 5% between each R wave, represented by each purple rectangle) in a retrospectively gated study (**A**), as well as single reconstructions obtained at end-systole (**B**) and end-diastole (**C**) representing single phases as would be acquired prospectively.

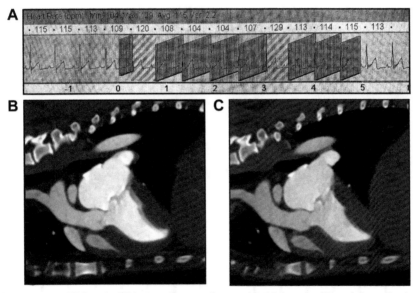

FIG. 5 Simultaneous ECG and cCT images from an 8-year-old, 4.3-kg mixed breed dog with sinus arrhythmia. In the ECG recording (**A**) at the time of acquisition there are 2 heart beats considerably faster than the underlying rhythm with instantaneous rates of 120 and 129 beats per minute. In the initial reconstruction (**B**), this heart rate variability results in blur motion artifact seen best along the caudal border of the left ventricle. After ECG editing to remove these 2 beats (seen as *dashed diagonal lines* on the ECG), the motion artifact is lessened and image quality improved (**C**).

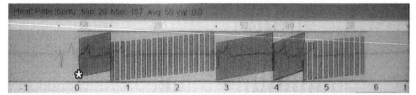

FIG. 6 In the ECG of this 9-month-old, 14-kg French bulldog a pronounced sinus arrhythmia leads to challenges with ECG gating. One short cycle is not detected by the scanner (*asterisk*) as evidenced the lack of a blue dot along the top of the trace. Further, the magnitude of cycle length variability makes percentage reconstructions unusable—note how the spacing of each purple rectangle differs across the R-R interval for each beat. In this situation, the 30% phase will represent a markedly different time in the cardiac cycle for each beat, resulting in poor image quality; this can be improved by reconstructing in milliseconds rather than by percentage.

- Prospective gating triggers the scanner to acquire images only during a portion of each cardiac cycle, typically when cardiac motion is least vigorous such as mid-diastole or end-systole. In humans, end-systole is preferred for higher heart rates, as diastolic time is compressed.
- Prospective gating is known as a move-and-shoot technique; the scanner is only activated for small windows of time and a single portion of the cardiac cycle is recorded, limiting radiation exposure but preventing dynamic analysis.

- Newer scanners have the ability to modulate dose during a retrospective scan such that the tube current is lower during systole, reducing dose by as much as half, and full tube current is applied during diastole or the portion of the scan least susceptible to artifact [23]. This approach mitigates some of the high-dose effects of retrospective gating, while retaining data in all phases of the cardiac cycle for reconstruction of any phase and for dynamic analysis.
- Respiratory gating or subjecting the animal to a breath-hold or apneic period during the scan is

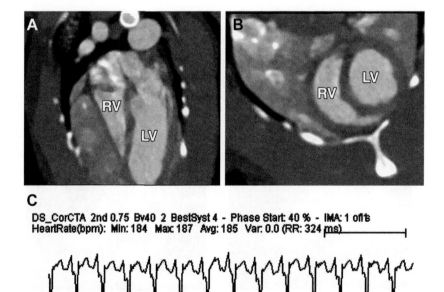

FIG. 7 Images obtained at high heart rate in a 2-year-old, 2.4-kg chicken demonstrating that dual-source cCT can resolve the intracardiac anatomy even at heart rates of 184 beats per minute in small patients. Both the left ventricle (LV) and right ventricle (RV) can be clearly delineated in both a 4-chamber plane (**A**) and a short-axis plane (**B**). The ECG at the time of acquisition is shown in (**C**).

also frequently used to avoid movement during scan acquisition. Although respiratory motion is less frequent than cardiac motion, an ill-timed breath can still result in substantial artifact.

- The ability of the scanner to appropriately gate the study relates to the temporal resolution of the scanner—at fast heart rates the scanner may not be able to acquire the images rapidly enough to adequately resolve the desired image.

HEART RATE AND RHYTHM

- Classically, cCT in humans was limited to patients with heart rates less than 60 or 65 beats per minute [24]. This target range would preclude most

veterinary patients (or human pediatric patients) from undergoing cCT.

- With the improved temporal resolution of new-generation scanners, much higher heart rates can be effectively scanned. In the author's experience using DSCT in animals, it is now the regularity of the heart rhythm that matters more than the absolute heart rate.
- With multibeat acquisitions, which will be required for all but the 16-cm z-axis scanners, a regular and consistent rhythm results in the best image quality. A regular heart rhythm allows the scanner to accurately predict when the next R wave will occur and results in the same phase of the cardiac cycle occurring at a consistent interval after each detected R wave.

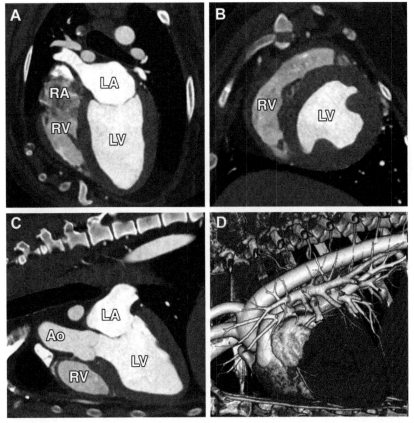

FIG. 8 A 4-chamber (**A**), short-axis (**B**), 3-chamber (**C**), and 3D volume rendering technique (**D**) obtained with a triphasic injection in a 4-year-old, 31-kg Labrador retriever. The injection parameters through a 20-gauge right cephalic catheter were 30 mL at 3 mL/s of iodinated contrast (iohexol 350 mg iodine/mL), followed by 30 mL at 3 mL/s of a 50:50 mixture of contrast:saline, followed by a 20 mL chase of saline at 3 mL/s. The scan was triggered on the aortic arch at a threshold of 150 HU. The intent of the triphasic injection is to have peak attenuation in the left heart and mixed contrast attenuation in the right heart, allowing delineation of all endocardial borders. Ao, aorta; LA, left atrium; LV, left ventricle; RA, right atrium; RV, right ventricle.

- Dogs natively have a pronounced sinus arrhythmia, with respiratory sinus arrhythmia estimated to be 3 times greater in dogs than humans [25]. This variability is exaggerated by sedation or anesthesia (Fig. 6) and can be even greater in certain breeds such as those with brachycephaly. The author frequently administers anticholinergic medications to dogs undergoing cCT to lessen heart rate variability. Usually, atropine at 0.01 mg/kg or glycopyrrolate at 0.005 mg/kg is given intravenously and the patient allowed to rest until the initial tachycardia abates and the rate begins to slow but remains regular. The dose may be repeated as needed until the desired heart rate is achieved.

- An optimal heart rate for cCT in small animals is not established and likely varies by scanner. Using DSCT, the author consistently obtains high-quality cCT images at heart rates from 50 to 150 beats per minute although has imaged at heart rates exceeding 200 per minute (Fig. 7) with still diagnostic quality.

- Advanced features on single source scanners such as arrhythmia detection may overcome many of the challenges of sinus arrhythmia seen in animals, but the magnitude of the cycle length variability in a sedated dog far exceeds that encountered in human medicine, and in the author's opinion maintaining a regular heart rhythm is more important than an optimal (slow) heart rate; this may not be true for scanners with a 16-cm z-axis, as the entire heart can be scanned in one gantry rotation.

DEVELOPMENT OF A CARDIAC COMPUTED TOMOGRAPHY PROTOCOL

- Determining a protocol to be used for cCT acquisition requires knowledge of the animal's heart rate, body weight, the site and gauge of vascular access, temporal resolution of the scanner, and the patient's specific heart defect to be imaged.

- Biphasic and triphasic injection protocols are preferable for cCT, which require the use of a dual-head

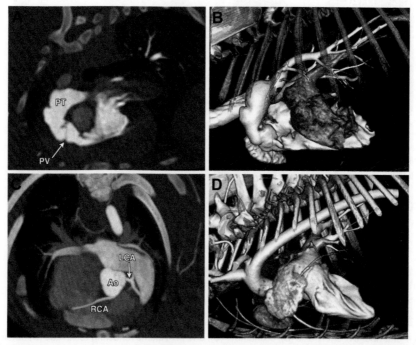

FIG. 9 Images from an 8-month-old, 6.6-kg French bulldog with severe pulmonary valve stenosis showing sequential cCT scans to capture peak attenuation in the right (**A, B**) and then left (**C, D**) sides of the heart using the same contrast bolus; this enables good visualization of the pulmonary valve (**A**) from one scan, with optimal imaging of the coronary arteries (**C**) in the second scan. The first scan was triggered on the pulmonary trunk (PT) with a programmed delay between scans of 4 seconds to account for the pulmonary transit time. Ao, aorta; LCA, left coronary artery; RCA, right coronary artery.

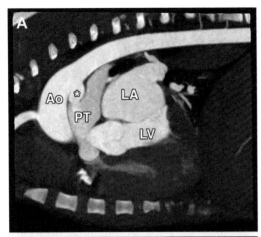

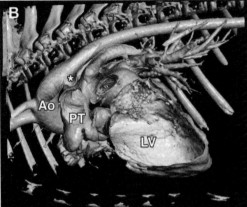

FIG. 10 cCT images in a sagittal maximum intensity projection (**A**) and a hollow 3D volume rendering technique (**B**) of a 4-month-old mixed breed dog with a left-to-right shunting patent arterial duct (*asterisk*). The scan is triggered on the aorta to allow opacification of the arterial duct as contrast passes from aorta (Ao) to pulmonary trunk (PT). The left atrium (LA) and left ventricle (LV) are also opacified.

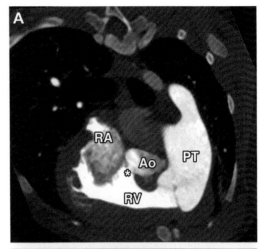

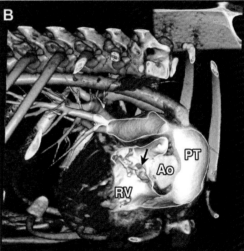

FIG. 11 cCT images obtained in a 7-month-old Bernedoodle with severe pulmonary hypertension and a right-to-left shunting perimembranous ventricular septal defect. The scan was triggered on the right atrium (RA) to optimize opacification of the right heart. The oblique transverse image (**A**) shows the septal defect (*asterisk*) with contrast streaming from the right ventricle (RV) to the aorta (Ao). There is also a dilated pulmonary trunk (PT). The 3D volume rendered image (**B**) was created by cropping much of the right atrium, and the defect (*arrow*) can be appreciated as a circular area of drop-out under the septal tricuspid valve leaflet and entering into the aorta.

power injector. The dual-head injector allows for simultaneous administration of contrast and saline, as well as a variable mixture of the 2 solutions.

- Optimally, vascular access is obtained in the right cephalic vein. Using the left cephalic vein results in potential contrast within the left brachiocephalic vein that lies just cranial to the heart and may result in streak artifact if opacified during cardiac imaging.
- For most studies, the author administers 1 mL/kg of iodinated contrast medium at 100% concentration, followed by 1 mL/kg of a 50:50 contrast-to-saline mixture, followed by 0.5 mL/kg of 100% saline.

The intent of this triphasic injection is to opacify the left heart with 100% contrast, whereas the right heart is filled with the 50:50 mixture, allowing endocardial border delineation of both sides but at

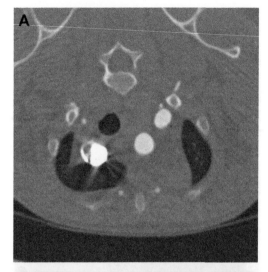

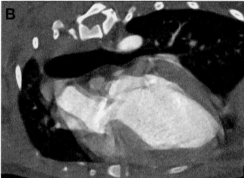

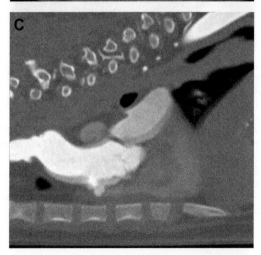

different attenuation values to clearly see the anatomic details of each chamber (Fig. 8). The saline chase allows the cranial vena cava to be cleared of contrast.

Left Heart Studies

o Left heart studies focused on left ventricular function, coronary artery anatomy, or aortic/ mitral valve anatomy are typically triggered on the aortic arch or in the left ventricular lumen similar to the protocol outlined earlier.

o In animals with mitral or aortic valve insufficiency, timing becomes less critical, as the contrast recirculates in the left heart.

o In very small patients, triggering on the aortic arch may still miss peak contrast filling, as there are a few seconds delay between the recognition that the threshold has been met and when the scan is commenced. To obtain a high-quality scan in these small patients, triggering earlier in the circulation (eg, the left atrium or pulmonary trunk) and using a slower injection rate to extend the contrast bolus through the circulation can be helpful.

Right Heart Studies

o When the right heart is the major focus of the study (eg, pulmonary valve stenosis, tricuspid valve disease), it can be advantageous to have peak contrast opacification of those structures. As such, triggering on the aortic arch may miss peak contrast of the right side and the author frequently triggers on the pulmonary trunk in such studies.

o Again, very small patients can pose a challenge with timing. Triggering on the pulmonary trunk may still miss peak contrast filling of the right heart. There are 2 ways to obtain a high-quality scan in this situation—triggering earlier in the circulation (eg, the cranial vena cava) and using a slower injection rate to extend the contrast bolus through the circulation as suggested in the earlier section on left heart studies.

Dual Heart Studies

o In some patients, it is advantageous to have high-quality scans of both the left and right sides of the heart, such as the dog with

FIG. 12 Artifacts seen during cCT imaging. In (**A**), beam hardening artifact can be seen as dark bands or streaks around the cranial vena cava associated with highly attenuating contrast. In (**B**), blur artifact is seen associated

with a vigorous cardiac motion exceeding the temporal resolution of the scanner. In (**C**), the appearance of 2 aortas offset from one another is an example of ghosting artifact.

pulmonary valve stenosis who may have an anomalous coronary artery (Fig. 9). There are 2 methods that may allow for peak opacification of both the left and right heart. First, a longer duration of contrast injection or greater volume may allow full opacification of all cardiac chambers; however, patient size may limit the volume that can be injected (the author avoids administering more than 875 mg iodine per kilogram body weight). Alternatively, the same bolus can be followed by sequential scanning. The author initiates the right heart scan first by triggering on the pulmonary trunk. A second scan is then programmed to occur based on the expected pulmonary transit time of the contrast bolus (see Fig. 9). This time varies by dog size, heart rate, and form of heart defect but is typically 2 to 4 seconds in normal dogs [26–28]. In cases of right heart obstructive lesions (eg, pulmonary valve stenosis) or poor right-sided output (eg, tricuspid valve dysplasia) this time should be extended.

Cardiac Shunts

○ cCT studies are typically pursued after other diagnostic tests such as echocardiography; these tests have likely led to a presumptive diagnosis with some understanding of the directionality of shunt flow. These data should be reviewed and considered when planning the cCT study.

○ For left-to-right shunts (Fig. 10), the author triggers on the aortic arch for most cases, as this will result in peak opacification of the shunt structure.

○ For right-to-left shunts (Fig. 11), the scan is often triggered from the pulmonary trunk (or upstream in the right ventricle or cranial cava for small patients).

○ If the shunt is bidirectional or the anatomy is complex, setting up 2 sequential scans can be beneficial to increase the chance of capturing peak opacification of the structures of interest, although this comes with the downside of increased radiation dose to the patient.

ARTIFACTS

• An understanding of potential imaging artifacts that can occur during cCT is necessary to prevent and cure nondiagnostic studies.

• The most common artifact seen in cCT is motion artifact, which may be related to cardiac motion, respiratory motion, or body motion (particularly during sedated scans).

• Motion artifact can be appreciated as misregistration or stair-stepping, streaking, ghosting, and blurring (Fig. 12) [29].

• Resolving cardiac motion artifact depends on the quality of the scanner available, although even the newest scanner can suffer from cardiac motion artifact if care is not paid to heart rate and rhythm.

○ Irregular heart rhythms (ie, sinus arrhythmia, premature complexes) result in discontinuity along the z-axis where the scanner fails to line up adjacent acquisitions.

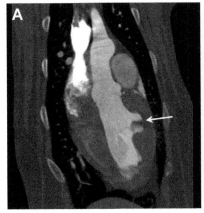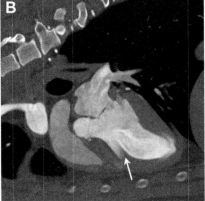

FIG. 13 In this scan, the dog took a breath during the cardiac acquisition, resulting in stair-step or misregistration artifact. Note in both the coronal (**A**) and sagittal (**B**) planes that there is discontinuity in the left ventricular endocardial border (*arrows*) consistent with misregistration of the acquisition in the z-axis.

- Motion associated with too rapid a heart rate causes blurring of the image and indistinct borders (see Fig. 12).
- If motion is a common issue encountered at a site having a scanner with low temporal resolution (eg, more than 250 msec), the only solution may be a change in equipment.
- If the study was retrospectively gated, selecting a different phase may eliminate cardiac motion artifact. At low heart rates, choosing a diastolic phase typically results in the least motion artifact, whereas at higher heart rates the end-systolic phase may show the least motion.
- ECG editing may also resolve motion artifact if there are 1 or 2 beats that are much more variable than the underlying rhythm (see Fig. 5).
- Normalizing the heart rhythm with anticholinergic medications can be helpful to avoid motion artifact if sinus arrhythmia is profound. Alternatively, slowing the heart rate with β-blockers can be considered so long as cycle length variability is not worsened, and the patient can tolerate β-blocker administration.

- Respiratory motion artifact occurs if the animal inhales or exhales at the time of the acquisition and may also result in misregistration artifact (Fig. 13).
  - Respiratory motion artifact can be limited by controlling respiration. If the animal is under general anesthesia, techniques to be used include hyperventilating the patient and then suspending ventilation during the acquisition. Some centers have used the use of an assistant in the room to hold positive pressure during the scan to limit respiratory artifact, but this increases radiation exposure to staff and should probably be avoided.

- Patient motion artifact is less a concern in animals, as CT imaging requires pharmacologic immobilization—either sedation or general anesthesia.
  - With the speed of new-generation scanners, the time that a patient needs to be immobile is lessened, and the author has achieved high-quality cCT scans in nonintubated dogs under sedation (Fig. 14) [9].
  - The trade-offs between nonintubated sedation and a deeper plane of anesthesia include an inability to control the airway or to mechanically suspend respiration. For some animals with complex or advanced heart disease, general anesthesia and control of the airway may be safer than a lighter plane of sedation.

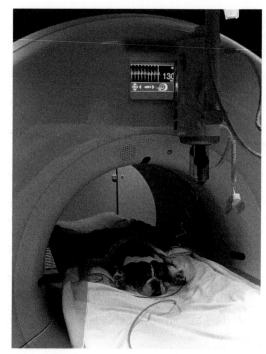

FIG. 14 A bulldog under sedation, nonintubated during cCT acquisition.

- Beam hardening (see Fig. 12) and metal streak (Fig. 15) artifacts may occur in cCT as they do when imaging other organs [30]; this occurs around very dense structures, which in the context of cCT typically means contrast or cardiac implants such as stents or pacing leads. Beam hardening may also be present due to retention of undiluted contrast in the right atrium that persists after the initial injection; this can be reduced or eliminated by use of a saline flush after the contrast administration [29].
- Mixing of contrast within the heart (Fig. 16) is not an artifact per se but can make interpretation of normal endocardial borders or vascular lumens difficult.
  - Contrast streaming occurs as contrast enters the vascular or cardiac chamber; this typically occurs if the scan is initiated early in the injection or when other vessels bring nonopacified blood into the same chamber (eg, mixing in the right atrium of opacified blood from the cranial vena cava with nonopacified blood from the caudal vena cava).
  - Increasing the delay to allow full circulation of contrast through the body can resolve mixing artifact as the contrast becomes homogenous

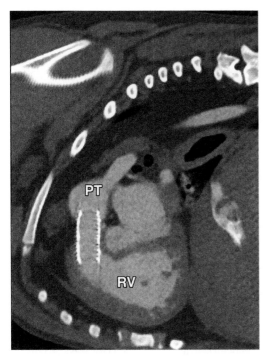

FIG. 15 cCT image from a 3-year-old English Bulldog demonstrating metallic streak artifact as lines emanating from the edges of a transpulmonary metallic stent. PT, pulmonary trunk; RV, right ventricle.

within the circulation but results in lower attenuation within the cardiac chambers that may result in suboptimal images.
○ Typically, a delay of 15 to 20 seconds after contrast is detected in the left heart allows full mixing of contrast throughout the cardiac chambers for small to medium size dogs.
• Poor contrast enhancement can be considered an artifact, although it usually relates to an improper protocol or technical errors. In the example in Fig. 17, the cCT scan was initiated with too great a delay before the monitoring (bolus-tracking) phase in a very small dog, and this resulted in the contrast having already passed the region of interest by the time the scanner started monitoring. The scan had to be manually triggered at which time the contrast was quite dilute within the cardiac chambers and the cCT study was of poor quality.

FUTURE AVENUES FOR RESEARCH
• cCT is in its infancy in veterinary medicine, and there is a large amount of optimization that still needs to occur. Greater understanding of preferred sedation protocols, contrast media (type, volume, injection rate), and scanning parameters across the various technologies are needed.
• There are many aspects of cCT not discussed in this article, including segmentation and 3-dimensional printing, dual-energy and spectral imaging, myocardial perfusion imaging, and dose-reduction strategies.

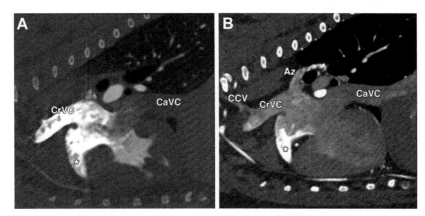

FIG. 16 cCT images of the right atrium from a 10-month-old English bulldog demonstrating nonopacified blood from the costocervical vein (CCV), azygos vein (Az), and caudal vena cava (CaVC) mixing with contrast in the cranial vena cava (CrVC) in an initial scan (**A**). This mixing complicates evaluation of the right atrial borders and may be misinterpreted as a filling defect such as a mass or thrombus in some cases. The same dog imaged a few seconds later (**B**) shows improved mixing in the right atrium with clear endocardial border delineation, albeit with persistence of contrast in the right auricular appendage (*asterisk*).

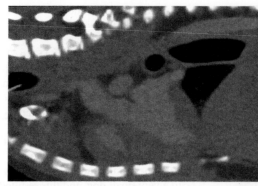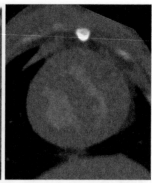

FIG. 17 cCT images in a sagittal plane (*left*) and a short-axis plane (*right*) from a 4-month-old, 4.9-kg French bulldog with severe pulmonary valve stenosis demonstrating poor contrast opacification related to improper timing. The protocol involved a trigger on the pulmonary trunk and administration of 6 mL of contrast at 3 mL/s, but the monitoring phase was not programmed to begin until 5 seconds after the injection. By the time the monitoring phase began, all contrast had passed the region of interest, and the scan was not triggered. Manual initiation of the scan was performed seconds after this was realized but the contrast in the cardiac chambers was very dilute, resulting in a poor-quality study; this could have been avoided by triggering upstream of the desired anatomy (eg, on the cranial vena cava), using a slower injection rate (eg, 1 mL/s), and shortening the delay before the monitoring phase.

Each of these areas of cCT imaging can be applied to animals and may enhance the diagnostic and treatment-planning benefits of this imaging modality.

SUMMARY

The heart has a complex spatial arrangement and is modified in unique and diverse ways by disease. Understanding the pathoanatomy of cardiac disease requires precise imaging, optimally in 3 dimensions. cCT provides remarkable detail without the limitations of echocardiography. The surge of cCT use in human medicine has led to technological improvements that benefit small animal imaging such as improved temporal resolution, submillimeter spatial resolution, and advanced arrhythmia management. Greater use of cCT in animals will help grow our understanding of the structure and function of this complex organ.

CLINICS CARE POINTS

- Perform a retrospectively acquired cardiac CT if you wish to reconstruct all cardiac phases and to view cardiac motion. Perform a prospectively acquired cardiac CT if you are interested in only a single phase of the cardiac cycle in order to limit radiation dose to the patient.

- Perform cardiac CT with a triphasic injection protocol consisting of 100% contrast, 50:50 dilution of contrast with saline, and a saline flush to visualize all cardiac chambers, separate right heart from left heart attenuation, and to minimize artifact from persistent contrast in the veins and right atrium.

- Sinus arrhythmia can complicate acquisition of a high-quality cardiac CT due to cycle length variability; consider administration of anticholinergic medications to normalize cycle length if the temporal resolution of your scanner is sufficient to resolve the higher heart rate.

DISCLOSURE

The author has no conflicts relevant to this material.

REFERENCES

[1] Abdelrahman KM, Chen MY, Dey AK, et al. Coronary computed tomography angiography from clinical uses to emerging technologies: JACC state-of-the-art review. J Am Coll Cardiol 2020;76(10):1226–43.

[2] Gulati M, Levy PD, Mukherjee D, et al. 2021 AHA/ACC/ASE/CHEST/SAEM/SCCT/SCMR Guideline for the Evaluation and Diagnosis of Chest Pain: A Report of the American College of Cardiology/American Heart Association Joint Committee on Clinical Practice Guidelines. Circulation 2021;144(22):e368–454.

[3] Bax JJ, Delgado V, Hahn RT, et al. Transcatheter aortic valve replacement: role of multimodality imaging in common and complex clinical scenarios. JACC Cardiovasc Imaging 2020;13(1 Pt 1):124–39.

[4] Ooms JF, Wang DD, Rajani R, et al. Computed tomography-derived 3D modeling to guide sizing and planning of transcatheter mitral valve interventions. JACC Cardiovasc Imaging 2021;14(8):1644–58.

[5] Ter-Pogossian MM, Weiss ES, Coleman RE, et al. Computed tomography of the heart. AJR Am J Roentgenol 1976;127(1):79–90.

[6] Drees R, Frydrychowicz A, Reeder SB, et al. 64-multidetector computed tomographic angiography of the canine coronary arteries. Vet Radiol Ultrasound 2011;52(5):507–15.

[7] Drees R, Johnson RA, Pinkerton M, et al. Effects of two different anesthetic protocols on 64-MDCT coronary angiography in dogs. Vet Radiol Ultrasound 2015;56(1):46–54.

[8] LeBlanc NL, Scollan KF. Quantification of right ventricular volume measured by use of real-time three-dimensional echocardiography and electrocardiography-gated 64-slice multidetector computed tomography in healthy dogs. Am J Vet Res 2018;79(4):404–10.

[9] Hostnik ET, Scansen BA, Habing AM, et al. Comparison of cardiac measurements by multi-detector computed tomography angiography and transthoracic echocardiography in English bulldogs. J Vet Cardiol 2017;19(6):480–91.

[10] To A, Hostnik ET, Rhinehart JD, et al. Electrocardiography-gated cardiac CT angiography can differentiate brachycephalic dogs with and without pulmonary valve stenosis and findings differ from transthoracic echocardiography. Vet Radiol Ultrasound 2018;48(5):797–817.

[11] Fries RC, Gordon SG, Saunders AB, et al. Quantitative assessment of two- and three-dimensional transthoracic and two-dimensional transesophageal echocardiography, computed tomography, and magnetic resonance imaging in normal canine hearts. J Vet Cardiol 2019;21:79–92.

[12] Owens EJ, LeBlanc NL, Scollan KF. Comparison of left and right atrial volumes determined by two- and three-dimensional echocardiography with those determined by multidetector computed tomography for healthy dogs. Am J Vet Res 2020;81(1):33–40.

[13] Henjes CR, Hungerbühler S, Bojarski IB, et al. Comparison of multi-detector row computed tomography with echocardiography for assessment of left ventricular function in healthy dogs. Am J Vet Res 2012;73(3):393–403.

[14] Scollan K, Sisson D. Multi-detector computed tomography of an aortic dissection in a cat. J Vet Cardiol 2014;16(1):67–72.

[15] Stieger-Vanegas SM, Scollan KF, Meadows L, et al. Cardiac-gated computed tomography angiography in three alpacas with complex congenital heart disease. J Vet Cardiol 2016;18(1):88–98.

[16] Stieger-Vanegas SM, Scollan KF, Riebold TW. Evaluation of non-ECG and ECG-gated computed tomographic angiography for three-dimensional printing of anomalous coronary arteries in dogs with pulmonic stenosis. J Vet Cardiol 2019;26:39–50.

[17] Laborda-Vidal P, Pedro B, Baker M, et al. Use of ECG-gated computed tomography, echocardiography and selective angiography in five dogs with pulmonic stenosis and one dog with pulmonic stenosis and aberrant coronary arteries. J Vet Cardiol 2016;18(4):418–26.

[18] Orvalho JS. Real-time three-dimensional echocardiography: from diagnosis to intervention. Vet Clin North Am Small Anim Pract 2017;47(5):1005–19.

[19] Eng J, Wilson RF, Subramaniam RM, et al. Comparative effect of contrast media type on the incidence of contrast-induced nephropathy: a systematic review and meta-analysis. Ann Intern Med 2016;164(6):417–24.

[20] Oda S, Utsunomiya D, Nakaura T, et al. Basic concepts of contrast injection protocols for coronary computed tomography angiography. Curr Cardiol Rev 2019;15(1):24–9.

[21] Behrendt FF, Bruners P, Keil S, et al. Impact of different vein catheter sizes for mechanical power injection in CT: in vitro evaluation with use of a circulation phantom. Cardiovasc Intervent Radiol 2009;32(1):25–31.

[22] Matsutani H, Sano T, Kondo T, et al. ECG-edit function in multidetector-row computed tomography coronary arteriography for patients with arrhythmias. Circ J 2008;72(7):1071–8.

[23] Sabarudin A, Sun Z. Coronary CT angiography: dose reduction strategies. World J Cardiol 2013;5(12):465–72.

[24] Brodoefel H, Reimann A, Burgstahler C, et al. Noninvasive coronary angiography using 64-slice spiral computed tomography in an unselected patient collective: effect of heart rate, heart rate variability and coronary calcifications on image quality and diagnostic accuracy. Eur J Radiol 2008;66(1):134–41.

[25] Grosso G, Vezzosi T, Briganti A, et al. Breath-by-breath analysis of respiratory sinus arrhythmia in dogs. Respir Physiolo Neurobiol 2021;294:103776.

[26] Capen RL, Latham LP, Wagner WW Jr. Comparison of direct and indirect measurements of pulmonary capillary transit times. J Appl Physiol (1985) 1987;62(3):1150–4.

[27] Slutsky RA, Carey PH, Bhargava V, et al. A comparison of peak-to-peak pulmonary transit time determined by digital intravenous angiography with standard dye-dilution techniques in anesthetized dogs. Invest Radiol 1982;17(4):362–6.

[28] Crosara S, Ljungvall I, Margiocco ML, et al. Use of contrast echocardiography for quantitative and qualitative evaluation of myocardial perfusion and pulmonary transit time in healthy dogs. Am J Vet Res 2012;73(2):194–201.

[29] Kalisz K, Buethe J, Saboo SS, et al. Artifacts at Cardiac CT: physics and solutions. Radiographics 2016;36(7):2064–83.

[30] Hathcock JT, Stickle RL. Principles and concepts of computed tomography. Vet Clin North Am Small Anim Pract 1993;23(2):399–415.

Advances in Small Animal Care 3 (2022) 57–71

ADVANCES IN SMALL ANIMAL CARE

Advanced Imaging of the Pancreas

Lauren von Stade, DVM, Angela J. Marolf, DVM, DACVR*

Department of Environmental and Radiological Health Sciences, Colorado State University Veterinary Teaching Hospital, College of Veterinary Medicine and Biomedical Sciences, Colorado State University, 300 West Drake Road, Fort Collins, CO 80525, USA

KEYWORDS
- Pancreatitis • Insulinoma • Pancreatic adenocarcinoma • Contrast-enhanced ultrasonography
- Computed tomography • Magnetic resonance imaging

KEY POINTS
- Computed tomography (CT) and magnetic resonance imaging (MRI) advantages in pancreatic imaging include detailed anatomic evaluation, decreased operator dependence, and lack of superimposition from overlying structures.
- Contrast-enhanced ultrasonography enables evaluation of pancreatic perfusion and improves detection of pancreatic nodules compared with conventional ultrasound.
- CT angiography is superior to ultrasound in identifying portal vein thrombosis, which has a high prevalence in dogs with pancreatitis and association with outcome.
- CT angiography is useful in the detection of canine insulinoma before surgery. Arterial phase hyperattenuation is a consistent feature.
- MRI shows promise for primary and metastatic insulinoma lesion detection and may be used in patients where contrast-induced nephropathy is a primary concern.

INTRODUCTION

The pancreas in dogs and cats is a thin organ in the right cranial abdomen composed of a left lobe, body, and right lobe; it shows both endocrine and exocrine functions. Although the normal pancreas has relatively nondescript imaging characteristics, pancreatic diseases including pancreatitis and pancreatic neoplasia have specific imaging features that make imaging an integral component of their diagnosis.

Ultrasound has traditionally been the diagnostic imaging modality of choice for evaluating the pancreas, in part due to its widespread availability, and because it is considered safe and noninvasive. Contrast-enhanced ultrasound (CEUS) is a newer tool that involves the use of intravenous (IV) contrast agents composed of gas microbubbles that remain within the intravascular space [1]. After injection of these contrast agents intravenously, ultrasound is used to evaluate the perfusion of organs [1].

In general, parenchyma with poor vascularity will be hypoechoic, whereas regions with high vascularity, such as highly vascular tumors, will be hyperechoic [1]. Tissue perfusion parameters can be evaluated using computer software with regions of interest placed over the organ in question to estimate the concentration or signal intensity of microbubbles in the blood flow [2]. However, CEUS is not widely performed at this time, and standard B-mode imaging continues to be the first-line imaging option for the pancreas. B-mode ultrasound can be disadvantageous in certain circumstances as it is highly operator dependent and evaluation of the whole pancreas may be difficult in large or uncomfortable patients or due to superimposition of overlying structures, in particular the presence of a full stomach or gas within gastrointestinal structures.

Advantages of more advanced imaging techniques such as computed tomography (CT) and magnetic

---

*Corresponding author, *E-mail address:* Angela.Marolf@colostate.edu

https://doi.org/10.1016/j.yasa.2022.05.003
2666-450X/22/

www.advancesinsmallanimalcare.com

57

resonance imaging (MRI) include complete anatomic evaluation including the ability to create multiplanar reconstructions to evaluate the anatomy in transverse, dorsal, sagittal, or oblique cross-sectional planes, the lack of superimposition of overlying structures, improved patient comfort, and decreased operator dependence. The use of IV contrast agents, iodinated contrast for CT, and gadolinium contrast for MRI, assists in evaluating organ blood flow and perfusion. Three-phase CT angiography has further refined the evaluation of the pancreas and other organs. With three-phase CT angiography, software is used to track the bolus of contrast administered for timing in the arterial, venous, and delayed phases of the study. This separation of vascular phases highlights arterial and venous blood flow and organ parenchymal enhancement. With abdominal MRI imaging, fat-saturation techniques can be used to darken intra-abdominal fat and highlight inflammation in organs such as the pancreas.

Advanced imaging technology is becoming increasingly more accessible due to factors such as decreased cost and increased availability. With better availability, an increasing amount of research is being published in veterinary medicine regarding the role of imaging in the diagnosis of pancreatic diseases in dogs and cats. As such, advanced imaging techniques, in particular contrast-enhanced CT, three-phase CT angiography, and MRI, play a more central role in the clinical diagnosis of pancreatic diseases. This article focuses on advanced imaging including CEUS, CT, and MRI of the pancreas in dogs and cats.

NORMAL PANCREAS
Contrast-enhanced Ultrasound
The use of CEUS to evaluate the normal pancreas has been performed in both dogs and cats [2–5]. In both species, the normal pancreas is sharply marginated and uniformly contrast enhances at peak intensity, with a progressive decrease in contrast enhancement during the washout phase [3–5]. In dogs, the cranial pancreaticoduodenal artery is well-defined and hyperechoic to the pancreatic parenchyma during peak intensity, whereas the adjacent cranial pancreaticoduodenal vein is anechoic and non-enhancing [4]. In cats, color and power Doppler ultrasonography pre- and post-contrast enhancement has been used to evaluate vascularity and blood volume of the normal pancreas, with contrast-enhanced Doppler ultrasonography measuring greater values of vascularity and blood volume than

pre-contrast Doppler ultrasonography [6]. Different techniques for contrast administration have been evaluated [2,7]. In a study comparing bolus to continuous infusion of contrast enhancement, continuous infusion provides a more gradual enhancement of the pancreas and has a slower washout phase, with less homogeneous contrast enhancement and altered perfusion parameters compared with bolus injection [5]. Most CEUS procedures are performed using bolus injection of contrast [2,7].

Computed Tomography
Computed tomography is increasingly used for evaluation of the pancreas, with advantages over radiology and ultrasound including improved contrast resolution, decreased reliance on operator ability, and lack of superimposition of adjacent structures. In addition, multiplanar reconstruction is useful for the evaluation of the pancreas in different planes and contributes to a more complete understanding of the relationship of the pancreas to adjacent structures. In dogs, the CT appearance and anatomy of the normal pancreas have been extensively described [8]. The pancreas is smoothly marginated and homogeneously isoattenuating to the liver pre-contrast, and the pancreatic duct is often difficult to identify [8]. In the arterial phase of an angiogram, the pancreas shows mild heterogeneous contrast enhancement [8]. In the venous and delayed phases of an angiogram, the pancreas is homogeneously enhancing (Fig. 1) [8]. On transverse images, the median height and normal range measurements of the pancreatic regions in the dog are as follows: body 1.4 cm (0.8–2.5 cm), left lobe 1.2 cm (0.8–1.9 cm), and right lobe 1.6 cm (1.2–2.1 cm) (Table 1) [8]. With angiography, much of the pancreatic triple arterial and venous blood supply vasculature originating from the splenic, hepatic, and right gastric arteries can be identified, in particular the cranial pancreaticoduodenal artery and vein [8]. In addition to the evaluation of associated vasculature and pancreatic contrast enhancement, pancreatic perfusion can be assessed with CT imaging [8–11]. A recent article prospectively evaluated the use of CT in determining pancreatic perfusion variables in normal dogs with the use of proprietary perfusion analysis software and found the methodology feasible for assessing pancreatic microcirculation (Fig. 2) [12]. The clinical utility of this technology in dogs with clinical pancreatic disease requires future research [12].

In cats, the pancreas is hypoattenuating to isoattenuating to both the liver and spleen, and homogeneously contrast enhances in all three phases (arterial, venous,

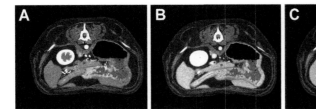

FIG. 1 Transverse computed tomography angiography images of a normal canine pancreas in arterial (A), venous (B), and delayed (C) phases. Note the location of the pancreatic body (P) dorsal to the pylorus and adjacent to the portal vein (* on venous phase image). The pancreas is thin, smoothly marginated, and homogenously enhancing. These features are similar in both dogs and cats.

and delayed phases) of an angiogram [13]. The left lobe of the pancreas is larger in height, width, and length compared with the right lobe in most cats, with no correlation of pancreatic volume to age or sex (Fig. 3) [13]. On transverse images, the average greatest height of the pancreatic body, left lobe, and right lobe are 7.1 to 7.7 mm, 6.5 to 6.6 mm, and 3.6 to 4.3 mm, respectively (Table 2) [13,14]. Cats with chronic diabetes mellitus have a larger pancreas than healthy cats with an average height of the pancreatic body, left lobe, and right lobe of 11.5 mm, 10 mm, and 7.5 mm, respectively [14]. The pancreatic duct is consistently visualized on CT, with best visualization in the portal phase of an angiogram likely because of the contrast between the enhanced parenchyma and the anechoic pancreatic duct [15]. On CT, the pancreatic duct typically has a tapered or tubular shape, with a mean diameter of 0.9 to 3.3 mm [15].

Magnetic Resonance Imaging

The normal appearance of the pancreas on MRI has been infrequently described, although several studies evaluating the pancreas in cats using MRI cholangiopancreatography have been performed [16,17]. In cats, the pancreas is homogeneously hyperintense on pre-contrast T1-weighted sequences relative to the liver with a hypointense, uniformly wide, and smoothly

marginated pancreatic duct [16]. On T2-weighted fat-saturated images, the pancreas is isointense to hypointense to both liver and fat (Fig. 4) [16,17]. The normal pancreatic duct measures 1.6 to 1.7 mm and is poorly visualized, although administering secretin can increase visualization of the pancreatic duct on T1 sequences by increasing its size [16].

PANCREATITIS

Acute pancreatitis can be difficult to diagnose in dogs, and a presumptive diagnosis is often made by consistent clinical signs, specific laboratory abnormalities, and diagnostic imaging findings. Clinical signs consistent with acute pancreatitis typically involve a combination of vomiting, diarrhea, lethargy, anorexia, and abdominal pain [18]. The specific canine pancreatic lipase (Spec cPL) assay is considered the most sensitive and specific test of acute pancreatitis and delivers quantitative results, whereas the SNAP canine pancreatic lipase (SNAP cPL) test is often used for rapid semiquantitative results in the hospital for quick results [18].

Pancreatitis is similarly challenging to diagnose in cats, with reliance on a combination of consistent clinical signs, blood work changes, and diagnostic imaging findings, and difficulty in differentiating between acute and chronic stages of pancreatitis [19]. Clinical signs

TABLE 1			
Computed tomography pancreatic measurements in dogs, transverse plane			
Normal Pancreas	**Body**	**Left Lobe**	**Right Lobe**
Median height (range)	1.4 (0.8–2.5) cm	1.2 (0.8–1.9) cm	1.6 (1.2–2.1) cm
Pancreatitis			
Median height (range)	1.97 (1.4–4.1) cm	2.05 (1.5–2.8) cm	2.26 (1.6–3.3) cm

Data from Refs. [8,28].

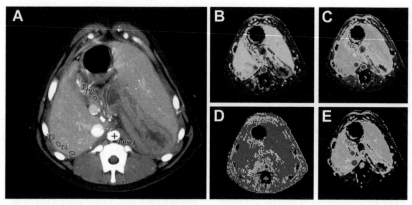

FIG. 2 Transverse CT images of the cranial abdomen in a healthy dog showing region of interest (ROI) placement for computer analysis of pancreatic and hepatic perfusion and generation of perfusion maps. (A) Initial transverse CT image with ROI placements on the abdominal aorta (+), pancreas (T1 and T2), and liver (T3 and T4). Perfusion maps generated include perfusion (B), peak enhancement index (C), time to peak enhancement (D), and blood volume (E).

most commonly include anorexia, lethargy, vomiting, and weight loss [19–22]. The serum feline pancreatic lipase immunoreactivity (fPLI) test has a high sensitivity for the diagnosis of feline pancreatitis, particularly in moderate-to-severe disease [22].

Contrast-enhanced Ultrasound

CEUS may be used to evaluate pancreatic perfusion, with particular enhancement patterns indicative of acute pancreatitis [23]. In a study evaluating dogs with acute abdominal signs, CEUS was able to identify multiple perfusion deficits in the pancreas of dogs with acute pancreatitis not visible with B-mode ultrasonography or contrast-enhanced CT, although lesion size underestimated that of lesions identified on CT [24]. In a study evaluating CEUS in healthy dogs and those with pancreatitis, mean and peak contrast enhancement were significantly higher in dogs with acute pancreatitis, occurred faster, and had a prolonged washout period [25]. In a study evaluating CEUS use in pancreatitis induced in dogs using IV infusion of Cerulein, dogs with pancreatitis had greater peak intensity of

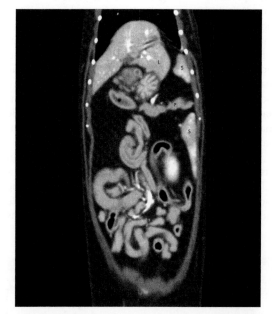

FIG. 3 Dorsal plane computed tomography angiography image of the left lobe of a normal cat pancreas (P) in the venous phase. Unlike in the dog, the left lobe of the pancreas in cats is more prominent than the right lobe. Note the smooth margins, homogeneous contrast-enhancement, and isoattenuation to the liver (L) and spleen (S).

TABLE 2			
Computed tomography pancreatic measurements in healthy cats, transverse plane			
Normal Pancreas	**Body**	**Left Lobe**	**Right Lobe**
Mean height range	7.1–7.7 mm	6.5–6.6 mm	3.6–4.3 mm

Data from Refs. [13,14].

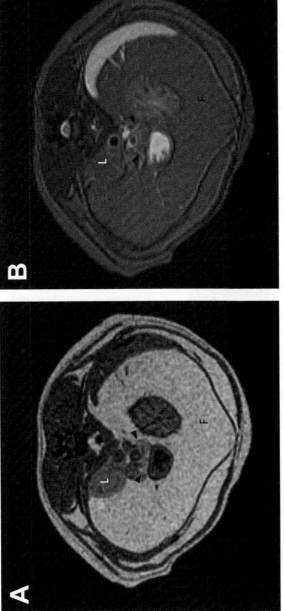

FIG. 4 Transverse MRI images of the cranial abdomen in a cat with a normal pancreas. (A) Pre-contrast T1W image. The pancreas (between *arrowheads*) is mildly hyperintense to the liver (L). Fat (F) surrounds the abdominal organs. (B) Fat-saturated T2W image. The pancreas is isointense to both liver (L) and fat (F). Note that fat is darker on this image compared with image A due to fat-saturation technique.

enhancement and a longer washout period compared with control dogs, with easier visualization of the pancreatic vasculature and interlobular edema [23]. These changes likely reflect both increased blood flow and congestion within the inflamed pancreas [23]. Hypoenhancing nodules within the parenchyma may represent regions of necrosis or abscessation (Fig. 5) [25]. Repeat CEUS studies in dogs with acute pancreatitis 10 to 15 days following the initial CEUS scan have shown a decrease in parenchymal enhancement compared with the initial study with comparable time to peak enhancement values of healthy dogs [25]. This indicates that CEUS may be used to evaluate therapeutic response in dogs with pancreatitis [25].

Computed Tomography

Pancreatitis in dogs and cats is increasingly being researched and evaluated through the use of CT with contrast-enhanced CT, CT angiography, and dynamic CT techniques used. Lack of superimposition and use of IV contrast are distinct advantages in the diagnosis of pancreatitis via CT. In a recent study, the entirety of the pancreas was visualized in 100% of dogs with CT

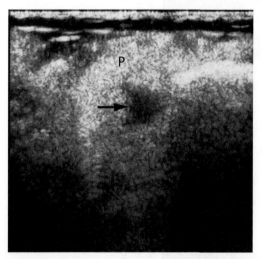

FIG. 5 Contrast-enhanced ultrasound image of a dog with necrotizing pancreatitis of the right pancreatic lobe. Most of the pancreatic parenchyma (P) is markedly hyperechoic, consistent with strong homogeneous contrast enhancement. There is a small moderately hypoechoic nodule (*arrow*), consistent with hypoperfusion secondary to necrosis. (*Adapted from* Rademacher N, Schur D, Gaschen F, Kearney M, Gaschen L. CONTRAST-ENHANCED ULTRASONOGRAPHY OF THE PANCREAS IN HEALTHY DOGS AND IN DOGS WITH ACUTE PANCREATITIS. *Vet Radiol Ultrasound*. 2016;57(1):58-64.)

angiography compared with only 73% of dogs with ultrasound [26]. In addition, CT angiography provides additional benefits including improved identification of vascular thrombosis, in particular portal vein thrombosis [26–28].

Computed tomography findings consistent with a diagnosis of pancreatitis in dogs include pancreatic enlargement, homogeneous to heterogeneous attenuation and contrast enhancement, ill-defined margination, and hyperattenuating surrounding mesentery (Figs. 6–8) [26,28,29]. The delayed phase of CT angiography is best for identifying heterogeneous pancreatic contrast enhancement including ring-like and patchy enhancement, which may indicate regions of necrosis or fibrosis [28]. Heterogeneous contrast enhancement is significantly associated with longer hospitalization, an increased frequency of hospitalization for 5 days or longer, portal vein thrombosis, and elevated Spec cPL [26]. CT size of the pancreas in dogs with pancreatitis is greater than is reported in normal dogs, with a median height and range measurements of body 1.97 cm (1.4–4.1 cm), left lobe 2.05 cm (1.5–2.8 cm), and right lobe 2.26 cm (1.6–3.3 cm) (see Table 1) [8,28]. Sequelae identified via CT include portal vein thrombosis, gastric and duodenal fluid distension or wall thickening, ascites, biliary duct dilatation, biliary mineralization, fat stranding/mesenteric inflammation, and regional lymphadenomegaly (Box 1) [26,28]. Pancreatic abscesses and pseudocysts may develop; these structures cannot be differentiated on imaging features alone, and fine-needle aspiration or biopsy should be performed for confirmation [30].

There is a high prevalence of portal vein thrombosis in dogs with acute pancreatitis compared with dogs with other abdominal or systemic disease, with a reported prevalence of 42% [27]. CT angiography is superior to ultrasound in identifying the presence of portal vein thrombosis and is considered the method of choice for evaluation of presence and extent of portal vein thrombi [26–28]. In a recent study, CT angiography diagnosed portal vein thrombosis in 10 dogs, whereas ultrasound identified its presence in only one of these 10 dogs (10%) [26]. In a separate study, ultrasound detected portal vein thrombosis in four of 21 cases identified by CT angiography (19%) [27]. This is clinically relevant in cases of acute pancreatitis as the presence of portal vein thrombosis is significantly associated with longer hospitalization, and its detection may help with clinical decision-making and therapeutic choices [26]. Most of the dogs develop portal vein thrombi in the main portal vein adjacent to the body of pancreas [26,27].

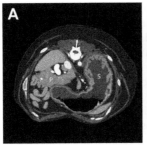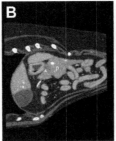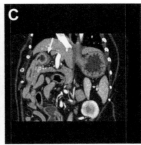

FIG. 6 Computed tomography angiography venous phase images of mild to moderate acute pancreatitis in a dog including transverse (A), sagittal (B), and dorsal (C) plane images. The pancreas is diffusely homogeneously contrast-enhancing. The body and right lobe of the pancreas are moderately enlarged and rounded with irregular margins, which is best appreciated on the transverse and sagittal plane images. Note the fluid distension of the stomach (S) consistent with gastric ileus secondary to pancreatitis as well as the thickened and irregular wall of the duodenum (*white arrow*), consistent with duodenitis secondary to pancreatitis.

Acute pancreatitis may lead to a pro-coagulable state through several pathways including cytokine activation leading to vascular endothelial damage and activation of the coagulation cascade [31]. This inflammatory state and proximity of the main portal vein to the body of the pancreas likely contributes to this predominant location.

Repeat CT imaging within 72 h of diagnosis has been investigated to determine if associated sequelae or heterogenous contrast enhancement may develop as pancreatic inflammation persists [29]. This investigation found that repeat CT did not show worsening imaging findings or further sequelae than the initial CT scan [29]. Repeat CT imaging of dogs with acute pancreatitis is not considered necessary unless clinical signs either do not improve or worsen.

Lastly, at the authors' institution, perfusion evaluation of dogs with presumed acute pancreatitis has been performed successfully using dynamic CT. This technology is being investigated for use in the evaluation of perfusion changes in mild-to-severe pancreatitis and its potential role in the prediction of the development of severe, necrotizing pancreatitis.

Computed tomography for the diagnosis of pancreatitis in cats has not been historically considered useful compared with other diagnostic tests such as ultrasound and serum fPLI [22]. In a previous study, only severe pancreatic changes were identified on contrast CT, with a reported sensitivity for pancreatitis diagnosis of 20% [20]. A separate study found no difference in size, margination, attenuation, or contrast enhancement between healthy cats and cats diagnosed with pancreatitis [22]. However, a recent article specifically evaluated the CT characteristics of the pancreatic duct in healthy cats and those with pancreatitis [15]. This study found that an enlarged pancreatic duct within

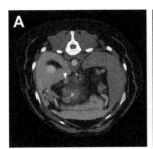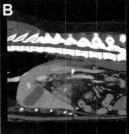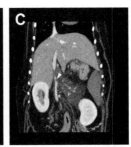

FIG. 7 Computed tomography angiography venous phase images of severe acute pancreatitis in a dog including transverse (A), sagittal (B), and dorsal (C) plane images. The pancreas (P) is heterogeneously contrast-enhancing with a large non-enhancing region in the left lobe, shown in the dorsal plane image. There is a portal vein thrombus (*white arrowhead*) adjacent to the pancreatic body. Note the hyperattenuating mesenteric fat stranding surrounding the pancreas.

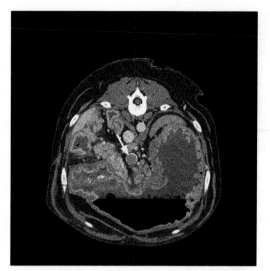

FIG. 8 Transverse post-contrast CT image of moderate acute, edematous pancreatitis in a dog. The pancreas (P) is moderately diffusely enlarged, with fluid dissecting between individual pancreatic lobules. A large portal vein thrombus (*white arrow*) is present adjacent to the pancreatic body. The stomach (S) contains a large volume of fluid and has thickened walls, consistent with gastric atony/ileus and gastritis.

the pancreatic body may be seen in cats with an elevated fPLI, with reported values of pancreatic duct width ranging from 1.3 to 5.6 mm [15]. Although there is overlap within this range with the pancreatic duct diameter in normal cats, significant dilation of the pancreatic duct on CT may support a diagnosis of pancreatitis in cats [15].

Magnetic Resonance Imaging

Magnetic resonance imaging has been evaluated as a tool for diagnosing pancreatitis in cats, with the added tool of MR cholangiopancreatography [17]. Magnetic resonance imaging does not require the use of ionizing radiation or IV contrast used with CT. In a study evaluating MRI in cats with chronic, chronic active, or acute pancreatitis and cholangitis or hepatitis, the pancreas was diffusely mildly to moderately enlarged with patchy and multifocal homogeneous hypointensity relative to liver on T1-weighted images and hyperintensity relative to liver on fat-saturated T2-weighted images indicating parenchymal edema and inflammation (Figs. 9–11) [17]. Most cats had a similar contrast enhancement pattern to normal pancreas, with only one cat having heterogeneous contrast enhancement [17]. Pancreatic duct measurements were increased both pre- and post-secretin administration [17]. Magnetic resonance imaging allowed for the evaluation of multifocal changes that were not identified on ultrasound [17]. Based on the review of the literature, MR imaging of the pancreas has not been well documented in dogs.

PANCREATIC NEOPLASIA
Insulinoma
Contrast-enhanced ultrasound

Pancreatic insulinoma is the most common endocrine tumor of the pancreas in dogs, arising from pancreatic beta cells and typically causing clinical signs associated with hypoglycemia. Insulinomas in cats are very rare, with few case reports describing ultrasonographic features [32–34]. Diagnosis can be difficult, and imaging is often used to detect pancreatic lesions before surgery,

---

BOX 1
Sequelae seen on computed tomography secondary to pancreatitis in dogs

Pancreatitis sequelae
  Portal vein thrombosis
  Fat stranding
  Ascites
  Gastric and/or duodenal fluid distension
  Gastric and/or duodenal wall thickening
  Biliary duct dilatation
  Biliary mineralization
  Pancreatic pseudocyst
  Pancreatic abscessation
  Regional lymphadenomegaly

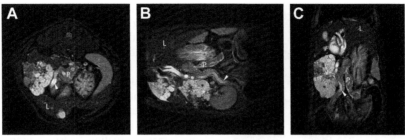

FIG. 9 Fat-saturated T2W transverse (A), sagittal (B), and dorsal (C) plane images of the cranial abdomen in a cat with pancreatitis. Note the hyperintensity of the pancreas (P) relative to the liver (L) as well as the distended pancreatic duct (*white arrowhead*). A hyperintense biliary cystadenoma is present in the right liver (*). This mass is hyperintense on T2 imaging due to its high fluid content.

as lesion localization can be helpful for surgical planning. B-mode ultrasound is often used as a first-line diagnostic evaluation for cause of hypoglycemia and for the potential detection of pancreatic nodules [35]. Ultrasonographic features are varied ranging from ill-defined to well-defined, round to oval, hypoechoic, or hyperechoic nodules within the parenchyma [36]. However, false-negative diagnosis with ultrasound is common [37].

Contrast-enhanced ultrasound has recently been used to evaluate canine insulinomas [7]. In a study evaluating pancreatic neoplasia in dogs with CEUS, insulinoma lesions were hypervascular and showed rapid wash-in of contrast in the arterial phase and rapid wash-out of contrast in the parenchymal phase, corresponding to the lesions appearing hyperechoic to surrounding pancreatic parenchyma in the arterial phase [7]. Contrast-enhanced ultrasound both improved detection of an increased number of nodules and anatomic localization and evaluation of nodules compared with B-mode ultrasound [7]. Although hyperenhancing lesions are most commonly detected, one dog has been reported to have a hypoenhancing lesion using CEUS [36].

In a separate case comparing conventional B-mode to CEUS in the evaluation of a pancreatic insulinoma in a cat, the pancreas was overall normal in size and echogenicity with a single focal, hypoechoic, and well-defined mass lesion and a suspected smaller lesion [33]. On CEUS, this mass showed lower contrast uptake as did two additional ill-defined smaller nodules, which is opposite of the hyperenhancing pattern seen in the majority of reported pancreatic insulinoma cases in dogs [7,33,36]. Importantly, the use of CEUS improved the detection of multifocal lesions in this case.

Computed tomography

Computed tomography is increasingly being used for the purposes of evaluation and detection of canine insulinomas before surgery and has been shown to

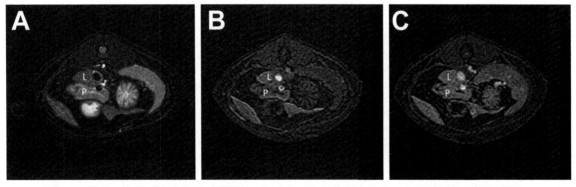

FIG. 10 (A) Transverse fat-saturated T2W image of the cranial abdomen in a cat with pancreatitis. The pancreas (P) is hyperintense relative to the liver (L) and has rounded margins. Transverse Fast Acquisition with Multiphase Efgre 3D images pre- (B) and post- (C) Gadolinium contrast administration. The pancreas (P) is hypointense relative to the liver (L) pre-contrast and hyperenhancing post-contrast.

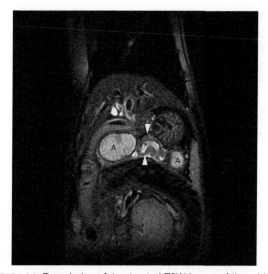

FIG. 11 Dorsal plane fat-saturated T2W image of the mid-to-cranial abdomen in a cat with pancreatitis. The pancreas (between *arrowheads*) is enlarged as is the pancreatic duct (*). Two abscesses (A) are present in the body and left lobe of the pancreas. These were aspirated and cytologically diagnosed as suppurative in nature.

have improved the detection of lesions compared with ultrasound [7,35,37,38]. The use of CT angiography is preferred to highlight arterial and venous enhancement patterns [37,38]. In a study evaluating 35 CT angiography studies in 34 dogs with insulinoma confirmed with histopathology or diagnosed with a combination of clinical signs, concurrent hypoglycemia, and inappropriately high insulin levels, pancreatic nodules or masses were identified in 33 out of 35 cases [39]. Most of these lesions were isoattenuating pre-contrast (32/33), hyperattenuating in the arterial phase (27/33), and isoattenuating (17/33) to hyperattenuating (15/33) in the venous phase [39]. This is consistent with previous reports describing marked hyperattenuation of canine insulinomas in the arterial phase with mild hyperattenuation to isoattenuation in venous and delayed phases [10,37]. Insulinoma masses and nodules may also be hypoattenuating pre-contrast [10,37]. In general, hyperattenuation in the arterial phase is a predominant feature of CT evaluation of canine insulinomas, attributed to their hypervascularity (Fig. 12) [38,39]. Sensitivity of the arterial phase for pancreatic insulinoma detection has been reported up to 94%, with an overall sensitivity of CT for canine insulinoma detection reported as up to 96% [39,40]. The use of bolus tracking for contrast administration and

capture of the arterial phase may increase the sensitivity of detecting pancreatic lesions in canine insulinoma [37,39]. Although hyperattenuation in the arterial phase is most common, arterial phase hypo-to isoattenuation is also reported [38,39]. One study evaluating nine dogs with insulinoma found hypoattenuation in the arterial phase more common than hyperattenuation [38]. A separate study found differing attenuation in all phases of the CT angiogram, with iso- to hyper-attenuation most common in the arterial phase [40]. Although the arterial phase is generally best for lesion detection, the portal and delayed phases have also been reported to have better lesion identification in some cases, making triple-phase angiography preferred to dual-phase angiography [38,39].

Other features of canine insulinoma may also be evaluated using CT. In the largest retrospective study of canine pancreatic insulinomas evaluated via CT angiography, lesions typically distorted the pancreatic shape with variable margination [39]. Cystic change and mineralization were not typically present, despite mineralization being frequently reported in human insulinomas [39]. This difference, as well as the difference in margination compared with human insulinomas, which are typically well marginated, has been attributed to the more aggressive biological behavior of canine insulinomas [39]. Lymph nodes with a similar enhancement pattern to the pancreatic lesions may represent metastatic lesions [38]. In multiple studies, lesion location on CT angiography correlated well with the anatomic location of pancreatic lesions at surgery [37,39]. However, one recent study showed only a 52% sensitivity of location detection using CT, although most of the major location error rates were with either single- or double-phase CT scans [40]. This lends further credence to the preferred use of triple-phase CT angiography for canine insulinoma detection [40]. Computed tomography angiography is superior to ultrasound for lesion identification, with hyperattenuation in the arterial phase the most consistent feature. Triple-phase CT angiography is now the gold standard for surgical planning.

The CT features of feline insulinoma have been reported to the authors' knowledge in a single case [32]. Dual-phase CT angiography showed a left pancreatic lobe nodule that was isoattenuating to adjacent pancreatic tissue pre-contrast, markedly homogeneously contrast enhancing in the arterial phase, and moderately contrast enhancing in the venous phase [32]. Computed tomography angiography additionally showed a separate mass adjacent to the pancreatic body with similar imaging characteristics, determined

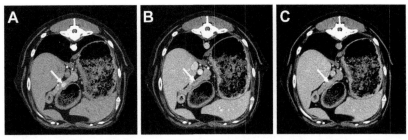

FIG. 12 Computed tomography angiography of a canine pancreatic insulinoma in arterial (A), venous (B), and delayed (C) phases. The insulinoma (*arrow*) can be seen best as a hyperattenuating nodule within the pancreas in the arterial phase.

on histopathology to be a metastatic lymph node [32]. Although further research is warranted on CT evaluation of feline insulinomas, this report supports that feline insulinomas have similar CT imaging features to that of dogs and humans with hyperattenuation in the arterial phase and CT may be similarly useful for surgical planning.

Magnetic resonance imaging

Recently, the appearance of canine insulinomas on MRI was described in four dogs [41]. In all dogs, insulinomas were homogeneous to heterogeneously hyperintense on T2-weighted sequences and isointense to normal pancreatic tissue on T1-weighted pre-contrast sequences, with variable contrast enhancement, which is similar to one previous MRI description (Fig. 13) [7,41]. The largest of these masses had a strong peripheral hyperintense rim on T2-weighted sequences [41]. Insulinoma metastases were also homogeneously to heterogeneously hyperintense on T2-weighted sequences [41]. All primary and metastatic lesions were identified without the use of contrast [41]. Magnetic resonance imaging is a promising tool for evaluation of both primary and metastatic insulinomas in veterinary patients, and may be considered in patients in which contrast-induced nephropathy is a concern.

Pancreatic Adenocarcinoma

Pancreatic adenocarcinoma is the most common exocrine tumor of the pancreas in dogs, although exocrine pancreatic tumors in both dogs and cats are rare [42]. Reports on imaging features are currently lacking and primarily limited to ultrasonographic descriptions [7,42–45]. On conventional ultrasound, canine pancreatic adenocarcinoma masses may appear hypoechoic or heterogeneous [7]. One study reported ultrasound features in 17 of 23 dogs with exocrine pancreatic neoplasia, with discrete masses typically

heterogeneous and well-defined or cavitated [44]. With diffuse pancreatic carcinoma, the pancreas ranged in appearance from normal to hypoechoic and enlarged, imaging characteristics that overlap that of acute pancreatitis [44]. Metastatic lymph nodes were hypoechoic and enlarged and metastatic hepatic lesions were either heterogeneous, hypoechoic, or targetoid in appearance [44]. In a separate study evaluating 13 cases of exocrine pancreatic neoplasia in dogs and cats, a pancreatic mass was identified with ultrasound in five cases, although specific features were not reported [42]. Other imaging findings in this study included hepatic and splenic nodules, diffusely abnormal hepatic echotexture, ascites, and a cystic abdominal mass, with metastasis frequently reported at necropsy [42]. In a study reviewing 34 cases of feline exocrine pancreatic carcinoma, ultrasound was performed in 33 cases and pancreatic nodules were identified in all of these cases; the features of these nodules were not reported [45]. Confirmed metastatic hepatic lesions had a targetoid appearance in one case, with diffuse hepatomegaly and nodules in a second case [45].

Contrast-enhanced ultrasound

Contrast-enhanced ultrasound increases the detection, localization, and evaluation of pancreatic carcinoma lesions [7]. Affected areas are hypovascular with poor enhancement and a hypoechoic appearance to surrounding pancreatic parenchyma on both arterial and parenchymal phases [7]. This is in contrast to the hypervascular appearance seen during the arterial phase in canine insulinomas [7].

Computed tomography

To the best of authors' knowledge, the CT features of pancreatic adenocarcinoma are not yet described. Anecdotally, at the authors' institution, CT characteristics of pancreatic adenocarcinoma include a large size

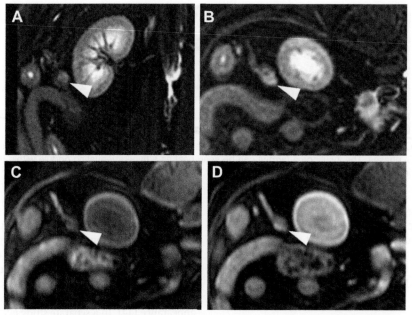

FIG. 13 Dorsal plane fat-saturated T2W (A) and transverse plane fat-saturated T2W (B), T1W pre-contrast (C), and T1W post-contrast (D) magnetic resonance images of the cranial abdomen in a dog with a pancreatic insulinoma. There is an ill-defined nodule within the right limb of the pancreas (*arrowhead*) that is hyperintense on fat-saturated T2W images (A + B), isointense to adjacent pancreas pre-contrast (C), with moderate ventral rim enhancement (D). (*From* Walczak R, Paek M, Uzzle M, Taylor J, Specchi S. Canine insulinomas appear hyperintense on MRI T2-weighted images and isointense on T1-weighted images. *Vet Radiol Ultrasound*. 2019;60(3):330-337.)

with heterogeneous contrast enhancement. This heterogeneous enhancement can include rim enhancement with non-enhancing, necrotic internal regions (Fig. 14).

Magnetic resonance imaging

A single case report briefly described MRI features of metastatic pancreatic adenocarcinoma as T1 isointense submandibular masses, intracranial growth, and

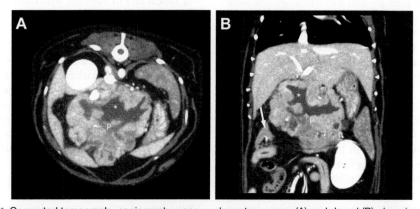

FIG. 14 Computed tomography angiography venous phase transverse (A) and dorsal (B) plane images of a canine pancreatic adenocarcinoma (P). Note the markedly enlarged size and heterogeneous contrast enhancement. This mass has a large non-enhancing necrotic internal central region (*asterisk*) with rim contrast enhancement. On the dorsal plane image, the normal right limb of the pancreas is seen (*white arrow*).

lymphadenopathy; however, the MRI features of the pancreas were not described [46].

SUMMARY AND FUTURE AVENUES

Although conventional ultrasound remains a practical initial diagnostic modality for the evaluation of pancreatic diseases, advanced imaging plays an increasingly important role in the detection of canine and feline pancreatic diseases and their associated sequelae. Contrast-enhanced ultrasonography is useful in the evaluation of pancreatic prefusion and improves the detection of pancreatic nodules in both dogs and cats, with differing contrast enhancement patterns in canine insulinoma and adenocarcinoma. Contrast-enhanced CT increases visualization of the pancreas and can provide prognostic information for clinicians in cases of canine acute pancreatitis, such as the presence of heterogeneous contrast enhancement and/or portal vein thrombosis. Computed tomography angiography improves the detection of canine insulinoma lesions compared with ultrasound. Magnetic resonance imaging may be used in cases with concern for contrast-induced nephropathy and has shown promise in the evaluation of pancreatic changes in cats with pancreatitis as well as detection of primary and metastatic canine insulinomas. Further research is needed using MRI in the evaluation of canine insulinomas as well as CT and MRI evaluation of pancreatic adenocarcinoma.

CLINICS CARE POINTS

- When using contrast-enhanced ultrasound to evaluate for acute pancreatitis in dogs, look for a high level of enhancement that occurs quickly and maintains over time.
- Prognostic imaging findings in dogs with acute pancreatitis include heterogeneous pancreatic contrast enhancement and the presence of portal vein thrombi.
- Computed tomography angiography is superior to ultrasound for the detection of portal vein thrombosis; the main portal vein is the most common location in dogs with pancreatitis, although thrombi may be seen in any of the portal venous branches.
- Triple-phase computed tomography angiography with the use of bolus tracking for timing is useful for insulinoma detection in both dogs and cats.

DISCLOSURE

The authors have no conflicts of interest or funding sources to disclose.

REFERENCES

[1] Haers H, Saunders JH. Review of clinical characteristics and applications of contrast-enhanced ultrasonography in dogs. J Am Vet Med Assoc 2009;234:460–70, 430.

[2] Leinonen MR, Raekallio MR, Vainio OM, et al. Quantitative contrast-enhanced ultrasonographic analysis of perfusion in the kidneys, liver, pancreas, small intestine, and mesenteric lymph nodes in healthy cats. Am J Vet Res 2010;71:1305–11.

[3] Diana A, Linta N, Cipone M, et al. Contrast-enhanced ultrasonography of the pancreas in healthy cats. BMC Vet Res 2015;11:64.

[4] Johnson-Neitman JL, O'Brien RT, Wallace JD. Quantitative perfusion analysis of the pancreas and duodenum in healthy dogs by use of contrast-enhanced ultrasonography. Am J Vet Res 2012;73:385–92.

[5] Lim SY, Nakamura K, Morishita K, et al. Qualitative and quantitative contrast enhanced ultrasonography of the pancreas using bolus injection and continuous infusion methods in normal dogs. J Vet Med Sci 2013;75: 1601–7.

[6] Rademacher N, Ohlerth S, Scharf G, et al. Contrast-enhanced power and color Doppler ultrasonography of the pancreas in healthy and diseased cats. J Vet Intern Med 2008;22:1310–6.

[7] Vanderperren K, Haers H, Van der Vekens E, et al. Description of the use of contrast-enhanced ultrasonography in four dogs with pancreatic tumours. J Small Anim Pract 2014;55:164–9.

[8] Caceres AV, Zwingenberger AL, Hardam E, et al. Helical computed tomographic angiography of the normal canine pancreas. Vet Radiol Ultrasound 2006;47:270–8.

[9] Zwingenberger AL, Shofer FS. Dynamic computed tomographic quantitation of hepatic perfusion in dogs with and without portal vascular anomalies. Am J Vet Res 2007;68:970–4.

[10] Iseri T, Yamada K, Chijiwa K, et al. Dynamic computed tomography of the pancreas in normal dogs and in a dog with pancreatic insulinoma. Vet Radiol Ultrasound 2007;48:328–31.

[11] Kishimoto M, Tsuji Y, Katabami N, et al. Measurement of canine pancreatic perfusion using dynamic computed tomography: influence of input-output vessels on deconvolution and maximum slope methods. Eur J Radiol 2011;77:175–81.

[12] Kloer TB, Rao S, Twedt DC, et al. Computed tomographic evaluation of pancreatic perfusion in healthy dogs. Am J Vet Res 2020;81:131–8.

[13] Secrest S, Sharma A, Bugbee A. Triple phase computed tomography of the pancreas in healthy cats. Vet Radiol Ultrasound 2018;59:163–8.

[14] Secrest S, Sharma A, Bugbee A. Computed Tomographic Angiography of the Pancreas in Cats with Chronic Diabetes Mellitus Compared to Normal Cats. J Vet Intern Med 2018;32:962–6.

[15] Park JY, Bugbee A, Sharma A, et al. Feline pancreatic ducts are consistently identified on CT and more likely to be dilated in the body of pancreas in cats with elevated feline pancreatic lipase immunoreactivity. Vet Radiol Ultrasound 2020;61:255–60.

[16] Marolf AJ, Stewart JA, Dunphy TR, et al. Hepatic and pancreaticobiliary MRI and mr cholangiopancreatography with and without secretin stimulation in normal cats. Vet Radiol Ultrasound 2011;52:415–21.

[17] Marolf AJ, Kraft SL, Dunphy TR, et al. Magnetic resonance (MR) imaging and MR cholangiopancreatography findings in cats with cholangitis and pancreatitis. J Feline Med Surg 2013;15:285–94.

[18] Leoni FP, Pelligra T, Citi S, et al. Ultrasonographic monitoring in 38 dogs with clinically suspected acute pancreatitis. Vet Sci 2020;7:180.

[19] Ferreri JA, Hardam E, Kimmel SE, et al. Clinical differentiation of acute necrotizing from chronic nonsuppurative pancreatitis in cats: 63 cases (1996-2001). J Am Vet Med Assoc 2003;223:469–74.

[20] Gerhardt A, Steiner JM, Williams DA, et al. Comparison of the sensitivity of different diagnostic tests for pancreatitis in cats. J Vet Intern Med 2001;15:329–33.

[21] Nivy R, Kaplanov A, Kuzi S, et al. A retrospective study of 157 hospitalized cats with pancreatitis in a tertiary care center: Clinical, imaging and laboratory findings, potential prognostic markers and outcome. J Vet Intern Med 2018;32:1874–85.

[22] Forman MA, Marks SL, De Cock HE, et al. Evaluation of serum feline pancreatic lipase immunoreactivity and helical computed tomography versus conventional testing for the diagnosis of feline pancreatitis. J Vet Intern Med 2004;18:807–15.

[23] Lim SY, Nakamura K, Morishita K, et al. Qualitative and quantitative contrast-enhanced ultrasonographic assessment of cerulein-induced acute pancreatitis in dogs. J Vet Intern Med 2014;28:496–503.

[24] Shanaman MM, Schwarz T, Gal A, et al. Comparison between survey radiography, B-mode ultrasonography, contrast-enhanced ultrasonography and contrast-enhanced multi-detector computed tomography findings in dogs with acute abdominal signs. Vet Radiol Ultrasound 2013;54:591–604.

[25] Rademacher N, Schur D, Gaschen F, et al. Contrast-Enhanced Ultrasonography of the Pancreas in Healthy Dogs and in Dogs with Acute Pancreatitis. Vet Radiol Ultrasound 2016;57:58–64.

[26] French JM, Twedt DC, Rao S, et al. Computed tomographic angiography and ultrasonography in the diagnosis and evaluation of acute pancreatitis in dogs. J Vet Intern Med 2019;33:79–88.

[27] von Stade LE, Shropshire SB, Rao S, et al. Prevalence of portal vein thrombosis detected by computed tomography angiography in dogs. J Small Anim Pract 2021;62:562–9.

[28] Adrian AM, Twedt DC, Kraft SL, et al. Computed tomographic angiography under sedation in the diagnosis of suspected canine pancreatitis: a pilot study. J Vet Intern Med 2015;29:97–103.

[29] French JM, Twedt DC, Rao S, et al. CT angiographic changes in dogs with acute pancreatitis: A prospective longitudinal study. Vet Radiol Ultrasound 2020;61:33–9.

[30] Scaglione M, Casciani E, Pinto A, et al. Imaging assessment of acute pancreatitis: a review. Semin Ultrasound CT MR 2008;29:322–40.

[31] Watson P. Pancreatitis in dogs and cats: definitions and pathophysiology. J Small Anim Pract 2015;56:3–12.

[32] Shorten E, Swallow A, McCallum KE, et al. Computed tomographic indings in a case of feline insulinoma. Vet Rec Case Rep 2020;8:1–4.

[33] Cervone M, Harel M, Segard-Weisse E, et al. Use of contrast-enhanced ultrasonography for the detection of a feline insulinoma. JFMS Open Rep 2019;5:2055116919876140.

[34] Gifford CH, Morris AP, Kenney KJ, et al. Diagnosis of insulinoma in a Maine Coon cat. JFMS Open Rep 2020;6:2055116919894782.

[35] Robben JH, Pollak YW, Kirpensteijn J, et al. Comparison of ultrasonography, computed tomography, and single-photon emission computed tomography for the detection and localization of canine insulinoma. J Vet Intern Med 2005;19:15–22.

[36] Nakamura K, Lim SY, Ochiai K, et al. Contrast-enhanced ultrasonographic findings in three dogs with pancreatic insulinoma. Vet Radiol Ultrasound 2015;56:55–62.

[37] Mai W, Caceres AV. Dual-phase computed tomographic angiography in three dogs with pancreatic insulinoma. Vet Radiol Ultrasound 2008;49:141–8.

[38] Fukushima K, Fujiwara R, Yamamoto K, et al. Characterization of triple-phase computed tomography in dogs with pancreatic insulinoma. J Vet Med Sci 2016;77:1549–53.

[39] Coss P, Gilman O, Warren-Smith C, et al. The appearance of canine insulinoma on dual phase computed tomographic angiography. J Small Anim Pract 2021;62(7):540–6.

[40] Buishand FO, Vilaplana Grosso FR, Kirpensteijn J, et al. Utility of contrast-enhanced computed tomography in the evaluation of canine insulinoma location. Vet Q 2018;38:53–62.

[41] Walczak R, Paek M, Uzzle M, et al. Canine insulinomas appear hyperintense on MRI T2-weighted images and isointense on T1-weighted images. Vet Radiol Ultrasound 2019;60:330–7.

[42] Bennett PF, Hahn KA, Toal RL, et al. Ultrasonographic and cytopathological diagnosis of exocrine pancreatic carcinoma in the dog and cat. J Am Anim Hosp Assoc 2001;37:466–73.

[43] Lamb CR. Ultrasonography of pancreatic neoplasia in the dog: a retrospective review of 16 cases. Vet Rec 1995;137:65–8.

[44] Pinard CJ, Hocker SE, Weishaar KM. Clinical outcome in 23 dogs with exocrine pancreatic carcinoma. Vet Comp Oncol 2021;19:109–14.

[45] Linderman MJ, Brodsky EM, de Lorimier LP, et al. Feline exocrine pancreatic carcinoma: a retrospective study of 34 cases. Vet Comp Oncol 2013;11:208–18.

[46] Chang SC, Liao JW, Lin YC, et al. Pancreatic acinar cell carcinoma with intracranial metastasis in a dog. J Vet Med Sci 2007;69:91–3.

Advances in Small Animal Care 3 (2022) 73–94

ADVANCES IN SMALL ANIMAL CARE

Update on Magnetic Resonance Imaging of the Brain and Spine

Silke Hecht, Dr med vet, DACVR, DECVDI

Department of Small Animal Clinical Sciences, University of Tennessee College of Veterinary Medicine, C247 Veterinary Medical Center, 2407 River Drive, Knoxville, TN 37996, USA

KEYWORDS

- Magnetic resonance imaging • MRI • Dog • Cat • Neurology • Central nervous system • Diagnostic imaging

KEY POINTS

- Magnetic resonance imaging (MRI) is generally considered the gold standard for the evaluation of diseases of the brain and spine in dogs and cats.
- Technical advances in MRI technology have led to the development of multiple new techniques and sequences.
- Some newer techniques and sequences routinely used in veterinary MRI include T2*-weighting, chemical fat suppression, MR myelography, 3D techniques, and diffusion-weighted imaging.
- Other techniques (eg, perfusion-weighted imaging, MR spectroscopy, and MR angiography) have shown initial promising results in research settings and may gain popularity for clinical veterinary MRI applications in the future.

INTRODUCTION

Compared to radiography, ultrasound and computed tomography (CT), magnetic resonance imaging (MRI) is considered a "newcomer" in the world of diagnostic imaging [1]. The first MR imaging-related articles were published in the late 1970s and early 1980s. Reports on the use of MRI in animals were largely limited to animal models at that point [2,3]. Over the following decades and with increasing recognition of the superb imaging capabilities of MRI in combination with the apparent low risk to patients, MRI research and clinical use especially in the area of neurology rapidly grew in both human and veterinary medicine. Today, with few exceptions, MRI is generally recognized as the gold standard for the evaluation of the central nervous system in people and animals [4,5].

MRI advances over time included improvement of available hardware (eg, type of magnet) and development/improvement of imaging techniques (eg, specialized MRI sequences). This article provides a brief comparison between low and high field MRI systems, gives an overview of over recent advances in imaging technology as it pertains to small animal neuroimaging, provides recommendations for MRI protocols for the imaging of the canine and feline brain and spine, and discusses possible limitations of MRI in the evaluation for certain neurologic diseases in dogs and cats.

MAGNETIC RESONANCE IMAGING HARDWARE
Magnetic Field Strength

Based on the magnetic field strength, MR systems have traditionally been subdivided into low, mid, and high fields. This subdivision is somewhat arbitrary, and definitions have changed over time. The following classification was suggested as being appropriate in 2020 [6]: Very low field (<0.1 T), low field (0.1–0.3 T), mid-field (0.3–1.0 T), high-field (1.0–3.0 T), very high-field (3.0–7.0 T), and ultra-high-field (≥7.0 T). Most

---

E-mail address: shecht@utk.edu

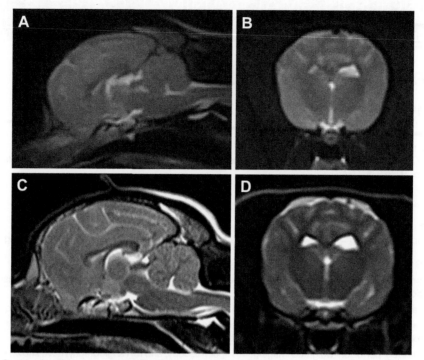

FIG. 1 Sagittal (**A, C**) and transverse (**B, D**) T2-weighted images of the brain in the same dog (2-year-old Boston Terrier) using a low-field MRI system (**A, B**) and a high-field MRI system (**C, D**). Note improved image quality and resolution with increasing field strength.

scanners in use in veterinary medicine fall into the low-to-mid field or high field category [7–9]. Advantages of low field MRI systems include lower cost (purchase price, installation, and maintenance) and less stringent room and installation requirements which has made them an attractive modality for use in private veterinary practices. Advantages of high field MRI systems include significant improvements in image quality due to an improved signal-to-noise ratio, decreased image acquisition times, and availability of advanced MRI sequences and techniques which may not be available for a low-field system. While low field MRI systems are generally capable of producing diagnostic-quality images of the canine and feline brain and spine (Fig. 1), imaging of the spine in very small and very large patients is challenging.

Gradients

Gradients in MRI refer to differences in magnitude or direction of the magnetic field [10]. The gradients of an MRI system affect both spatial resolution and the speed of image acquisition. While gradient strength cannot be influenced during day-to-day operations of the scanner,

it is an important factor to take into consideration along with the overall magnetic field strength when purchasing a new MR system.

Radiofrequency Coils

Radiofrequency coils are an essential MRI hardware component that directly impacts the spatial and temporal resolution, sensitivity, and uniformity in MRI. These coils transmit and/or receive radiofrequency pulses, making them an important component in the MR image acquisition process [11]. Coils commonly used in veterinary neuroimaging include head, neck, and spine coils. To improve image quality when imaging the brain or spine in small veterinary patients, coils intended for imaging small structures such as joints in people (orthopedic or small flex coils) may be used as long as they fit the anatomic area of interest.

MAGNETIC RESONANCE IMAGING TECHNIQUES

MR imaging technology is a constantly evolving field, and new MRI techniques and sequences are being developed and brought to market on a regular basis. While the terminology used for standard spin-echo and inversion recovery MRI sequences is fairly consistent between vendors, terms and acronyms used for newer and advanced techniques often vary significantly. For example, vendor-specific abbreviations used for a similar new gradient-echo sequence include E Short (Elscint), Field Echo (Fonar), SSFP/DE FGR (GE), Timed Reversed Sarge (Hitachi), T2 FFE (Philips), CE FAST (Picker), STERF (Shimadzu) and PSIF (Siemens). An assessment of the respective quality of these sequences for different systems, evaluation of the diagnostic yield of new sequences compared to a gold standard, and comparison of similar sequences between vendors is difficult at best. For this article, generic sequence names will be used whenever possible except in instances where the use of vendor-specific acronyms is common.

Spin-Echo Sequences and Modified Spin-Echo Sequences

Spin-echo (SE) sequences were developed early and are still widely used. They are characterized by successive and repetitive application of 2 radiofrequency pulses (typically, 90° and 180°) and can be modified (weighted) by a modification of the repetition time (TR) between successive 90° pulses and the echo time (TE) between the initial 90° pulse and the MRI signal [12]. T1-weighted and T2-weighted images are the "bread and butter" sequences when performing MRI of the small animal brain and spine [13–15]. Proton density (PD)-weighted images round out the group of classic SE sequences.

- *T2-weighting:* Fluid and tissues with an abnormal content, distribution, or binding of hydrogen protons appear bright (hyperintense), rendering this sequence the classic "pathology scan" (Fig. 2A).
- *T1-weighting:* Fluid is hypointense and fat is hyperintense. The value of this sequence lies in its good anatomic detail and in it being used for the acquisition of postcontrast images (Fig. 2B, D).
- *PD-weighting:* T1 and T2 effects are minimized, and the signal intensity of a given tissue depends on its content of mobile hydrogen protons. Images are characterized by superb anatomic detail (Fig. 2C). This sequence has proven superior to other sequences in the imaging of cortical bone, supporting its inclusion in the MRI protocol if bony lesions of the skull or spine are of concern [16].

Original SE sequences (especially T2-weighting) were characterized by long acquisition times and have largely been replaced with *fast or turbo spin-echo (FSE/ TSE)* techniques [17,18]. T2-weighted FSE sequences are not only faster, they also provide improved T2 contrast compared to conventional sequences. Fat appears hyper- rather than hypointense on T2-weighted FSE/TSE images, which may represent a possible pitfall when imaging the canine and feline spine as the subarachnoid space and epidural fat are unable to be distinguished. For this reason, evaluation of T2-weighted FSE/ TSE images of the spine is usually conducted in conjunction with the evaluation of fat-suppressed images (eg, STIR) and/or MR myelograms (see later in discussion).

Ultrafast spin-echo sequences have gained popularity in neuroimaging due to the ability of improved visualization of noncirculating liquids such as CSF [19,20]. When imaging the spine, these sequences effectively result in an *MR myelogram* without the need for contrast medium injection as required for conventional myelography. Vendor-specific names/acronyms for these sequences include SSH-TSE and UFSE (Philips), SSTSE and HASTE (Siemens), SS-FSE (GE), FSE–ADA (Hitachi), and (Super)FASE and DIET (Toshiba). MR myelograms are tremendously useful in the localization of a lesion within the vertebral canal in relation to the spinal cord (extradural, intradural-extramedullary, intramedullary), in the identification or exclusion of compressive myelopathies such as intervertebral disc herniation, and in the differentiation between acute and chronic lesions [21,22] (Fig. 3). MR myelogram has proven superior to other MR sequences in the identification of subarachnoid diverticula [23] (Fig. 4). A decrease in or loss of the normal strongly hyperintense CSF signal can be seen with extradural compressive lesions (eg, intervertebral disc extrusion and hemorrhage), spinal cord swelling (eg, trauma), alteration of CSF composition (eg, increased protein and cell content with meningomyelitis), and infiltrative diseases affecting the subarachnoid space (Fig. 5). These sequences have a certain prognostic value as an increasing length of CSF attenuation is associated with an increasing risk of the development of myelomalacia [24].

Recently, *3D fast spin-echo techniques optimized for isotropic 3D imaging* have been introduced [25]. Examples include isoFSE (Hitachi), CUBE (GE), SPACE (Siemens), VISTA (Philips), and FASE3D mVox (Canon). Voxels generated with these sequences have the same dimension in each direction (eg, 0.5 mm × 0.5 mm × 0.5 mm). These techniques allow the acquisition of high-resolution, contiguous, thin section images which can be reformatted into additional planes. Initial studies indicate improved evaluation of

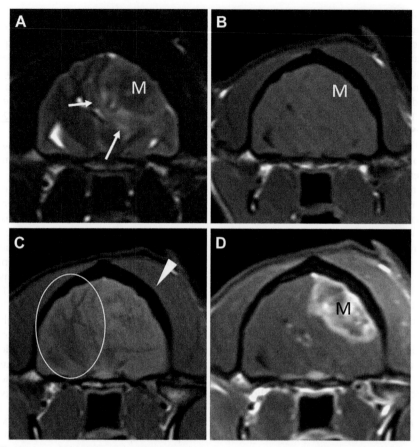

FIG. 2 Transverse spin-echo images of the brain in a 9-year-old cat with a large extra-axial mass (meningioma, confirmed). (**A**) On the T2-weighted image, the mass (M) is bordered by perilesional hyperintensity (*arrows*), consistent with vasogenic edema. An associated mass effect and midline shift is evident. (**B**) On the T1-weighted image, the mass is isointense to brain parenchyma. (**C**) On the proton density-weighted image, there is thickening of the skull adjacent to the mass (hyperostosis; *arrowhead*). Note excellent anatomic detail with a clear distinction between the right-sided cerebral gray and white matter (*circle*). (**D**) On postcontrast T1-weighted image, the mass is strongly and heterogeneously contrast enhancing.

intervertebral disc disease especially in small patients using this technique rather than conventional sequences [26] (Fig. 6).

Inversion Recovery Sequences

Inversion recovery sequences employ an inversion pulse before the initiation of a spin-echo sequence with the goal of suppressing signal from a certain tissue/material. This adds an additional factor affecting image weighting to TR and TE (time of inversion; TI).

With *fluid-attenuated inversion recovery (FLAIR)*, pure fluid (eg, CSF) is attenuated. This sequence is routinely used with T2-weighting (*T2-FLAIR*) when imaging the canine and feline brain and allows differentiation

between fluid-filled (cystic) structures and solid T2 hyperintense lesions (eg, edema, inflammation, neoplasia) which will remain hyperintense on T2-FLAIR (Fig. 7) [27]. An additional advantage of this sequence includes increased conspicuity of lesions bordering the ventricular system or subarachnoid space (Fig. 8). FLAIR has proven valuable in the evaluation of dogs with suspected otitis media/interna due to lack of suppression of signal in the affected inner ear [28]. A possible pitfall of this technique is the presence of proteinaceous or cellular fluid which will not reliably attenuate. Opinions differ as to the value of postcontrast FLAIR imaging compared to conventional postcontrast spin-echo sequences [29,30].

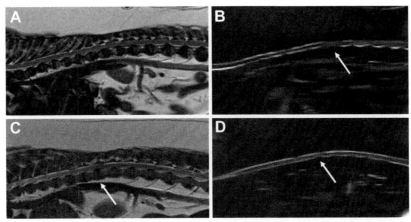

FIG. 3 Acute versus chronic intervertebral disc disease. (**A, C**) Sagittal T2-weighted FSE images, (**B, D**) sagittal MR myelogram. (**A, B**) Acute intervertebral disc extrusion at T13-L1 with multifocal chronic intervertebral disc disease in a 12-year-old dachshund. (**A**) There is a decrease in normal T2 hyperintensity of the intervertebral discs and multifocal variable degree intervertebral disc herniation into the vertebral canal. As both fat and CSF are hyperintense obscuring any sites of CSF attenuation, a site explaining the acute neurologic signs is not identified. (**B**) On MR myelogram there is focal circumferential attenuation of the subarachnoid space at T13-L1 (*arrow*), consistent with acute disc herniation. (**C, D**) Multifocal chronic intervertebral disc disease in a 3-year-old dachshund. (**C**) There is multifocal variable degree decrease in normal T2 hyperintensity of the intervertebral discs. A possible acute site of compressive myelopathy is noted at T11-12 (*arrow*). (**D**) On MR myelogram there is a minor dorsal deviation of the ventral subarachnoid space at this level (*arrow*); however, the CSF signal is circumferentially maintained, consistent with a chronic disease process.

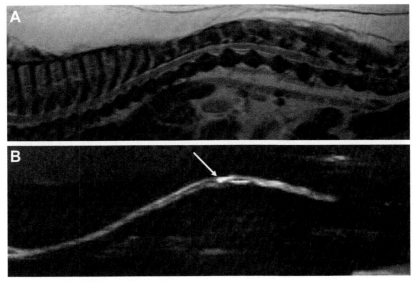

FIG. 4 Subarachnoid diverticulum in a 10-year-old pug. (**A**) On sagittal T2-weighted FSE image, there is evidence of multifocal intervertebral disc degeneration with protrusions into the vertebral canal. (**B**) On MR myelogram there is a focal tear-drop shape dilatation of the dorsal subarachnoid space at T13-L1 (*arrow*), not seen on other sequences.

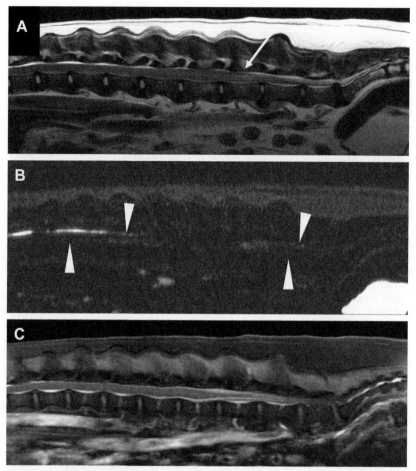

FIG. 5 Diffuse infiltrative meningeal disease in a 7-year-old Golden retriever. (**A**) On sagittal T2-weighted FSE images, no significant abnormalities are identified. The focal intramedullary hyperintensity (*arrow*) was attributed to the previous attempt unsuccessful lumbar CSF tap. (**B**) On sagittal MR myelogram, there is a complete loss of signal from CSF throughout nearly the entire lumbar spine (*arrowheads*). (**C**) On postcontrast T1-weighted images with fat saturation, there is marked diffuse contrast enhancement and thickening of the meninges. Postmortem diagnosis was extensive meningeal histiocytic sarcoma.

A *short tau inversion recovery (STIR)* sequence suppresses the signal from fat. This sequence is especially valuable in the evaluation of the spine where suppression of signal from bone marrow fat allows improved visualization of bone marrow edema or infiltrative disease [13,31,32] (Fig. 9). The sequence is valuable in the evaluation of paraspinal soft tissue abnormalities including muscle changes in dogs with intervertebral disc disease [13,33], and it is indispensable in the evaluation of possible brachial or lumbosacral plexus abnormalities (Fig. 10). STIR is not commonly used for brain imaging, but has been shown to provide a very good contrast between gray and white matter [34].

Similar to the situation for the spine, this technique may be beneficial when evaluating the osseous skull or soft tissues of the head including the orbits.

Phase corrected or phase-sensitive inversion recovery sequences (PSIR) have shown value, especially in the evaluation of white matter lesions such as those seen with multiple sclerosis in people [35]. Corresponding studies in animals are lacking to date.

Gradient-Echo Sequences

Gradient-echo (GRE) sequences use gradients rather than radiofrequency pulses to manipulate protons and generate transverse magnetization. The flip angle

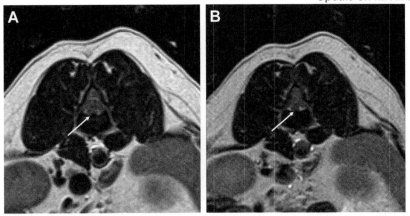

FIG. 6 Intervertebral disc extrusion in a small (5kg) 8-year-old mixed-breed dog. (**A**) On standard transverse T2-weighted FSE image (slice thickness 2.5 mm) extruded disc material is only faintly visible (*arrow*) and is difficult to delineate from the spinal cord. (**B**) On transverse isotropic 3D FSE sequence (slice thickness < 1 mm) the extradural material within the right ventral aspect of the vertebral canal (*arrow*) is clearly visible and results in moderate spinal cord compression.

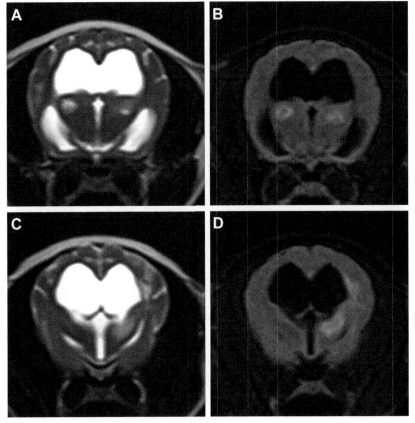

FIG. 7 Meningoencephalitis of undetermined etiology (likely necrotizing meningoencephalitis) in a 6-year-old dachshund. (**A**, **C**) On transverse T2-weighted images, there are multifocal variable size and shape intra-axial T2 hyperintense lesions. There is also generalized ventriculomegaly. (**B**, **D**) On corresponding transverse T2-FLAIR images, some lesions remain homogeneously hyperintense, while others have a central less intense center, consistent with cavitation.

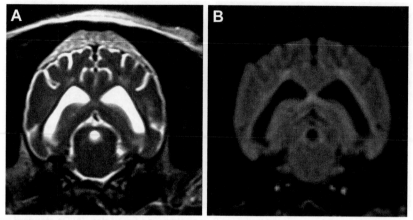

FIG. 8 Brain atrophy and leukoaraiosis (age-related white matter changes) in a 15-year-old West Highland White Terrier. (**A**) On transverse T2-weighted image, there is evidence of mild ventriculomegaly and increased conspicuity of the cerebral sulci. (**B**) On T2-FLAIR image, there is bilaterally symmetric T2 hyperintensity associated with the white matter bordering the lateral ventricles.

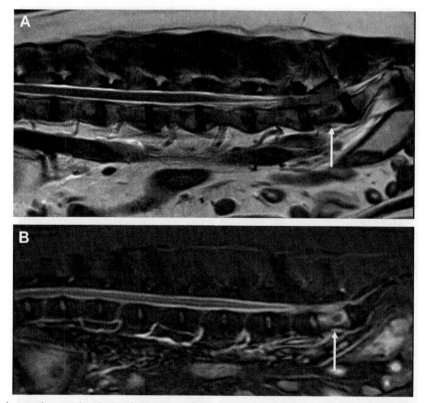

FIG. 9 Aggressive vertebral lesion (sarcoma confirmed) in an 11-year-old mixed-breed dog. (**A**) On sagittal T2-weighted FSE image, the L7 vertebra is of heterogeneous intensity, with hyper- and hypointense regions (*arrow*). There is evidence of abnormal extradural material within the vertebral canal at this level. The remaining lumbar vertebrae in the field of view are also of mixed signal intensity and there is evidence of multifocal degenerative intervertebral disc disease. (**B**) On sagittal STIR the majority of the L7 vertebra is hyperintense (*arrow*), consistent with an infiltrative lesion within the medullary cavity. The remaining lumbar vertebrae are homogeneously hypointense, consistent with successful suppression of bone marrow fat.

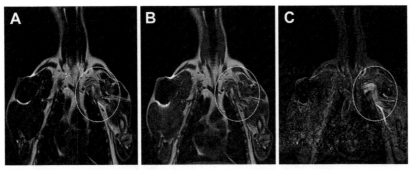

FIG. 10 Dorsal T2-weighted FSE (**A**), T1-weighted (**B**), and STIR (**C**) images of the axillary region in an 8-year-old mixed-breed dog with a brachial plexus tumor. There is a large tubular mass lesion (*circle*) associated with the left caudal neck and axilla, better visible on STIR than in other sequences. Note also muscle atrophy of the left forelimb.

is typically less than 90°, which, in addition to TR and TE, has an effect on image weighting. GRE sequences lack the 180° refocusing pulse employed in spin-echo imaging. As a result, external field inhomogeneities are not reversed and have an increased influence on the spinning protons which dephase more rapidly (T2 is shortened to T2*) [12]. Practically, this means that anatomic regions that contain magnetically heterogeneous material will appear hypointense or even distorted ("susceptibility artifact"). This can be beneficial (eg, in the identification of hemorrhagic lesions, mineral, and intralesional gas) or detrimental (increased severity of artifacts related to the presence of metallic material [36]). A large number of GRE sequences exists, and new sequences are continuously being developed. Sequences can be divided into 2 categories–*incoherent or spoiled and coherent or steady-state techniques* [37]. A detailed discussion of the physics behind those techniques is beyond the scope of this article. GRE sequences important from a small animal neuroimaging perspective include T2*-weighting, susceptibility-weighted imaging, 3D-volumetric sequences, and some steady-state techniques.

T2-weighted imaging* increases the sensitivity of MRI for the identification of hemorrhagic lesions associated with the brain and spine and allows the refinement of a given list of differential diagnoses for MRI abnormalities dependent on the presence or absence of intralesional hemorrhage (Figs. 11–13 [38–40]). The utility of this sequence has been documented in canine and feline patients, and it is now routinely included in veterinary brain (and to a lesser degree spine) MRI protocols.

Susceptibility-weighted imaging (SWI) is a high-resolution three-dimensional GRE technique believed to be superior to T2*-weighted imaging in the identification of hemorrhagic lesions and venous structures. This technique may allow the differentiation of paramagnetic (hemorrhagic) and diamagnetic (calcification) brain lesions (Fig. 14) and may provide additional information in patients with traumatic brain injury [41–43].

3D-volumetric MRI sequences allow the acquisition of very thin (submillimeter) slices without an interslice gap which can be reconstructed into other planes. Examples include TIGRE (GE), LAVA-XL (GE), VIBE (Siemens), THRIVE (Philips), and 3D Quick (Canon). These types of sequences are beneficial in the evaluation of small structures such as cranial nerves and pituitary gland (Fig. 15) and allow improved evaluation of cortical bone compared to other MRI sequences [16,44–46].

3D constructive interference in steady-state sequences (eg, Siemens CISS; GE FIESTA-C; Hitachi PBSG) are considered superior to other sequences in evaluating structures surrounded by CSF due to their inherently high signal-to-noise and contrast-to-noise ratio. They have shown initial promise in the evaluation of spinal arachnoid diverticula and adhesions as well as intradural-extramedullary neoplasia in dogs [47,48].

Functional Magnetic Resonance Imaging Techniques

Diffusion-weighted imaging (DWI) highlights the microscopic (Brownian) motion of water molecules in tissues. In normal tissues, there is no restriction to water movement ("free diffusion"). Certain pathologic processes result in barriers to the movement of water ("restricted diffusion") which can be visualized by means of DWI [12]. The most important application of this technique is in the imaging of ischemic brain

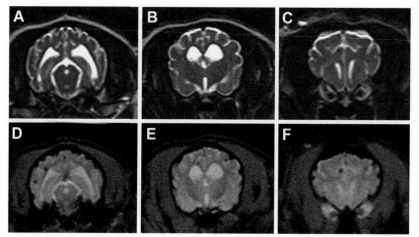

FIG. 11 Transverse T2-weighted FSE (**A–C**) and corresponding T2*-weighted (**D–F**) GRE images of the brain in a 15-year-old Shi Tzu. Only seen on T2*-weighted images, there are multifocal punctate hypointense foci (susceptibility artifacts) associated with the brain parenchyma, consistent with cerebral microbleeds. There is also evidence of generalized ventriculomegaly and increased conspicuity of the cerebral sulci, consistent with brain atrophy.

disease (stroke) [49–51]. An acute ischemic stroke quickly results in cytotoxic edema. DWI is significantly more sensitive than conventional pulse sequences in the peracute stage, when standard MRI sequences may be normal. With acute stroke, increased signal of the infarcted brain parenchyma becomes evident on DWI. As other lesions may also result in DWI hyperintense lesions ("T2 shine through"), DWI images are evaluated in conjunction with a calculated *apparent diffusion coefficient (ADC)* map. A lesion that is hyperintense on DWI and hypointense on ADC is consistent with an acute ischemic event (Fig. 16). It is important to understand that DWI is typically of less importance in veterinary patients with stroke than in people, as imaging is often

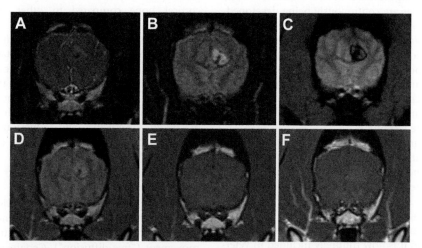

FIG. 12 Brain MRI study in a 4-year-old Rottweiler with a hemorrhagic stroke due to immune-mediated thrombocytopenia. Transverse T2-weighted (**A**), T2-FLAIR (**B**), T2*-weighted (**C**), proton density-weighted (**D**), T1-weighted (**E**) and postcontrast T1-weighted (**F**) images show a focal heterogeneous intra-axial lesion associated with the left forebrain. This lesion is strongly hypointense on T2*-weighted image, consistent with hemorrhage and allowing the refinement of the list of differential diagnoses.

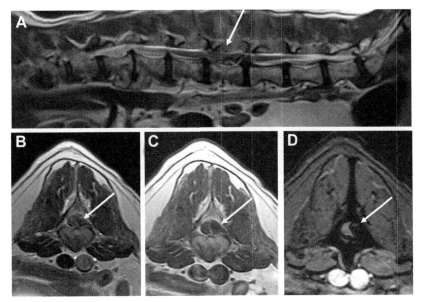

FIG. 13 Extradural hematoma secondary to intervertebral disc extrusion in a 12-year-old Labrador retriever. On sagittal T2-weighted FSE image (**A**), transverse T2-weighted FSE image (**B**), and transverse T1-weighted image (**C**) there is a heterogeneous left-sided extradural mass lesion centered over the L4 vertebral body (*arrows*). There is also evidence of multifocal intervertebral disc disease. On transverse T2*-weighted GRE image (**D**) the extradural material is homogeneously hypointense, consistent with extradural hemorrhage. The imaging diagnosis of an extradural hematoma secondary to L4-5 intervertebral disc extrusion was confirmed surgically.

performed with a significant delay and as thrombolytic therapy is typically not performed in animals. ADC values will remain low for approximately 1 week following the stroke before pseudo-normalizing and subsequently increasing [52]. In animals that are typically imaged with a delay following the onset of neurologic signs, the diagnostic value of DWI/ADC is often limited. DWI/ADC has shown promise in the imaging

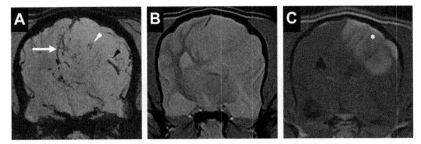

FIG. 14 Transverse susceptibility-weighted imaging (SWI) minimum intensity (mIP) projection (**A**), T2*-weighted gradient-echo (**B**), and T1-weighted postcontrast images (**C**) of an 11-year-old Yorkshire Terrier with a confirmed histiocytic sarcoma of the left parietal lobe. On SWI mIP sequences (**A**), there is a displacement of venous structures within the falx cerebri (*white arrow*). Neovascular structures are infiltrating the mass (*black arrowhead*). Intra-lesional micro-hemorrhages are identified (white *arrowhead*). No signal voids are noted on T2*-weighted GE sequences (**B**). Homogeneous enhancement is noted on T1w postcontrast sequences (**C**) (*asterisk*). (*From* Weston P, Morales C, Dunning M, Parry A, Carrera I. Susceptibility weighted imaging at 1.5 Tesla magnetic resonance imaging in dogs: Comparison with T2*-weighted gradient echo sequence and its clinical indications. Vet Radiol Ultrasound 2020;61(5):566-76; with permission.)

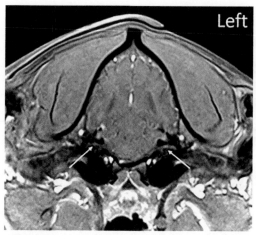

FIG. 15 Left-sided facial neuritis in a 7-year-old boxer. On this transverse postcontrast T1-weighted 3-D volumetric GRE image (slice thickness < 1 mm) the left facial nerve (*arrow*) is thickened and has increased contrast medium uptake compared to the right.

of other neurologic conditions in small animals including ischemic myelopathy [53] (Fig. 17), idiopathic epilepsy [54], brain tumors [55], and intracranial abscesses [56].

Diffusion tensor imaging (DTI) is a specialized diffusion technique that is based on motion restriction in tissues that have a longitudinal fiber orientation such as the brain and spine white matter tracts [49] (Fig. 18). Even though initial studies in normal animals and dogs with various spinal diseases yielded promising results [57–61], this technique is not routinely used in the diagnostic workup of small animal neurology cases to date.

Perfusion-weighted imaging (PWI) encompasses several different techniques which allow the evaluation of brain perfusion including cerebral blood volume and cerebral blood flow [62]. Contrast-based techniques

measure signal intensity changes following the bolus administration of gadolinium-based contrast agents. With noncontrast-based techniques such as arterial spin labeling, arterial blood water protons are selectively excited and used as an endogenous tracer (Fig. 19). Measurement of brain perfusion is used extensively in various neuroimaging applications in people (eg, cerebrovascular disease and brain neoplasia). Initial studies proved the feasibility of these techniques in dogs [63–65], and they are likely to increase in popularity in the future.

Additional advanced MR techniques including *Magnetic Resonance Spectroscopy (MRS)*, *Magnetization Transfer Imaging (MTI)*, and *Functional MR Imaging (fMRI)* are at this point limited to research settings, and readers interested in learning more are referred to specialized publications [66–68].

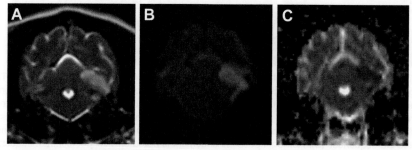

FIG. 16 Acute ischemic infarct of the left rostral cerebellar artery in a 9-year-old pug. The lesion is associated with the left dorsal cerebellar hemisphere, is sharply marginated and wedge-shaped, hyperintense on T2-weighted image (**A**), hyperintense on DWI (**B**), and hypointense on the ADC map (**C**).

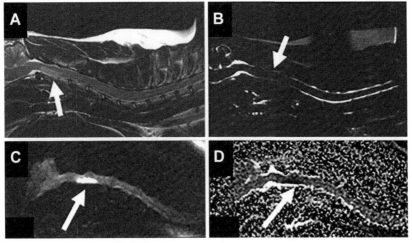

FIG. 17 Sagittal T2-weighted (**A**), single-shot FSE (**B**), and diffusion-weighted (**C**) images and apparent diffusion coefficient map (**D**) of the cervical spine in a 16-year-old female spayed domestic shorthair cat with acute ambulatory tetraparesis. There is a focal area of T2-weighted hyperintensity in the ventral aspect of the spinal cord with a longitudinal extension (*arrow*, **A**), corresponding to loss of cerebrospinal fluid signal over the C2-C3-C4 length consistent with spinal cord swelling (*arrow*, **B**). On diffusion-weighted imaging, there is markedly hyperintense signal corresponding to the same area as seen on T2-weighted images (*arrow*, **C**) and on the apparent diffusion coefficient map there is a marked signal drop indicative of restricted diffusion (*arrow*, **D**). (*Modified from* Mai W. Reduced field-of-view diffusion-weighted MRI can identify restricted diffusion in the spinal cord of dogs and cats with presumptive clinical and high-field MRI diagnosis of acute ischemic myelopathy. *Vet Radiol Ultrasound* 2020; 61(6): 688-95; with permission.)

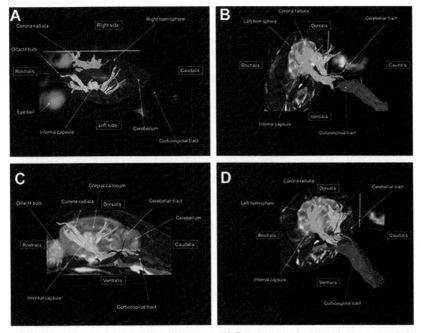

FIG. 18 Diffusion tensor imaging of the brain in a cat. (**A**) Cat corticospinal tract in transversal view. (**B**) Cat corticospinal tract in coronal view. (**C**) Cat corticospinal tract in sagittal view. (**D**) Cat corticospinal tract in coronal view. (*From* Jacqmot O, Van Thielen B, Michotte A, et al. Comparison of several white matter tracts in feline and canine brain by using magnetic resonance diffusion tensor imaging. *Anat Rec* 2017;300(7):1270-89; with permission.)

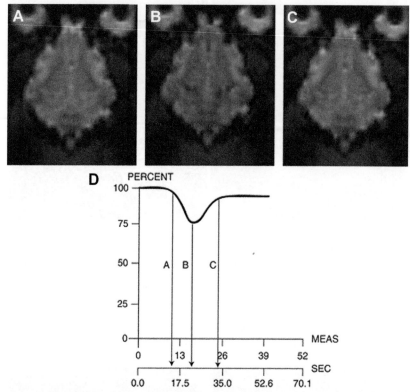

FIG. 19 Perfusion-weighted imaging in a normal dog. (**A–C**) Composite of sequential dorsal T2*-EPI images acquired dynamically during the intravascular transit of a bolus of gadolinium and (**D**) plot of pixel signal intensity levels (relative to a preinjection baseline) over time. Because paramagnetic gadolinium is present within the microvasculature, magnetic field heterogeneity within the voxel leads to susceptibility losses in the EPI image. Note how the signal intensity drops (**B**), corresponding to the susceptibility loss that occurs during normal perfusion of the brain. Also note that during the clinical application, regions of interest placed over the suspected ischemic tissue and compared with a region of normal tissue in the contralateral hemisphere would permit the assessment of time to peak enhancement, relative cerebral blood volume, mean transit time, and relative cerebral blood flow. (*From* Tidwell AS, Robertson ID. Magnetic resonance imaging of normal and abnormal brain perfusion. *Vet Radiol Ultrasound* 2011;52(1 Suppl 1):S62-71; with permission.)

Magnetic Resonance Angiography

MRI-based vascular imaging techniques (*MR Angiography; MRA*) maximize vascular contrast by enhancing the signal from spins in flowing blood and/or suppressing the signal from surrounding stationary tissues [69–72]. This can be accomplished without contrast medium administration (*time-of-flight MRI, phase-contrast MRA, or digital subtraction MRA*); however, *contrast-enhanced MRA* provides improved image quality and is thus considered a superior technique. While imaging of larger vascular structures of the head and spine in small animals can be achieved using standard high-field MRI systems, image resolution appears insufficient for imaging of smaller arteries at this point. MRA is,

therefore, of limited use when assessing a canine or feline patient for an acute ischemic event. However, MRA may aid in the identification of vascular anomalies such as arteriovenous fistulas or aberrant vessels, or help in the identification of venous thrombosis. Additionally, MRA may allow a diagnosis of aortic thromboembolism or other large vessel conditions mimicking neurologic disease (Fig. 20).

Other Technical Modifications and Postprocessing Options

Fat saturation (FatSat) is an add-on technique that can be applied to any sequence to suppress the signal from fat without affecting signal from other tissues

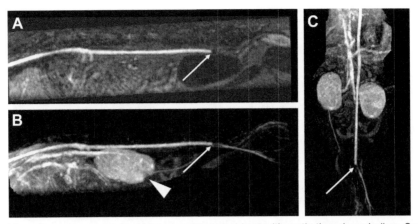

FIG. 20 Magnetic resonance angiography in an 11-year-old cat with aortic thromboembolism. Sagittal arterial phase image (**A**) and venous phase images in sagittal (**B**) and dorsal (**C**) planes. Note abrupt termination of intravascular signal at the level of the caudal aorta on the arterial phase image, and near-complete occlusion of the right external iliac and median sacral arteries and marked narrowing of the origin of the left external artery on venous phase images (*arrows*). Note also evidence of a focal indentation within the caudal aspect of the left kidney (*arrowhead*), consistent with a renal cortical infarct.

[73]. It is different from STIR as it is not a stand-alone sequence. The most common application in veterinary neuroimaging is postcontrast T1-weighted imaging of the spine (and less commonly the brain) [74,75]. By suppressing the signal from subcutaneous and bone marrow fat, any hyperintense structure on postcontrast images will truly represent contrast-enhancing tissue. Postcontrast FatSat improves the visualization of meningeal enhancement, bone marrow lesions, and lesions within the paraspinal tissues (Figs. 21 and 22).

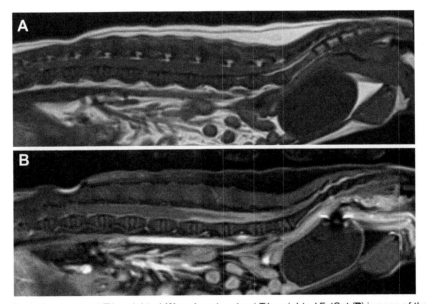

FIG. 21 Sagittal precontrast T1-weighted (**A**) and postcontrast T1-weighted FatSat (**B**) images of the lumbar spine in an 8-month-old Maltese with meningomyelitis of undetermined etiology. Note marked thickening and contrast enhancement of the meninges in the caudal lumbar spine.

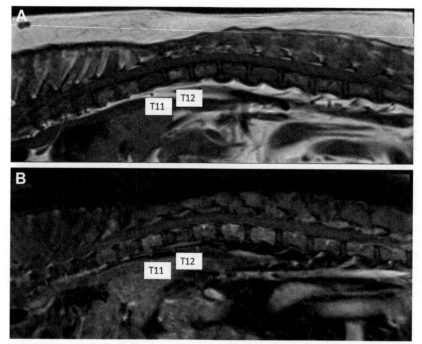

FIG. 22 Sagittal precontrast T1-weighted (**A**) and postcontrast T1-weighted FatSat images of the thoracolumbar spine in a 7-year-old Boston Terrier with multifocal infiltrative bone marrow neoplasia (strongly suspected multiple myeloma). (**A**) The thoracic and lumbar vertebrae are heterogeneous in intensity on precontrast images. (**B**) In postcontrast images, there is patchy contrast enhancement of multiple vertebrae (eg, T11) and suppression of precontrast hyperintense bone marrow fat (eg, T12).

Subtraction techniques may be used to document differences in tissues at certain points in time. In addition to digital subtraction MRA briefly mentioned above, these have been described as a means to evaluate contrast-enhancing lesions and especially meningeal enhancement in small animals. By subtracting precontrast T1-weighted images from postcontrast T1-weighted images, contrast-enhancing tissues and lesions are accentuated (Fig. 23). It is unclear at this point if these techniques truly increase accuracy in the diagnosis of meningitis and other meningeal diseases [76,77].

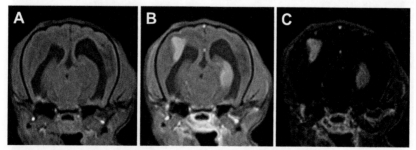

FIG. 23 Transverse pre and postcontrast T1-weighted 3D volumetric GRE images (**A, B**) and subtraction image (**C**) of a 7-year-old Pomeranian with meningoencephalitis of undetermined etiology. There are multifocal strongly contrast-enhancing intra-axial brain lesions. While these are accentuated on the subtraction image (**C**), the regular postcontrast image (**B**) provides improved delineation of other anatomic structures including the lateral ventricles.

BOX 1
Suggested Brain MRI Protocol

Sagittal T2-weighted

Transverse T1-weighted, T2-weighted, T2-FLAIR and T2*-weighted

T1-weighted images (+/− fat saturation) following contrast medium administration in transverse (+/− sagittal and dorsal) planes

+/− dorsal T2-weighted, proton density weighted, DWI/ADC, Volumetric GRE, and others dependent on clinical suspicion and initial findings on routine MRI sequences

---

MAGNETIC RESONANCE IMAGING PROTOCOL RECOMMENDATIONS

Factors to consider when designing an MRI protocol include that it should provide an answer to a given clinical question, that the examination time should be kept as short as possible, and that study results should be reproducible. Imaging protocols must be adapted to the equipment available and are often adjusted to radiologist/clinician preference. For example, diagnosis of a disc extrusion in the cervical spine in a chondrodystrophic dog may be accomplished with only T1-weighted and T2-weighted images, while the full evaluation of a patient with a focal intramedullary lesion may require the inclusion of multiple additional sequences. Consensus recommendations for standardized MRI protocols have been published for veterinary patients with epilepsy and for patients included in multicenter canine brain tumor clinical trials [78,79]. The following suggestions (Boxes 1 and 2) are supported by protocol recommendations found in the veterinary imaging literature [13,14,80,81].

POSSIBLE LIMITATIONS OF MAGNETIC RESONANCE IMAGING

As mentioned above, MRI is generally considered the gold standard for diagnostic imaging of the canine and feline brain and spine. Very small or very large patient size may be a problem when imaging the spine, especially when using a low field system, and alternate techniques (myelography, CT, CT-myelography) may be preferable in cases where adequate image quality cannot be achieved by means of MRI. Metallic material in the area of interest (eg, surgical implants, identification microchips, or ballistic projectiles) may render an MRI study nondiagnostic and necessitate the use of alternate imaging modalities (Fig. 24). Even though the advancement in MRI techniques and sequences has improved the capabilities of MRI for the imaging of cortical bone and osseous/mineralized lesions, CT remains superior to MRI in the evaluation of patients with acute osseous head and spinal trauma (Fig. 25), bone anomalies and malformations, and certain mineralized lesions including some cases of foraminal or far lateral herniation of mineralized disc material.

BOX 2
Suggested Spine MRI Protocol

Dorsal STIR

Sagittal T2-weighted, T1-weighted, STIR, and MR myelogram

Transverse T2-weighted images (if possible isotropic) through the entire area of lesion localization

+/− T1-weighted and T2*-weighted images of abnormal areas

+/− proton density weighted, DWI/ADC, Volumetric GRE, and others dependent on clinical suspicion and initial findings on routine MRI sequences

+/− T1-weighted images (with fat saturation) following contrast medium administration in sagittal (+/− transverse and dorsal) planes

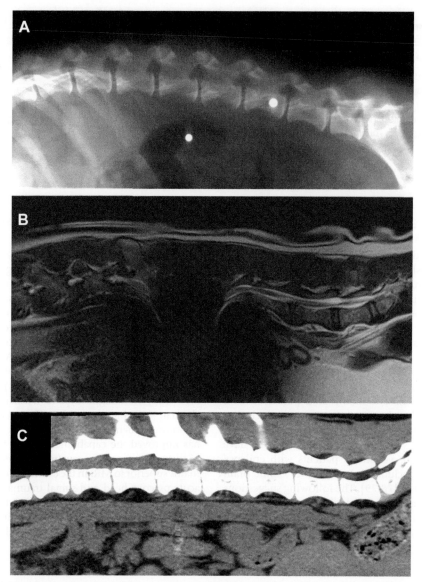

FIG. 24 Intervertebral disc extrusion in a 4-year-old mixed-breed dog with a previous history of ballistic injury. The lateral radiograph of the lumbar spine (**A**) shows 2 large metallic projectiles in the vicinity of the lumbar spine. These projectiles result in severe susceptibility artifacts and a nondiagnostic MRI study (**B**). A diagnosis of L3-4 intervertebral disc extrusion and associated hemorrhage is made on CT (**C**).

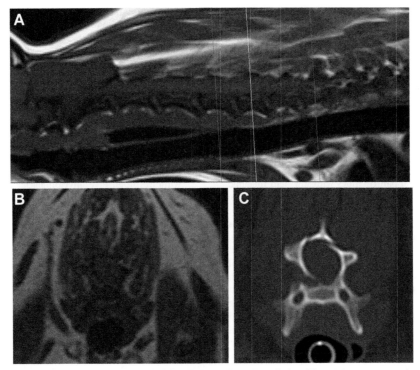

FIG. 25 Vertebral fracture in a 10-year-old Chihuahua. Even though the C6 vertebra appears abnormally shaped on sagittal (**A**) and transverse (**B**) T1-weighted MR images, exact fracture delineation is not possible in this small patient. The transverse CT image (**C**) allows much improved evaluation of the comminuted fracture.

CLINICS CARE POINTS

- Magnetic resonance imaging (MRI) is the gold standard for the diagnostic imaging evaluation of most small animal neurology patients.
- Other techniques (myelography, CT, CT-myelography) may be preferable in instances where adequate image quality cannot be achieved due to patient size, in cases where metallic material is present in the area of interest, and in cases where a detailed evaluation of cortical bone is desired (such as acute osseous head and spinal trauma and congenital anomalies).
- The MRI protocol depends on the available equipment, clinical question to be answered, and findings on initial MRI sequences.
- The minimum sequences for the evaluation of the brain should include sagittal T2-weighted, transverse T1-weighted, T2-weighted, T2-FLAIR, and T2*-weighted, and transverse T1-weighted images following contrast medium administration.

- The minimum sequences for the evaluation of the spine should include dorsal STIR, sagittal T2-weighted, T1-weighted, STIR and MR myelogram, and transverse T2-weighted images (if possible isotropic) through the entire area of lesion localization.
- Additional sequences should be added dependent on the clinical indication and initial imaging findings.

REFERENCES

[1] Edelman RR. The history of MR imaging as seen through the pages of radiology. Radiology 2014;273:181–200.

[2] Alfidi RJ, Haaga JR, El-Yousef SJ, et al. Preliminary experimental results in humans and animals with a superconducting, whole-body, nuclear magnetic resonance scanner. Radiology 1982;143:175–81.

[3] Runge VM, Price AC, Wehr CJ, et al. Contrast enhanced MRI. Evaluation of a canine model of osmotic blood-brain barrier disruption. Invest Radiol 1985;20:830–44.

[4] Gavin PR. Growth of clinical veterinary magnetic resonance imaging. Vet Radiol Ultrasound 2011;52(1 Suppl 1):S2–4.

[5] Symms M, Jager HR, Schmierer K, et al. A review of structural magnetic resonance neuroimaging. J Neurol Neurosurg Psychiatr 2004;75:1235–44.

[6] Elster AD. Characterizing field strength. In: Questions and answers in MRI. Available at: https://mriquestions.com/low-v-mid-v-high-field.html. Accessed January 20, 2022.

[7] Konar M, Lang J. Pros and cons of low-field magnetic resonance imaging in veterinary practice. Vet Radiol Ultrasound 2011;52(1 Suppl 1):S5–14.

[8] Martin-Vaquero P, da Costa RC, Echandi RL, et al. Magnetic resonance spectroscopy of the canine brain at 3.0 T and 7.0 T. Res Vet Sci 2012;93:427–9.

[9] Mai W. Technical particularities with low-field imaging. In: Mai W, editor. Diagnostic MRI in dogs and cats. Boca Raton: CRC Press; 2018. p. 153–60.

[10] Elster AD. Magnetic field gradient defined. In: Questions and answers in MRI. Available at: https://mriquestions.com/what-is-a-gradient.html. Accessed January 20, 2022.

[11] Gruber B, Froeling M, Leiner T, et al. RF coils: a practical guide for nonphysicists. J Magn Reson Imaging 2018; 48(3):590–604.

[12] Mai W. Image characteristics in MRI and principal pulse sequences. In: Mai W, editor. Diagnostic MRI in dogs and cats. Boca Raton: CRC Press; 2018. p. 36–69.

[13] Dennis R. Optimized technique: spine. In: Mai W, editor. Diagnostic MRI in dogs and cats. Boca Raton: CRC Press; 2018. p. 106–29.

[14] Hecht S. Optimized technique: brain. In: Mai W, editor. Diagnostic MRI in dogs and cats. Boca Raton: CRC Press; 2018. p. 88–105.

[15] Zhalniarovich Y, Adamiak Z, Pomianowski A, et al. Most commonly used sequences and clinical protocols for brain and spine magnetic resonance imaging allowing better identification of pathological changes in dogs. Pol J Vet Sci 2013;16:157–63.

[16] Hecht S, Anderson KM, Castel A, et al. Agreement of magnetic resonance imaging with computed tomography in the assessment for acute skull fractures in a canine and feline cadaver model. Front Vet Sci 2021. https://doi.org/10.3389/fvets.2021.603775.

[17] Miyabayashi T, Smith M, Tsuruno Y. Comparison of fast spin-echo and conventional spin-echo magnetic resonance spinal imaging techniques in four normal dogs. Vet Radiol Ultrasound 2000;41:308–12.

[18] Sage JE, Samii VF, Abramson CJ, et al. Comparison of conventional spin-echo and fast spin-echo magnetic resonance imaging in the canine brain. Vet Radiol Ultrasound 2006;47:249–53.

[19] Castillo M, Mukherji SK. Clinical applications of FLAIR, HASTE, and magnetization transfer in neuroimaging. Semin Ultrasound CT MR 2000;21:417–27.

[20] Rumboldt Z, Marotti M. Magnetization transfer, HASTE, and FLAIR imaging. Magn Reson Imaging Clin N Am 2003;11:471–92.

[21] Pease A, Sullivan S, Olby N, et al. Value of a single-shot turbo spin-echo pulse sequence for assessing the architecture of the subarachnoid space and the constitutive nature of cerebrospinal fluid. Vet Radiol Ultrasound 2006;47:254–9.

[22] Mankin JM, Hecht S, Thomas WB. Agreement between T2 and Haste sequences in the evaluation of thoracolumbar intervertebral disc disease in dogs. Vet Radiol Ultrasound 2012;53:162–6.

[23] Seiler GS, Robertson ID, Mai W, et al. Usefulness of a half-Fourier acquisition single-shot turbo spin-echo pulse sequence in identifying arachnoid diverticula in dogs. Vet Radiol Ultrasound 2012;53:157–61.

[24] Gilmour LJ, Jeffery ND, Miles K, et al. Single-shot turbo spin echo pulse sequence findings in dogs with and without progressive myelomalacia. Vet Radiol Ultrasound 2017;58:197–205.

[25] Mugler JP. Optimized three-dimensional fast-spin-echo MRI. J Magn Reson Imaging 2014;39:745–67.

[26] Lee S, Hwang J, Ko J, et al. Comparison between T2-weighted two-dimensional and three-dimensional fast spin-echo MRI sequences for characterizing thoracolumbar intervertebral disc disease in small-breed dogs. Vet Radiol Ultrasound 2022. https://doi.org/10.1111/vru.13049.

[27] Cherubini GB, Platt SR, Howson S, et al. Comparison of magnetic resonance imaging sequences in dogs with multi-focal intracranial disease. J Small Anim Pract 2008;49:634–40.

[28] Castillo G, Parmentier T, Monteith G, et al. Inner ear fluid-attenuated inversion recovery MRI signal intensity in dogs with vestibular disease. Vet Radiol Ultrasound 2020;61:531–9.

[29] Falzone C, Rossi F, Calistri M, et al. Contrast-enhanced fluid-attenuated inversion recovery vs. contrast-enhanced spin echo T1-weighted brain imaging. Vet Radiol Ultrasound 2008;49:333–8.

[30] Merhof K, Lang J, Durr S, et al. Use of contrast-enhanced fluid-attenuated inversion recovery sequence to detect brain lesions in dogs and cats. J Vet Intern Med 2014; 28:1263–7.

[31] Allett B, Hecht S. Magnetic resonance imaging findings in the spine of six dogs diagnosed with lymphoma. Vet Radiol Ultrasound 2016;57:154–61.

[32] Auger M, Hecht S, Springer CM. Magnetic resonance imaging features of extradural spinal neoplasia in 60 dogs and 7 cats. Front Vet Sci 2020. https://doi.org/10.3389/fvets.2020.610490.

[33] Morrison EJ, Baron-Chapman ML, Chalkley M. MRI T2/STIR epaxial muscle hyperintensity in some dogs with intervertebral disc extrusion corresponds to histologic patterns of muscle degeneration and inflammation. Vet Radiol Ultrasound 2021;62:150–60.

[34] Young BD, Mankin JM, Griffin JF, et al. Comparison of two fat-suppressed magnetic resonance imaging pulse sequences to standard T2-weighted images for brain parenchymal contrast and lesion detection in dogs with inflammatory intracranial disease. Vet Radiol Ultrasound 2015;56:204–11.

[35] Feger J, Baba Y. Phase-sensitive inversion recovery. In: Radiopaedia. Available at: https://radiopaedia.org/articles/phase-sensitive-inversion-recovery?lang=us. Accessed January 26, 2022.

[36] Hecht S, Adams WH, Narak J, et al. Magnetic resonance imaging susceptibility artifacts due to metallic foreign bodies. Vet Radiol Ultrasound 2011;52:409–14.

[37] Chavhan GB, Babyn PS, Jankharia BG, et al. Steady-state MR imaging sequences: physics, classification, and clinical applications. Radiographics 2008;28:1147–60.

[38] Hammond LJ, Hecht S. Susceptibility artifacts on T2*-weighted magnetic resonance imaging of the canine and feline spine. Vet Radiol Ultrasound 2015;56:398–406.

[39] Hodshon AW, Hecht S, Thomas WB. Use of the T2*-weighted gradient recalled echo sequence for magnetic resonance imaging of the canine and feline brain. Vet Radiol Ultrasound 2014;55:599–606.

[40] Kerwin SC, Levine JM, Budke CM, et al. Putative cerebral microbleeds in dogs undergoing magnetic resonance imaging of the head: A retrospective study of demographics, clinical associations, and relationship to case outcome. J Vet Intern Med 2017;31:1140–8.

[41] Noh D, Choi S, Choi H, et al. Evaluating traumatic brain injury using conventional magnetic resonance imaging and susceptibility-weighted imaging in dogs. J Vet Sci 2019. https://doi.org/10.4142/jvs.2019.20.e10.

[42] Weston P, Morales C, Dunning M, et al. Susceptibility weighted imaging at 1.5 Tesla magnetic resonance imaging in dogs: Comparison with T2*-weighted gradient echo sequence and its clinical indications. Vet Radiol Ultrasound 2020;61:566–76.

[43] Wolfer N, Wang-Leandro A, Beckmann KM, et al. Intracranial lesion detection and artifact characterization: Comparative study of susceptibility and T2*-weighted imaging in dogs and cats. Front Vet Sci 2021. https://doi.org/10.3389/fvets.2021.779515.

[44] van der Vlugt-Meijer RH, Meij BP, Voorhout G. Thin-slice three-dimensional gradient-echo magnetic resonance imaging of the pituitary gland in healthy dogs. Am J Vet Res 2006;67:1865–72.

[45] Fleming KL, Maddox TW, Warren-Smith CMR. Three-dimensional T1-weighted gradient echo is a suitable alternative to two-dimensional T1-weighted spin echo for imaging the canine brain. Vet Radiol Ultrasound 2019;60:543–51.

[46] Smith PM, Goncalves R, McConnell JF. Sensitivity and specificity of MRI for detecting facial nerve abnormalities in dogs with facial neuropathy. Vet Rec 2012;171:349.

[47] Tauro A, Di Dona F, Garosi LS. "Golf-tee sign" on 3D-CISS MRI sequences in a dog with spinal nephroblastoma. J Small Anim Pract 2021;62:610.

[48] Tauro A, Jovanovik J, Driver CJ, et al. Clinical application of 3D-CISS MRI sequences for diagnosis and surgical planning of spinal arachnoid diverticula and adhesions in dogs. Vet Comp Orthop Traumatol 2018;31:83–94.

[49] Baliyan V, Das CJ, Sharma R, et al. Diffusion weighted imaging: technique and applications. World J Radiol 2016;8:785–98.

[50] McConnell JF. Ischemic brain disease and vascular anomalies. In: Mai W, editor. Diagnostic MRI in dogs and cats. Boca Raton: CRC Press; 2018. p. 251–81.

[51] Garosi LS, McConnell JF. Ischaemic stroke in dogs and humans: a comparative review. J Small Anim Pract 2005;46:521–9.

[52] Bhuta S, Saber M. Diffusion weighted MRI in acute stroke Radiopaedia. Available at: https://radiopaedia.org/articles/diffusion-weighted-mri-in-acute-stroke-1?lang=us. Accessed January 26th 2022.

[53] Mai W. Reduced field-of-view diffusion-weighted MRI can identify restricted diffusion in the spinal cord of dogs and cats with presumptive clinical and high-field MRI diagnosis of acute ischemic myelopathy. Vet Radiol Ultrasound 2020;61:688–95.

[54] Hartmann A, Sager S, Failing K, et al. Diffusion-weighted imaging of the brains of dogs with idiopathic epilepsy. BMC Vet Res 2017;13(1):338.

[55] Fages J, Oura TJ, Sutherland-Smith J, et al. Atypical and malignant canine intracranial meningiomas may have lower apparent diffusion coefficient values than benign tumors. Vet Radiol Ultrasound 2020;61:40–7.

[56] Scherf G, Sutherland-Smith J, Uriarte A. Dogs and cats with presumed or confirmed intracranial abscessation have low apparent diffusion coefficient values. Vet Radiol Ultrasound 2022. https://doi.org/10.1111/vru.13064.

[57] Anaya Garcia MS, Hernandez Anaya JS, Marrufo Melendez O, et al. In vivo study of cerebral white matter in the dog using diffusion tensor tractography. Vet Radiol Ultrasound 2015;56:188–95.

[58] Pease A, Miller R. The use of diffusion tensor imaging to evaluate the spinal cord in normal and abnormal dogs. Vet Radiol Ultrasound 2011;52:492–7.

[59] Jacqmot O, Van Thielen B, Fierens Y, et al. Diffusion tensor imaging of white matter tracts in the dog brain. Anat Rec 2013;296:340–9.

[60] Jacqmot O, Van Thielen B, Michotte A, et al. Neuroanatomical reconstruction of the canine visual pathway using diffusion tensor imaging. Front Neuroanat 2020;14:54. https://doi.org/10.3389/fnana.2020.00054.

[61] Jacqmot O, Van Thielen B, Michotte A, et al. Comparison of several white matter tracts in feline and canine brain by using magnetic resonance diffusion tensor imaging. Anat Rec 2017;300:1270–89.

[62] Tidwell AS, Robertson ID. Magnetic resonance imaging of normal and abnormal brain perfusion. Vet Radiol Ultrasound 2011;52(1 Suppl 1):S62–71.

[63] Hartmann A, Driesen A, Lautenschlager IE, et al. Quantitative analysis of brain perfusion in healthy dogs by means of magnetic resonance imaging. Am J Vet Res 2016;77:1227–35.

[64] Hartmann A, von Klopmann C, Lautenschlager IE, et al. Quantitative analysis of brain perfusion parameters in

dogs with idiopathic epilepsy by use of magnetic resonance imaging. Am J Vet Res 2018;79:433–42.

[65] Hoffmann AC, Ruel Y, Gnirs K, et al. Brain perfusion magnetic resonance imaging using pseudocontinuous arterial spin labeling in 314 dogs and cats. J Vet Intern Med 2021;35:2327–41.

[66] Carrera I, Richter H, Meier D, et al. Regional metabolite concentrations in the brain of healthy dogs measured by use of short echo time, single voxel proton magnetic resonance spectroscopy at 3.0 Tesla. Am J Vet Res 2015;76:129–41.

[67] Vite CH, McGowan JC. Magnetization transfer imaging of the canine brain: a review. Vet Radiol Ultrasound 2001;42:5–8.

[68] Berns GS, Brooks AM, Spivak M. Scent of the familiar: an fMRI study of canine brain responses to familiar and unfamiliar human and dog odors. Behav Processes 2015; 110:37–46.

[69] Ishikawa C, Ito D, Kitagawa M, et al. Comparison of conventional magnetic resonance imaging and nonenhanced three dimensional time-of-flight magnetic resonance angiography findings between dogs with meningioma and dogs with intracranial histiocytic sarcoma: 19 cases (2010-2014). J Am Vet Med Assoc 2016;248:1139–47.

[70] Ishikawa C, Ito D, Tanaka N, et al. Use of three-dimensional time-of-flight magnetic resonance angiography at 1.5 Tesla to evaluate the intracranial arteries of 39 dogs with idiopathic epilepsy. Am J Vet Res 2019; 80:480–9.

[71] Martin-Vaquero P, da Costa RC, Echandi RL, et al. Time-of-flight magnetic resonance angiography of the canine brain at 3.0 Tesla and 7.0 Tesla. Am J Vet Res 2011;72:350–6.

[72] Sager M, Assheuer J, Trummler H, et al. Contrast-enhanced magnetic resonance angiography (CE-MRA) of intra- and extra-cranial vessels in dogs. Vet J 2009; 179:92–100.

[73] Delfaut EM, Beltran J, Johnson G, et al. Fat suppression in MR imaging: techniques and pitfalls. Radiographics 1999;19:373–82.

[74] D'Anjou MA, Carmel EN, Tidwell AS. Value of fat suppression in gadolinium-enhanced magnetic resonance neuroimaging. Vet Radiol Ultrasound 2011;52(1 Suppl 1):S85–90.

[75] Freeman AC, Platt SR, Kent M, et al. Magnetic resonance imaging enhancement of intervertebral disc disease in 30 dogs following chemical fat saturation. J Small Anim Pract 2012;53:120–5.

[76] Keenihan EK, Summers BA, David FH, et al. Canine meningeal disease: associations between magnetic resonance imaging signs and histologic findings. Vet Radiol Ultrasound 2013;54:504–15.

[77] Lamb CR, Lam R, Keenihan EK, et al. Appearance of the canine meninges in subtraction magnetic resonance images. Vet Radiol Ultrasound 2014;55:607–13.

[78] Packer RA, Rossmeisl JH, Kent MS, et al. Consensus recommendations on standardized magnetic resonance imaging protocols for multicenter canine brain tumor clinical trials. Vet Radiol Ultrasound 2018;59:796.

[79] Rusbridge C, Long S, Jovanovik J, et al. International Veterinary Epilepsy Task Force recommendations for a veterinary epilepsy-specific MRI protocol. BMC Vet Res 2015; 11:194. https://doi.org/10.1186/s12917-015-0466-x.

[80] Dennis R. Optimal magnetic resonance imaging of the spine. Vet Radiol Ultrasound 2011;52(1 Suppl 1): S72–80.

[81] Robertson I. Optimal magnetic resonance imaging of the brain. Vet Radiol Ultrasound 2011;52(1 Suppl 1): S15–22.

SECTION III: GASTROENTEROLOGY

Advances in Small Animal Care 3 (2022) 95–107

ADVANCES IN SMALL ANIMAL CARE

Modifying the Gut Microbiota – An Update on the Evidence for Dietary Interventions, Probiotics, and Fecal Microbiota Transplantation in Chronic Gastrointestinal Diseases of Dogs and Cats

Silke Salavati Schmitz, Dr med vet, Dipl ECVIM-CA, FHEA, PhD, FRCVS

Hospital for Small Animals, Royal (Dick) School of Veterinary Studies, College of Medicine and Veterinary Medicine, University of Edinburgh, Easter Bush, Midlothian EH25 9RG, United Kingdom

KEYWORDS

- Dogs • Cats • Synbiotics • Microbiome • Chronic enteropathy • Diarrhea • Transfaunation
- Inflammatory bowel disease

KEY POINTS

- Microbiota disturbance (dysbiosis) is not a feature of a specific disease, but can be seen with many conditions inside and outside of the gastrointestinal tract.
- Even though there is abundant evidence that dietary changes (including supplementation with dietary fiber and other prebiotics) lead to changes in the microbiota composition and richness in healthy dogs and cats, evidence in disease is more mixed.
- Data on the benefit of probiotics in acute and chronic GI diseases in dogs and cats are inconsistent, with some single strains and mixtures showing clinical as well as functional benefits, but overall, the number and quality of studies are low.
- FMT is a novel procedure with the aim to largely change or replace the existing intestinal microbiota, but its use (indication, application, success rates, complications) is largely unexplored in small animals.

INTRODUCTION

The gut microbiota, the trillions of microorganisms inhabiting the intestine, is a complex ecological system. Through its collective metabolic activities (eg, providing molecules for epithelial health) and interactions with the host (eg, via the mucosal immune system, or specific receptors that allow it to affect organ systems distant to the gastrointestinal tract [GIT]), it influences both normal physiology and disease susceptibility or maintenance.

The attempt of understanding these complex interplays with the goal of applying and developing therapies that target the microbiota is immense, particularly as in companion animals very little is yet known about individual variations, environmental influences, or temporal fluctuations in composition and changes during disease development.

In addition, microbial community composition based on next-generation sequencing (NGS) techniques alone does not necessarily provide an understanding of

---

E-mail address: Silke.Salavati@ed.ac.uk

https://doi.org/10.1016/j.yasa.2022.05.010
2666-450X/22/

microbiota function. While the existence of a "core microbiota composition" is questionable even in humans [1], "core microbiota functions" are likely to exist in both people and small animals, despite any divergence in composition or richness between individuals. Equally, many microbial genes might only be expressed under specific circumstances, that is, there might be functional variation with disease, diet, physiologic processes such as aging, drug administration, environmental exposures, or other factors that DNA sequencing studies overlook. While there is some data on this microbiota "resilience" (or lack thereof) in people [1], this has not been assessed in sufficient depth in dogs or cats.

The concept of "dysbiosis" (disturbance of microbiota homeostasis) is also generally loosely applied to a variety of situations (eg, the likely vastly flawed definition of Small Intestinal Bacterial Overgrowth [SIBO] based on fecal cultures [2]), while a true definition of it and how to best "diagnose" it in a clinical setting is lacking in small animal gastroenterology. This, and the fact that a plethora of different diseases within the GIT, acute or chronic, infectious and noninfectious, as well as diseases outside the GIT are associated with degrees of intestinal "dysbiosis," makes it difficult to use microbiota composition as a "marker" of any specific pathology. This calls the clinical usefulness of tools such as the dysbiosis index (DI) for both diagnosing specific GIT diseases and guiding treatment aimed at microbiota modification into question [3].

From a clinical perspective, approaches to modify the intestinal microbiota in dogs and cats can be divided into 3 main categories (Fig. 1). The first consists of dietary manipulations that change the macronutrient profile in a way that encourages the growth of specific (assumed beneficial) bacterial populations or their functions. This includes restricted or hydrolyzed protein sources, the addition of dietary fiber (DF), and other prebiotics. The second involves the administration of preselected live microorganisms (probiotics) with the aim to improve microbiota composition (eg, treating "dysbiosis") or function (eg, stimulating the mucosal immune system in "overgrowth" or infection or dampening it in conditions such as inflammatory bowel disease [IBD] or chronic enteropathy [CE]). Thirdly, bacteriotherapy or fecal microbiota transplantation (FMT), sometimes also called transfaunation, is an attempt to fully exchange a "dysbiotic" microbiota with a healthy one. This treatment has been performed in one way or another for its perceived health benefits in rather for people and animals for centuries [4]. However, its more stringent and scientifically guided

applications and benefits for specific conditions have only been explored recently, when it has initially been used to treat *Clostridium difficile* infection (CDI) in people [5]. It is one of the most novel and potentially exciting treatment options for several canine and feline GIT conditions, but knowledge about its most appropriate application is lacking, as are standardized protocols [6]. The following paragraphs will examine the evidence (or lack thereof) for these 3 ways to influence the small animal gut microbiota in more detail.

DIETARY MODIFICATIONS AND PREBIOTICS

There is ample scientific literature about the most appropriate composition of canine and feline feed, and it is generally accepted that changes to the microbiota occur quickly in response to dietary interventions [7], even though some studies suggest that a rather drastic food change is necessary to allow significant changes of bacterial phyla [8], and not every intervention results in a change of microbiota composition [9,10]. These differences in study results might be due to the types of diet chosen or variations in the resilience of the canine and feline microbiota to dietary change in health versus disease, but this has not been directly compared or futher examined. Food components that "bypass" the upper GIT as they are incompletely digested likely serve as the most significant nutrient source for the intestinal microbiota, and exert a certain selective pressure on their composition and function, namely *dietary fiber* (DF) and other *prebiotics*. The latter have traditionally been defined as "nondigestible food ingredients that beneficially affect the host by selectively stimulating the growth and/or activity of one or a limited number of bacterial species already established in the colon, and thus in effect improve host health" [11], but it is now understood that any substance available to the gut microbiota for fermentation, such as carbohydrates, protein, amino acids, fat, and polyphenols, can serve as a prebiotic [7].

Numerous studies have examined the impact of complex carbohydrates, selected DF, and prebiotics on the intestinal/fecal microbiota composition in healthy dogs, while far fewer studies have evaluated the effect of DF on the microbiota in cats [7]. The reader is referred to more detailed literature on this elsewhere.

As outlined in a recent review about dietary interventions in dogs with conditions such as CE, it is important to understand that not all DF is the same and that the benefits and side effects of fiber vary according to their

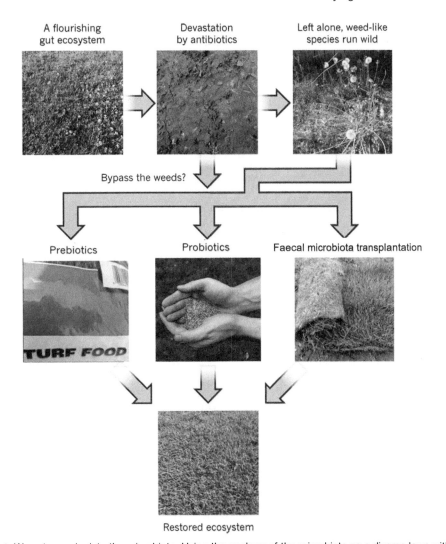

A flourishing gut ecosystem

Devastation by antibiotics

Left alone, weed-like species run wild

Bypass the weeds?

Prebiotics

TURF FOOD

Probiotics

Faecal microbiota transplantation

Restored ecosystem

FIG. 1 Ways to manipulate the microbiota. Using the analogy of the microbiota as a diverse lawn with different grasses, mosses, and herbs, dysbiosis or microbiota "devastation" can occur with disease (or with antibiotics), and if left untreated, unwanted "weeds" can grow. To either prevent or treat this dysbiosis, strategies include to "feed the lawn" (eg, to give prebiotics that will promote the growth of desirable species), to sow new lawn seed (eg, to administer probiotics that have known beneficial effects) or to roll out a completely new fully functional and diverse lawn (eg, to perform a fecal microbiota transplantation). All of these strategies could potentially lead to the restauration of the previously established ecosystem. (*Modified from* Lozupone CA, Stombaugh JI, Gordon JI, Jansson JK, Knight R. Diversity, stability and resilience of the human gut microbiota. *Nature.* 2012;489(7415):220-230.)

characteristics (Fig. 2) [12]. This wide range of benefits can include immune system stimulation, vitamin production, creation of an antiinflammatory environment, increased colonocyte absorptive capacity, reduction in toxic metabolites, improvement of intestinal barrier function, and healing (eg, via production of short-chain fatty acids [SCFAs]), but also slowed or accelerated GIT transit time, reduced nutrient absorption, increased gas production, and stool bulking [12].

Nutrition has the potential to affect disease conditions of the GIT directly through the provision of macro- and micronutrients, as well as indirectly by changing the microbiota. Dogs with CE have been shown to have lower concentrations and altered

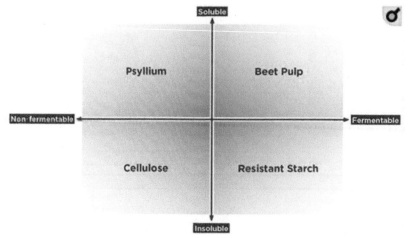

FIG. 2 Spectrum of solubility and fermentability of complex carbohydrates and fiber. Common fiber sources used in pet food, vary in their degree of solubility and fermentability (upper quadrants: more soluble; lower quadrants: less soluble; left quadrants: less fermentable; right quadrants: more fermentable). Examples are fibers that generally represent each combination of solubility and fermentability are named. (*From* Wernimont SM, Radosevich J, Jackson MI, et al. The Effects of Nutrition on the Gastrointestinal Microbiome of Cats and Dogs: Impact on Health and Disease. Front Microbiol. 2020;11:1266. Published 2020 Jun 25.)

patterns of SCFAs, while both dogs and cats with CE demonstrate significant fecal microbiota alterations compared to healthy controls [13]. In dogs, alpha diversity, which represents the number of taxonomic groups, is decreased, and beta diversity, which represents community similarity is significantly different from healthy dogs [14]. Alterations of intestinal microbiota composition in dogs with CE are similar to what is seen in people with IBD, namely an increase in Proteobacteria, especially the class of Gammaproteobacteria and within that the family of Enterobacteriaceae (including *Escherichia coli*), with a concurrent decrease in Firmicutes (including *Clostridia* and *Faecalibacterium*), Fusobacteria and Bacteroidetes (Fig. 3) [15,16].

Two studies found that dogs with food-responsive CE (FRE), as defined by clinical improvement on change in an elimination diet, experienced an alteration of the microbiota composition within the mucosal layer of the duodenum and colon, while another study showed a small increase in bacterial species (alpha) diversity, in response to a hydrolyzed diet, but no change in microbial composition (beta diversity) [10,17]. Another study, in which nearly 70% of dogs with CE were found to have FRE, demonstrated that remission of clinical signs was associated with an improvement in the composition of the microbiota as well as increased levels of secondary bile acids [18]. Those dogs who responded to the diet had a predominance of *Bilophila* and *Burkholderia* and enrichment in

Bacteriodes, while those that did not improve had a greater abundance of *Neisseriaceae*.

There are few studies investigating microbiota composition in cats with GI diseases. Similar to dogs, cats with IBD have increased numbers of *Enterobacteriaceaea*. Mucosally adherent *Clostridium* spp also correlates with intestinal inflammation. Luminal microbiota in feline IBD are characterized by decreased *Bifidobacteria* and increased *Desulfovibrio*, but the significance of this is unclear [19].

The impact of different types of DF on microbiota composition has mostly been evaluated in healthy dogs and cats [7]. One study assessing the effects of chondroitin sulfate and several prebiotics, including resistant starch, beta-glucan, and mannan-oligosaccharides in dogs with IBD as an additional treatment to dietary intervention showed no difference in clinical IBD activity or microbiome composition, while the histology severity score was significantly reduced in the supplement, but not the placebo group [20]. Further studies with different types of DF and prebiotics are required to assess their usefulness in managing CE in dogs and cats.

PROBIOTICS IN CANINE AND FELINE GASTROINTESTINAL DISEASE

The definition of *probiotics* as live microorganisms benefiting the host is originally derived from the

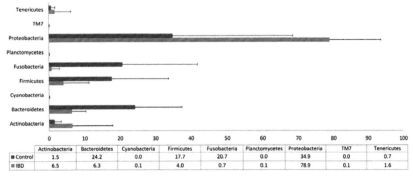

	Actinobacteria	Bacteroidetes	Cyanobacteria	Firmicutes	Fusobacteria	Planctomycetes	Proteobacteria	TM7	Tenericutes
■ Control	1.5	24.2	0.0	17.7	20.7	0.0	34.9	0.0	0.7
■ IBD	6.5	6.3	0.1	4.0	0.7	0.1	78.9	0.1	1.6

FIG. 3 Differences in microbiota composition in healthy dogs (*red*) and dogs with Inflammatory Bowel Disease (IBD) (*blue*). A significant increase in Proteobacteria and Actinobacteria with a concurrent decrease in Fusobacteria, Firmicutes, and Bacteroidetes can be observed. (*From* Suchodolski JS, Dowd SE, Wilke V, Steiner JM, Jergens AE. 16S rRNA gene pyrosequencing reveals bacterial dysbiosis in the duodenum of dogs with idiopathic inflammatory bowel disease. PLoS One. 2012;7(6):e39333.)

observation by Eli Metchnikoff at the beginning of the last century that specific bacteria and their metabolites could be harnessed to "replace" harmful microbes in the intestine [21]. This eventually resulted in the definition still used by the FAO/WHO today [22,23]. In addition, *synbiotics* are defined as mixtures of probiotics and prebiotics.[23].

Several mechanisms of probiotic action within the GI tract and the gut-associated immune system have been proposed (Fig. 4), including the displacement of intestinal pathogens, production of antimicrobial substances, and enhancement of immune responses, for example, promoting the proliferation of regulatory T-cells and associated tolerogenic cytokines [23]. However, very few of them have been confirmed to take place specifically in dogs or cats. Generally, peer-reviewed studies investigating *in vivo* use of pro- or synbiotics in the prevention or treatment of GI disease in dogs and cats are sparse, and have been summarized in recent reviews [23,24].

In animals with acute uncomplicated diarrhea, evidence of the effects of probiotics are contradictory, even when similar bacterial strains have been used. Beneficial effects reported include significantly shorter duration of diarrhea, possible prevention of mild diarrhea and better fecal scores (Table 1). In canine acute hemorrhagic diarrhea syndrome (AHDS), a commercial mixture of lactic acid bacteria (LAB) reduced clinical severity, and increased fecal amounts of *Faecalibacterium* spp., while reducing numbers of *Clostridium perfringens* and their enterotoxins. In infectious enteritis, probiotics give equally mixed results, with no effects observed on *Giardia* cyst or ancylostoma egg shedding, while a specific LAB mixture added to the standard treatment of

dogs with parvovirosis reduced mortality from 30% to 10% in one study (see Table 1) [23]. The addition of *Enterococcus faecium* (EF) reduced relapses of *Tritrichomonas blagburni* (previously *Tritrichomonas fetus*) infections in cats when given alongside ronidazole compared with placebo (Table 2) [25]. There are no other studies of probiotics in acute GI conditions in cats, apart from 2 studies assessing their effect on antibiotic-induced diarrhea in otherwise healthy cats, which showed that there was no difference in diarrhea occurrence or severity and that the pro- or synbiotics were unable to "rescue" the antibiotic-induced fecal dysbiosis [26,27].

The most commonly used probiotic in studies for CE in small animals is EF, but LAB mixtures have also been trialed. In canine immunosuppressive-responsive enteropathy (IRE), specific probiotics seem to be a promising adjunctive or possibly even sole treatment (see Table 2). One study administered the commercial "de Simone" LAB mixture (*L. plantarum* DSM24730, *Scc. thermophilus* DSM24731, *B. breve* DSM24732, *L.paracasei* DSM24733, *L. delbrueckii* subsp. *bulgaricus* DSM24734, *L. acidophilus* DSM24735, *B. longum* 120 DSM24736, *B. infantis* DSM24737) and demonstrated that it was not inferior to the control treatment (metronidazole + prednisolone) in inducing clinical remission [28]. In addition, only in probiotic-treated dogs an increase in tissue markers of a tolerogenic micro-environment (TGFß, FoxP3) was observed, but not in the control treatment group [28]. Probiotics also modulate intestinal epithelial permeability via the expression of tight junction proteins in dogs [28,29]. In another probiotic study, a small number of dogs with inflammatory protein-losing enteropathy

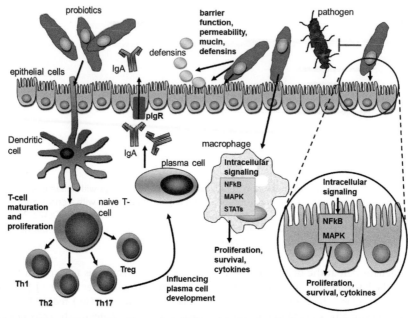

FIG. 4 Proposed mechanisms of actions of probiotics. Intestinal epithelial cells (IECs) are represented in green; the upper part of the panel shows the luminal side of the intestine with both probiotics/commensals and pathogens, and the lower panel shows the mucosal immune system in the lamina propria. Effects depicted include the stimulation of the innate (macrophages, dendritic cells) and adaptive (T-cells, plasma cells) immune system as well as interactions with the IECs themselves through intracellular signaling. IgA, immunoglobulin A; MAPK, MAP kinase; NFkB, nuclear factor-kappa B; STATs, signal transducer and activator of transcription; Treg, regulatory T-lymphocyte.

(PLE) was included, which showed a significant improvement in clinical severity (Canine Chronic Enteropathy Clinical Activity Index; CCECAI) and serum albumin values when given *Saccharomyces boulardii* as adjunctive treatment [30]. The only study assessing the use of probiotics in cats with chronic GI problems found evidence that the "Slab51" LAB mixture (*Scc. thermophilus* DSM32245, *L acidophilus* DSM32241, *L plantarum* DSM32244, *L. casei* DSM32243, *L.helveticus*, DSM32242, *L. brevis* DSM27961, *B. lactis* DSM32246, *B lactis* DSM32247) reduced clinical severity score of constipation (see Table 2). However, as the study population was small (n = 10) and not all cats had a confirmed diagnosis for the cause of constipation (only 3 cats with idiopathic megacolon were included), the results seem preliminary [31].

FECAL MICROBIOTA TRANSPLANTATION

Fecal microbiota transplantation (FMT) is the transfer of feces from a healthy donor into the gut of a recipient, with the goal of modulating or replacing the recipients'

entire microbiota (see Fig. 1) [6]. It is now an integral part of treating recurrent *C difficile* infection (CDI) in people [32] and investigated as a sole or ancillary treatment in a number of GI disorders in people (eg, Crohn's disease [33], ulcerative colitis [34], colorectal cancer [35]) as well as in disorders of other organ systems [36] with some promising but mixed results. In contrast, there are only few peer-reviewed studies describing the use of FMT in dogs or cats. Even though the beneficial effects of FMT on the intestinal microbiota composition or function have not been clearly identified, evidence is mounting that FMT can be possibly helpful in acute noninfectious diarrhea in dogs [6], as ancillary treatment in parvovirosis [37] as well as correcting antibiotic-induced dysbiosis [38] (Fig. 5). An increase in microbiota richness and a shift of the recipient's microbiota profile toward those more commonly associated with healthy animals are likely essential benefits in many acute GI diseases and are in line with what is seen in CDI in people. FMT is likely to create less favorable conditions for the growth of pathogens and create an improved

TABLE 1
Pro- or Synbiotics with an Effect in Acute and Infectious Gastrointestinal Conditions in Dogs (D) and Cats (C)

Pro- or Synbiotic Used	Dose	Animals (n)	Disorder	Observed Outcomes
B. animalis AHC7	1×10^{10} cfu BID	31 (D)	Acute idiopathic diarrhea	• Resolution of diarrhea in probiotic group 3.9 ± 2.3 d compared with placebo group (6.6 ± 2.7 d)
B. animalis AHC7	1×10^7 cfu/day to 1×10^9 cfu/day	121 (D)	Kennel-stress associated diarrhea	• Better fecal score for all probiotic groups compared with placebo at week 3 (not before)
E. faecium DSM 10663 NCIMB 10415 4 b/E1707 + FOS and gum arabic	2×10^9 cfu/day	399 treated, 374 placebo (D&C)	Shelter-associated diarrhea	• On synbiotic 2% have diarrhea vs 3% in placebo group • On synbiotic, 18.8% have >1 d of diarrhea vs 27.2% in placebo group
E. faecium DSM 10663 NCIMB 10415 4 b/E1707 + FOS and gum Arabic, kaolin, montmorillonite, pectin, alpha-glucan butyrogenic, patented mucopolysaccharide starch	n/a	13 ronidazole & placebo; 13 ronidazole & synbiotic (C)	Natural *Tritrichomonas fetus* infection	• Significantly less relapses (2/13) compared with placebo (8/13)
LAB mixture: L. *acidophilus*, *Pediococcus acidilactici*, *Bacillus subtilis*, *Bacillus licheniformis*, L. *farciminis*	n/a	15 treated, 21 placebo (D)	Acute gastroenteritis	• Days to last abnormal feces: probiotic 1.3 d (0.5–2.1 d); placebo 2.2 d (1.3–3.1 d)
LAB mixture: "de Simone[a]" formulation	4.5×10^{10} cfu/day	10 standard treatment alone, 10 standard treatment & probiotics (D)	Parvoviral enteritis	• Significant improvement in clinical scores between groups on day 3 and day 5
LAB mixture: "de Simone[a]" formulation	225×10^9 cfu for 1–10 kg dogs; 450×10^9 cfu for 10–20 kg dogs; 900×10^9 cfu for 20–40 kg dogs	13 treated, 12 control (D)	AHDS	• Lower clinical severity on day 3 and 4 in the probiotic group • Increased abundances of *Turicibacter* sp. and *Faecalibacterium* sp. on day • Lower abundance of *C. perfringens* on day 7 • Lower *C. perfringens* enterotoxins on day 7

Abbreviations: Cfu, colony-forming units; EF, *Enterococcus (E.) faecium*; FOS, fructo-oligosaccharides; LAB, lactic acid bacteria.

[a] The "de Simone" formulation was previously marketed as VSL#3, but is now available as Visbiome (US & Canada) or VivoMixx (Europe). More details can be found in Salavati, 2021 [23].

TABLE 2
Pro- or Synbiotics with an Effect in Chronic Gastrointestinal Conditions in Dogs (D) and Cats (C)

Pro- or synbiotic used	Dose	Animals (n)	Disorder	Observed outcome differences
E. faecium DSM 10663 NCIMB 10415 4 b/E1707 + FOS and gum Arabic	1×10^9 cfu/day	7 treated, 5 placebo (all on hydrolyzed protein diet) (D)	FRE	• Small increase in fecal microbiota diversity in dogs treated with synbiotic
L. acidophilus DSM13241	6×10^6 cfu/g dry food	6 (D)	Nonspecific dietary sensitivity	• Fecal dry matter higher during probiotic administration
LAB mixture: L. acidophilus NCC2628, L. acidophilus NCC2766, L. johnsonii NCC2767	1×10^{10} cfu/day	11 probiotic, 10 placebo (all on diet) (D)	FRE	• TNFα mRNA levels in colonic biopsies increased during placebo-treatment (but not LAB treatment)
Saccharomyces boulardii	1×10^{10} cfu/day	6 treated, 7 placebo (all on other treatments) (D)	IRE with or without PLE	• CCECAI improved significantly more in dogs receiving S boulardii compared with placebo on day 45 and day 60 • Stool frequency was significantly reduced in the S boulardii group on days 30, 45, and 60 • In the subgroup of PLE dogs, serum albumin was >2 g/dL in 3/3 dogs in the treatment and 2/3 dogs in the placebo group
LAB mixture: "de Simone[a]" formulation	112–225 $\times 10^9$ cfu/10 kg BW/day	10 treated, 10 control (D)	IRE	• clinical improvement was faster with control treatment (range 2.5–7 d) compared with probiotic (range 5–15 d) • TGFβ expression increased more in the probiotic group • FoxP3+ cells increased only in the probiotic group

LAB mixture: SLAB51 blend	2×10^{11} cfu lyophilized bacteria per 5 kg body weight	10 (C)	Chronic constipation (7/10)/idiopathic megacolon (3/10)	• *Faecalibacterium* spp. increased only in the probiotic group • Clinical severity score significantly reduced at end of probiotic treatment • Number of ICC increased significantly • Significant increase in fecal streptococci and lactobacilli after treatment (of total of 9 analyzed taxa)
LAB mixture "de Simone"[a] formulation	$112–225 \times 10^{9}$ cfu/10 kg BW/day	14 treated, 12 placebo (all on standard treatment) (D)	IRE	• Total number of mucosal bacteria increased in probiotic group • Increased *Lactobacillus* spp., decreased *Bifidobacteria* spp. • Intestinal tight junction proteins up-regulated

More details can be found in Salavati, 2021 [23].

Abbreviations: BW, body weight; CCECAI, canine chronic enteropathy clinical activity index; CE, chronic enteropathy; cfu, colony-forming units; CIBDAI, canine inflammatory bowel disease activity index; EF, *Enterococcus* (*E.*) *faecium*; FISH, fluorescent in situ hybridization; FOS, fructo-oligosaccharides; FRE, food-responsive chronic enteropathy; IEC, intestinal epithelial cells; IHC, immunohistochemistry; IL, interleukin; IRE, immunosuppressive-responsive enteropathy; LAB, lactic acid bacteria; TGFβ, transforming growth factor-beta; TNFα, tumour-necrosis factor-alpha.

[a] The "de Simone" formulation was marketed under the trade name VSL#3 until 2016. Since then, the composition of VLS#3 has changed and the "de Simone" blend is available under the trade name of Visbiome in the US & Canada and VivoMixx in Europe.

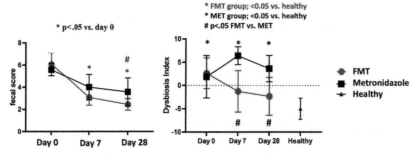

FIG. 5 Fecal scores and dysbiosis index (DI) in dogs with acute diarrhea treated with either FMT as a single enema or with metronidazole for 7 days. A lower fecal score indicates a more normal stool consistency. Left panel: In both groups, a significant decrease in fecal scores was observed o day 7, and fecal scores were significantly lower in the FMT group compared with metronidazole group on day 28. Right panel: Dogs after FMT showed a significant decrease (= improvement) in DI, which were no longer different from healthy dogs on day 7 and 28, while dogs treated with metronidazole retained a high DI that was different from healthy dogs at both timepoints. (*Modified from* Chaitman J, Ziese AL, Pilla R, et al. Fecal Microbial and Metabolic Profiles in Dogs With Acute Diarrhea Receiving Either Fecal Microbiota Transplantation or Oral Metronidazole. Front Vet Sci. 2020;7:192. Published 2020 Apr 16.)

microenvironment, not only by the sheer change in composition, but by transferring additional "postbiotic" components (like butyrate, which can induce regulatory T-cells and antiinflammatory cytokines), mucins, bacteriocins and secondary bile acid (or bacteria with the capacity to transform primary into secondary bile acids), as well as possible bacteriophages from the donor [6].

Unfortunately, the available evidence is less compelling in dogs with CE, possibly in line with variable responses to FMT in human IBD [33]. Another factor is likely a large variety of different protocols used for administering FMT in dogs, ranging from endoscopic delivery, oral routes, or rectally via enema. When dogs with either Giardia infection or CE were given a single FMT via enema, they responded within 1 week, but long-term follow-up is lacking. In another study 16 dogs with refractory CE, and CCECAI improved at 1 and 3 months after endoscopic & oral FMT delivery combined. In the author's experience, responses of dogs with CE that failed dietary or antibiotic treatment trials, responses can be very mixed and are most often short-lived (several weeks). Other very recent data support this observation and suggest that dogs with a relatively quick resolution of dysbiosis after a single FMT are more likely to have a favorable long-term response [39]. Remaining data on FMT in dogs with chronic intestinal diseases consist of case reports or case series [6]. A recent survey has revealed that there is a lack of consensus among veterinary practitioners and specialists not only about the indications for FMT in dogs but also about the most appropriate way of

administering FMT, with a vast number of different protocols reported [40]. There is a clear need for guidelines on the use and practicalities of FMT in small animals, which will in turn allow prospective studies to be more comparable and deliver much-needed information on how to optimize all aspects of this potentially revolutionary treatment modality for both dogs and cats: from donor selection and screening, optimal recipient-donor "matching," to route, "dose" and frequency of administration and the appropriate assessment of treatment "success."

SUMMARY

With the intestinal microbiota being linked to an increasing number of conditions inside and outside of the GIT in people as well as in small animals, microbiota manipulation is an exciting treatment opportunity, both as definitive as well as an adjunctive therapy. However, how drastic or targeted any potential treatment addressing microbiota "dysbiosis" needs to be to be deemed successful, and how this relates to the underlying condition addressed (eg, is the temporary introduction of a small shift via pre or probiotic sufficient? Is FMT in an attempt to cause major microbiota changes required? Are long-term treatments of the microbiota needed?), remains unknown. The questions on how to identify the ideal combination of host factors, intervention goals and characteristics, microbiota compositional or functional targets, and how to achieve them, remain unanswered, as the matter is complex and studies specific to small animals are too few to make generalized recommendations. In addition, practical considerations (dose, duration of treatment, outcome measures to be assessed) in any of these contexts remain undefined. Even though many prescription diets, DF, pro, or synbiotics are available for use in small animals and are well embedded into small animal veterinary practice, many of them do not strictly fulfill the criteria required for their evidence-based use. On the contrary, much of their use remains empirical, and their specific effects and mechanisms of action still remain to be elucidated. Unfortunately, studies on probiotics in both acute and chronic GI conditions suffer from significant limitations; for example, lack of control group, ill-defined disease phenotypes, and inappropriate and nonspecific inclusion criteria. In addition, the wide range of different potential probiotics used at different dosages and in various conditions as well as a huge discrepancy in measured outcomes is problematic and does not allow comparisons. Preliminary evidence suggests that certain pro or synbiotics could be beneficial in acute or infectious GI conditions, namely parvovirus infection and AHDS, while little benefit was observed with adjunctive administration of probiotics to dogs with FRE [10,41,42] or tylosin-responsive diarrhea [43]. In IRE, specific probiotic strains (*S boulardii* [30]) or mixtures ("de Simone" formulation [28,29]) can reduce clinical severity as well as induce a more tolerogenic microenvironment and improved permeability of the intestinal mucosa.

FMT is likely a more "complete" and hence possibly more effective way to alter or exchange the intestinal microbiota, but the indications for its use are even less clear. The risk to cause harm is potentially higher with FMT than with DF or probiotic supplements, as evidenced by serious health alerts issued in 2020 in the face of infections with pathogenic *E. coli* in 6 people after FMT, 4 of which required hospitalization and 2 of which subsequently died[a]. No such side effects have been observed in animals [40], even though this could be due to underreporting, and needs to be reassessed once this becomes a more common procedure in small animals.

Despite the limitations of available information, preliminary evidence is emerging that FMT is possibly more beneficial (and with an immediate visible and measurable effect) when administered as adjunctive treatment to animals with infectious GIT disease or antibiotic-induced diarrhea/dysbiosis. Even in dogs and cats with chronic conditions, there may be a benefit of FMT, but this likely requires careful donor and recipient selection and characterization, and the monitoring of effects that go beyond simple visible clinical outcomes (eg, improvement or resolution of diarrhea), but concentrate on "deep remission" as defined by the molecular resolution of dysbiosis and microscopic resolution of inflammation (tissue remission).

CONCLUSION

Well-designed studies evaluating the potential benefit of dietary interventions including DF, pre-, pro, and synbiotics as well as FMT to achieve desired microbiota-related outcomes in small animals are needed. These studies should be designed to include animals with well-defined clinical phenotypes, have sufficient statistical power, and should focus on assessing outcomes that go beyond clinical parameters. Elucidating mechanisms of action and assessing microbiota-related targets that can further the understanding of interactions between the commensal or dysbiotic microbiota and macro- and micronutrients as well as administered live microorganisms (probiotics or FMT) will drive rational and evidence-based clinical use of these modalities and inform new treatments recommendations in the future.

CLINICS CARE POINTS

- while dietary interventions are still important in a lot of gastrointestinal conditions, their impact on the intestinal microbiota is less clear and somewhat variable
- knowledge and evidence about the best use of pre- and probiotics in a clinical setting is still limited in small animals
- probiotics cannot be used interchangeably, as they are likely specific to individual hosts and conditions
- FMT is an emerging treatment modality for acute and chronic gastrointestinal conditions in dogs and cats, but protocols for its most appropriate use are lacking

---

[a]U.S. Food & Drug Administration Fecal Microbiota for Transplantation: Safety Alert – Risk of Serious Adverse Events Likely Due to Transmission of Pathogenic Organisms. Issued 3/12/2020, updated 04/07/2020. Available on: https://edin.ac/34Fjkhr.

DISCLOSURE

The author declares no conflict of interest. This article was not supported by any third parties.

REFERENCES

[1] Lozupone CA, Stombaugh JI, Gordon JI, et al. Diversity, stability and resilience of the human gut microbiota. Nature 2012;489(7415):220–30.

[2] German AJ, Day MJ, Ruaux CG, et al. Comparison of Direct and Indirect Tests for Small Intestinal Bacterial Overgrowth and Antibiotic-Responsive Diarrhea in Dogs. J Vet Intern Med 2003;17(1):33–43.

[3] AlShawaqfeh MK, Wajid B, Minamoto Y, et al. A dysbiosis index to assess microbial changes in fecal samples of dogs with chronic inflammatory enteropathy. FEMS Microbiol Ecol 2017;93(11). https://doi.org/10.1093/FEMSEC/FIX136.

[4] Neyen C. Foundational Article: Mechnikov I, 1909: Intestinal Bacteriotherapy. J Leukoc Biol 2021;109(3):519–33.

[5] Brandt LJ, Reddy SS. Fecal microbiota transplantation for recurrent Clostridium difficile infection. J Clin Gastroenterol 2011;45(SUPPL. 3). https://doi.org/10.1097/MCG.0B013E318222E603.

[6] Chaitman J, Gaschen F. Fecal Microbiota Transplantation in Dogs. Vet Clin Small Anim Pract 2021;51(1):219–33.

[7] Wernimont SM, Radosevich J, Jackson MI, et al. The Effects of Nutrition on the Gastrointestinal Microbiome of Cats and Dogs: Impact on Health and Disease. Front Microbiol 2020;11. https://doi.org/10.3389/FMICB.2020.01266.

[8] Herstad KMV, Gajardo K, Bakke AM, et al. A diet change from dry food to beef induces reversible changes on the faecal microbiota in healthy, adult client-owned dogs. BMC Vet Res 2017;13(1):1–13.

[9] Bresciani F, Minamoto Y, Suchodolski JS, et al. Effect of an extruded animal protein-free diet on fecal microbiota of dogs with food-responsive enteropathy. J Vet Intern Med 2018;32(6):1903–10.

[10] Pilla R, Guard BC, Steiner JM, et al. Administration of a synbiotic containing enterococcus faecium does not significantly alter fecal microbiota richness or diversity in dogs with and without food-responsive chronic enteropathy. Front Vet Sci 2019;6(AUG). https://doi.org/10.3389/fvets.2019.00277.

[11] Gibson GR, Roberfroid MB. Dietary modulation of the human colonic microbiota: introducing the concept of prebiotics. J Nutr 1995;125(6):1401–12.

[12] Tolbert MK, Murphy M, Gaylord L, et al. Dietary management of chronic enteropathy in dogs. J Small Anim Pract 2022. https://doi.org/10.1111/JSAP.13471.

[13] Minamoto Y, Minamoto T, Isaiah A, et al. Fecal short-chain fatty acid concentrations and dysbiosis in dogs with chronic enteropathy. J Vet Intern Med 2019;33(4):1608–18.

[14] Hashimoto-Hill S, Alenghat T. Inflammation-Associated Microbiota Composition Across Domestic Animals. Front Genet 2021;12. https://doi.org/10.3389/FGENE.2021.649599/PDF.

[15] Suchodolski JS, Dowd SE, Wilke V, et al. 16S rRNA gene pyrosequencing reveals bacterial dysbiosis in the duodenum of dogs with idiopathic inflammatory bowel disease. PLoS One 2012;7(6):e39333.

[16] Vázquez-Baeza Y, Hyde ER, Suchodolski JS, et al. Dog and human inflammatory bowel disease rely on overlapping yet distinct dysbiosis networks. Nat Microbiol 2016;1. https://doi.org/10.1038/NMICROBIOL.2016.177.

[17] Marchesi MC, Timpano CC, Buschian S, et al. The role of diet in managing inflamatory bowel disease affected dogs: a retrospective cohort study on 76 cases. Vet Ital 2017;53(4):297–302.

[18] Wang S, Martins R, Sullivan MC, et al. Diet-induced remission in chronic enteropathy is associated with altered microbial community structure and synthesis of secondary bile acids. Microbiome 2019;7(1). https://doi.org/10.1186/S40168-019-0740-4.

[19] Ziese AL, Suchodolski JS. Impact of Changes in Gastrointestinal Microbiota in Canine and Feline Digestive Diseases | Elsevier Enhanced Reader. Vet Clin North Am Small Anim Pract 2021;51:155–69.

[20] Segarra S, Martínez-Subiela S, Cerdà-Cuéllar M, et al. Oral chondroitin sulfate and prebiotics for the treatment of canine Inflammatory Bowel Disease: a randomized, controlled clinical trial. BMC Vet Res 2016;12(1). https://doi.org/10.1186/S12917-016-0676-X.

[21] Metchnikoff E. Lactic acid as inhibiting intestinal putrefaction. In: Heinemann W, editor. The Prolongation of Life; Optimistic Studies. London: Heinemann; 1907. p. 161–83.

[22] FAO/WHO. Probiotics in food - Report of a Joint FAO/WHO Expert Consultation on Evaluation of Health and Nutritional Properties of Probiotics in Food inlcuding Powder Milk with Live Lactic Acid Bacteria - Cordoba, Argentina, 1-4 October 2001. Published online 2006. doi:ISBN 92-5-105513-0.

[23] Salavati Schmitz S. Value of Probiotics in Canine and Feline Gastroenterology. Vet Clin North Am Small Anim Pract 2021;51(1):171–217.

[24] Jensen AP, Bjørnvad CR. Clinical effect of probiotics in prevention or treatment of gastrointestinal disease in dogs: A systematic review. J Vet Intern Med 2019;33(5):1849–64.

[25] Lalor S, Gunn-Moore D. Effects of concurrent ronidazole and probiotic therapy in cats with Tritrichomonas foetus-associated diarrhoea. J Feline Med Surg 2012;14(9):650–8.

[26] Whittemore JC, Stokes JE, Price JM, et al. Effects of a synbiotic on the fecal microbiome and metabolomic profiles of healthy research cats administered clindamycin: a randomized, controlled trial. Gut Microbes 2019;10(4):521–39.

[27] Torres-Henderson C, Summers S, Suchodolski J, et al. Effect of Enterococcus Faecium Strain SF68 on Gastrointestinal Signs and Fecal Microbiome in Cats Administered Amoxicillin-Clavulanate. Top Companion Anim Med 2017;32(3):104–8.

[28] Rossi G, Pengo G, Caldin M, et al. Comparison of microbiological, histological, and immunomodulatory

parameters in response to treatment with either combination therapy with prednisone and metronidazole or probiotic VSL#3 strains in dogs with idiopathic inflammatory bowel disease. PLoS One 2014;9(4). https://doi.org/10.1371/journal.pone.0094699.

[29] White R, Atherly T, Guard B, et al. Randomized, controlled trial evaluating the effect of multi-strain probiotic on the mucosal microbiota in canine idiopathic inflammatory bowel disease. Gut Microbes 2017;8(5):451–66.

[30] Angelo SD', Fracassi F, Bresciani F, et al. Effect of Saccharomyces boulardii in dogs with chronic enteropathies: double-blinded, placebo-controlled study. Vet Rec 2018;182(9):258.

[31] Rossi G, Jergens A, Cerquetella M, et al. Effects of a probiotic (SLAB51™) on clinical and histologic variables and microbiota of cats with chronic constipation/megacolon: A pilot study. Benef Microbes 2018;9(1):101–10.

[32] Waller KMJ, Leong RW, Paramsothy S. An update on fecal microbiota transplantation for the treatment of gastrointestinal diseases. J Gastroenterol Hepatol 2021. https://doi.org/10.1111/JGH.15731.

[33] Tan P, Li X, Shen J, et al. Fecal Microbiota Transplantation for the Treatment of Inflammatory Bowel Disease: An Update. Front Pharmacol 2020;11:1409.

[34] Blanchaert C, Strubbe B, Peeters H. Fecal microbiota transplantation in ulcerative colitis. Acta Gastroenterol Belg 2019;82(4):519–28.

[35] Park R, Umar S, Kasi A. Immunotherapy in Colorectal Cancer: Potential of Fecal Transplant and Microbiota-Augmented Clinical Trials. Curr Colorectal Cancer Rep 2020;16(4):81–8.

[36] Zhou Y, Xu H, Huang H, et al. Are There Potential Applications of Fecal Microbiota Transplantation beyond Intestinal Disorders? Biomed Res Int 2019;2019:3469754.

[37] Pereira GQ, Gomes LA, Santos IS, et al. Fecal microbiota transplantation in puppies with canine parvovirus infection. J Vet Intern Med 2018;32(2):707–11.

[38] Chaitman J, Ziese AL, Pilla R, et al. Fecal Microbial and Metabolic Profiles in Dogs With Acute Diarrhea Receiving Either Fecal Microbiota Transplantation or Oral Metronidazole. Front Vet Sci 2020;7(April 16):192.

[39] Toresson L, Steiner JM, Spillmann T, Lidbury JA, Ludvigsson U, Suchodolski JS. Clinical effects of fecal microbiota transplantation in dogs with chronic enteropathies. Uniwersytet śląski. doi:10.2/JQUERY.MIN.JS.

[40] Salavati Schmitz S. Observational study of small animal practitioners' awareness, clinical practice and experience with faecal microbiota transplantation in dogs. Top Companion Anim Med 2022;100630. https://doi.org/10.1016/J.TCAM.2022.100630.

[41] Schmitz S, Glanemann B, Garden OA, et al. A Prospective, Randomized, Blinded, Placebo-Controlled Pilot Study on the Effect of Enterococcus faecium on Clinical Activity and Intestinal Gene Expression in Canine Food-Responsive Chronic Enteropathy. J Vet Intern Med 2015;29:533–43.

[42] Sauter SN, Benyacoub J, Allenspach K, et al. Effects of probiotic bacteria in dogs with food responsive diarrhoea treated with an elimination diet. J Anim Physiol Anim Nutr (Berl) 2006;90(7–8):269–77.

[43] Westermarck E, Skrzypczak T, Harmoinen J, et al. Tylosin-Responsive Chronic Diarrhea in Dogs. J Vet Intern Med 2005;19(2):177–86.

Advances in Small Animal Care 3 (2022) 109–119

ADVANCES IN SMALL ANIMAL CARE

Nutrition in Canine and Feline Gastrointestinal Disease

Aarti Kathrani, BVetMed (Hons), PhD, FHEA, MRCVS
Royal Veterinary College, Hawkshead Lane, Hatfield, Hertfordshire AL9 7TA, United Kingdom

---

KEYWORDS

• Diet • Food • Enteropathy • Lymphangiectasia • Fat • Hydrolyzed • Constipation • Fiber

KEY POINTS

- Nutritional assessment allows determination of the animal's nutritional status, to help identify malnutrition, as well as allow for monitoring of any changes to this status.
- Nutritional assessment involves assessment of the animal, diet, feeding strategy, environment, and reassessment and monitoring once the chosen dietary strategy has been implemented.
- Nutrition has many positive effects on the gastrointestinal (GI) tract and is therefore important in the management of various canine and feline GI diseases.
- Several GI diseases such as acute gastroenteritis, GI adverse reaction to food, chronic inflammatory enteropathy, and constipation benefit from specific nutritional strategies.

INTRODUCTION

Nutritional assessment is considered the fifth vital sign, after the assessment of temperature, pulse, respiration, and pain [1]. The objectives of nutritional assessment are to ascertain the animal's nutritional status and identify malnutrition, which then allows for monitoring of any changes to this status. Malnutrition is defined by the World Health Organization as a deficiency, excess, or imbalance in a person's intake of energy and/or nutrients. Malnutrition can develop quickly even in adequately nourished dogs and cats. In dogs and cats with gastrointestinal (GI) disease, the following may serve as risk factors for malnutrition:

- Severity and length of the GI disease
- Impaired digestion and absorption of nutrients due to the GI disease
- Comorbidities
- Complications from the GI disease and associated treatment
- An incomplete and unbalanced diet

Adequate nutritional support can preserve lean body mass, reverse the maladaptive metabolic response to injury, maintain organ function, and decrease morbidity [2]. Therefore, nutritional assessment should be performed in all dogs and cats to help identify and address any deficiencies. Nutritional assessment involves assessment of the animal, the diet, the feeding strategy and the environment [3], as well as reassessment and monitoring once the chosen dietary strategy is implemented.

Nutrition has many direct beneficial effects on the different functions of the GI tract. Certain nutritional strategies can [4]

- Beneficially affect the intestinal microbiota
- Modulate the intestinal mucosal immune system
- Regulate gene expression and epigenetics
- Promote intestinal epithelial barrier function
- Normalize GI motility

E-mail address: akathrani@rvc.ac.uk

https://doi.org/10.1016/j.yasa.2022.05.004
2666-450X/22/

Therefore, diet plays a central role in the therapeutic intervention of dogs and cats with different GI diseases.

SIGNIFICANCE
Principles of Nutritional Management of Canine and Feline Gastrointestinal Diseases
Assessment of the nutritional status of the patient

Assessing body weight, as well as trends, is not only important for nutritional assessment but also may provide prognostic information. Weight loss should be quantified as mild (less than 5% of body weight loss), moderate (5%–10% of body weight loss), or severe (more than 10% of body weight loss) to help determine the severity of the loss [5,6].

Examination of the following is important to assess the overall nutritional health of the animal [3]:
- Animal's stature
- Body condition
- Muscle condition
- Hair coat and foot pads
- Ocular system
- Cardiovascular system
- Neurologic system
- Orthopedic system

In addition, dental examination should be performed to assess for any disease. Assessment for poor wound healing is important, because this may be an indication of inadequate nutritional intake [7].

Assessment of body condition score (BCS) should be performed using a standardized scoring system. The World Small Animal Veterinary Association (WSAVA) Global Nutrition Committee recommends use of the 9-point scale for assessment, which is based on characterization of body silhouette and palpation of body fat.

Unlike the assessment of BCS, there is currently no standardized scoring system for muscle mass in dogs and cats. Assessment of muscle condition can be performed subjectively by using the 4-point scale recommended by the WSAVA Global Nutrition Committee or by assessing the muscle mass as adequate or mild, moderate, or severe loss together with the location and distribution of this loss.

Unfortunately, there are currently no laboratory tests available to definitively determine the nutritional status of dogs or cats. However, a minimum database consisting of a complete blood cell count, serum biochemistry and urinalysis, and serum cobalamin and folate in dogs and cats with chronic GI signs will likely help to provide a gross overview of the nutritional status of the patient.

Assessment of diet, feeding plan, and the environment

A complete and thorough diet history will help to determine if the animal is consuming sufficient energy and nutrients, as well as the need for dietary intervention. The diet history should encompass all foods that the animal is eating, and this includes all
- Commercial pet foods
- Commercial treats
- Human foods
- Dietary supplements
- Foods used to administer medications

The manufacturer, brand, dry or tinned formula, and flavor should be specified for all of the aforementioned where applicable.

Feeding of smaller meals more frequently throughout the day is advantageous in GI disease to prevent overloading of the GI tract. If the animal has an ideal BCS, then the number of daily calories that were previously fed can be continued. If the animal is underconditioned, then the daily number of calories should be increased by 10% increments, to account for any malassimilation from the GI disease until an ideal condition is reached.

Diet may act as a significant environmental risk factor in susceptible animals with chronic inflammatory enteropathy. Therefore, an assessment of the diet just before or at the onset of chronic GI signs is important to identify any potential dietary triggers, which can then be avoided.

Reassessment and monitoring

Reassessment and monitoring are important after any new diet has been implemented to ensure compliance and evaluate the effects, as well as to determine if any adjustments to the feeding plan are needed. The owner should regularly assess the animal's body weight and BCS to ensure an ideal body condition is maintained or achieved with the new diet, appetite and food intake, overall appearance and activity, as well as GI signs.

Possible explanations for failure to respond favorably to the new diet include:
- The need for a different dietary strategy to control the GI signs
- The need for medication in addition to diet to control the signs
- Owner noncompliance with feeding
- Interconcurrent diseases, such as pancreatitis or hepatic disease
- Misdiagnosis of the underlying GI condition

Nutritional Strategies for Canine and Feline Gastrointestinal Diseases

Acute gastroenteritis

Unfortunately, studies determining the ideal dietary composition for animals with acute gastroenteritis are currently lacking. However, the following nutritional strategies are likely beneficial for this condition: high digestibility, low fat, or high dietary fiber. These strategies can be implemented using either a commercial therapeutic diet or a complete and balanced home-prepared diet formulated by a board-certified veterinary nutritionist. Probiotics may also be beneficial in the therapy for acute gastroenteritis.

Acute gastroenteritis may compromise the digestion and absorption of nutrients, therefore diets with high digestibility may be beneficial for these cases. Also, because diets with high digestibility produce fewer residues in the GI tract, this can help to lessen overloading of the gut and subsequent osmotic diarrhea.

The digestibility of a diet, which is usually expressed as a percentage, refers to the degree to which food or macronutrients present in the diet is digested and absorbed by the GI tract. However, because digestibility is impacted by many factors, this is not a constant value. The following factors can impact digestibility:

- Ingredients used in the diet
- The processing of the diet; for example, heat processing generally increases the digestibility of starch but decreases the digestibility of protein
- Animal factors, such as breed, age, GI health, and physiologic status
- The amount of food fed

The size of the dog has been shown to have an effect on digestion, with larger breed dogs typically displaying lower digestibility of food compared with smaller breed dogs [8]. Age also impacts digestibility, with approximately 20% of cats older than 12 years having decreased protein digestibility [9]. Although there are no absolute criteria that define a highly digestible diet, a diet with a total digestibility of at least 80% and digestibility of macronutrients of at least 90% are considered to meet this criterion.

High dietary fat can have adverse effects on the GI tract, such as delayed gastric emptying, colonic dysbiosis, increased intestinal permeability, and detrimental effects on the GI mucosal immune response in genetically susceptible individuals [10–12]. In animals with acute gastroenteritis leading to nausea, regurgitation, or vomiting, feeding a diet with low fat may help to improve these clinical signs due to hastened gastric transit. In addition, in those animals in which acute gastroenteritis leads to reduced fat digestion and absorption, increased passage of the undigested fat into the colon may result in dysbiosis, as well as secretory diarrhea [10,12], and therefore these animals are likely to also benefit from a low-fat diet.

Dietary fibers are mainly plant-based carbohydrates, which can neither be digested by mammalian enzymes nor absorbed by their GI tract [13]. Their advantageous effects are numerous and include the following [14,15]:

- Modifying gastric emptying by altering the viscosity of ingesta
- Normalizing intestinal motility
- Optimizing intestinal mucosal barrier function
- Homeostasis within the colon via the generation of short-chain fatty acids, which have anti-inflammatory effects
- Buffering of toxins
- Binding excess water
- Promoting the growth of beneficial bacteria

Owing to these advantageous effects, animals with acute gastroenteritis with exclusively or predominantly large intestinal signs may benefit from a high-fiber diet. However, because not all animals with large intestinal signs may respond favorably to high dietary fiber, trial and error with this approach may be needed and should be prioritized for those cases with large intestinal signs that do not respond to a highly digestible diet, and especially before the use of empirical antimicrobials.

Several studies investigating probiotics in dogs and cats with acute gastroenteritis have shown beneficial effects:

- A randomized double-blinded single-center study showed that a probiotic cocktail significantly decreased the mean number of days of abnormal stool from 2.2 days to 1.3 days in dogs with acute self-limiting gastroenteritis [16].
- A double-blinded placebo-controlled study showed that a canine-specific probiotic had a normalizing effect on stool consistency in dogs with acute or intermittent diarrhea [17].
- The probiotic *Bifidobacterium animalis* strain AHCS (IAMS Veterinary Formula Prostora) was able to significantly reduce the time to resolution of acute idiopathic diarrhea in dogs, as well as decrease the percentage of dogs that were administered metronidazole compared with dogs receiving placebo [18].
- *Lactobacillus murinus* LbP2 was shown to improve stool consistency as well as appetite in dogs with distemper-associated diarrhea [19].
- Probiotic treatment with Visbiome was shown to accelerate the normalization of the intestinal microbiome in dogs with acute hemorrhagic diarrhea [20].

- A specific antidiarrheal probiotic paste was shown to significantly shorten the duration of diarrhea and the rate of resolution of diarrhea in dogs with acute uncomplicated diarrhea compared with placebo [21].
- Cats with acute diarrhea in an animal rescue center were shown to benefit from *Enterococcus faecium* SF68 probiotic (Purina Pro Plan Veterinary Diets FortiFlora Nutritional Supplement) by having fewer episodes of diarrhea for 2 or more days when compared with controls [22].

Although these studies suggest that probiotics may be beneficial for dogs and cats with acute gastroenteritis, the effects are likely strain specific, and therefore the efficacy and safety of each, particularly in younger or immunocompromised animals, should be investigated in larger scale studies.

Food should be offered as soon as possible to dogs and cats with acute gastroenteritis, once they have been appropriately stabilized and rehydrated. Feedings should be initiated at 25% of the calculated resting energy requirement (RER; $70 \times BW$ (kg)$^{0.75}$) split into multiple meals throughout the day to help with gastric emptying and intestinal motility. Vomiting has been shown to be an adverse effect of enteral nutrition in the initial phase in dogs with hemorrhagic gastroenteritis [23]. Therefore, if the animal demonstrates intolerance to the food initially, food should be withheld for as short a time as possible, and then offered again at a reduced amount of 10% to 15% of RER. If the animal tolerates 25% of RER, then this should be slowly increased by 25% increments daily until 100% of RER is reached on day 4. A slow transition to 100% of RER over 4 days will help to prevent overloading of the GI tract and therefore worsening of signs, as well as allow for the assessment of tolerance to the new diet. Feeding more than 100% of RER per day should be avoided in hospital to prevent complications associated with overfeeding [24].

The regular diet can be slowly reintroduced over the next 7 to 10 days, once the GI signs have fully resolved. The daily number of calories that was previously fed can be continued if the animal is at an ideal body condition.

Adverse reaction to food

Gastrointestinal adverse reaction to food (GI ARF) includes conditions with a wide range of causes, such as toxic and nontoxic [25]. The nontoxic causes include non–immune-mediated and immune-mediated causes, with the non–immune-mediated causes comprising enzymatic and pharmacologic causes (dietary intolerance) and the immune-mediated causes mainly including diseases with an IgE-mediated, non-IgE-mediated, or mixed IgE- and non-IgE-mediated cause (food allergy or food hypersensitivity).

Unfortunately, the diagnosis of food allergy or food hypersensitivity in dogs and cats is challenging, because currently there are no laboratory tests commercially available that allow for a definitive diagnosis [26]. As such, the gold-standard diagnostic test currently remains an exclusion diet trial with provocation testing [26]. However, provocation testing is commonly not performed due to low owner compliance, and therefore, the definitive diagnosis of food allergy or food hypersensitivity remains tentative in most cases.

Commercial therapeutic hydrolyzed diets may be effective for food allergy or food hypersensitivity [27], because they contain proteins that are considered small enough to theoretically avoid a type 1 IgE-mediated hypersensitivity, by preventing cross-linking of 2 IgE antibody receptors on a mast cell. However, because it is unknown what proportion of dogs and cats with GI food allergy or food hypersensitivity have a type 1 IgE-mediated hypersensitivity, some dogs and cats with this condition may fail to respond adequately to these diets. This fact was demonstrated in one study, in which a significant proportion (21%) of dogs sensitized to the intact protein still reacted adversely to the hydrolyzed diet [28]. Therefore, persistent GI signs may be anticipated with hydrolyzed diets, particularly in dogs and cats with a non-IgE-mediated cause for their food allergy or food hypersensitivity. If the dog or cat's GI signs do not adequately respond to feeding with a hydrolyzed diet, then a limited-ingredient novel protein diet, either commercially or home prepared, should be trialed.

Limited-ingredient novel protein diets may be beneficial for cases of GI food allergy or food hypersensitivity in dogs and cats, because the animal has not been previously sensitized to the novel proteins. A comprehensive antigen exposure list compiled from the ingredients of all currently and previously fed diets, including treats, snacks, and table foods, is needed to ascertain which ingredients would be truly novel for the animal. Over-the-counter diets that claim to contain novel ingredients should be avoided, due to the concern for contamination with commonly fed antigens [29].

Some dogs and cats may experience an allergy or hypersensitivity to an antigen that was unmasked or developed during the commercialization process of the dry or canned pet food. In this scenario, the dog or cat may be intolerant to any commercial pet foods, whether over the counter or therapeutic. Therefore, a home-prepared diet would be needed to help diagnose and manage these cases.

For those dogs and cats with suspected food allergy or food hypersensitivity, a strict exclusion diet trial should be performed for at least 8 to 12 weeks, especially if dermatologic signs are concurrently present. After this time, a provocation challenge with the original diet or single ingredients would be needed to confirm the culpable source. Unfortunately, because this is not frequently performed, the diagnosis of food allergy or food hypersensitivity remains tentative in most cases. However, some cases of food intolerance may also relapse with provocation testing and therefore may not be specific for a diagnosis of food allergy or food hypersensitivity.

Chronic inflammatory enteropathy

Chronic inflammatory enteropathy in dogs and cats is commonly subclassified retrospectively depending on the response to specific treatment [30]. For example, food-responsive enteropathy (FRE) includes those cases of chronic inflammatory enteropathy that respond favorably to dietary treatment alone [30]. Studies have shown that FRE comprises approximately two-thirds of dogs presenting with chronic inflammatory enteropathy in a secondary to tertiary referral population [6,31]. Although the underlying cause of FRE is unknown, chronic inflammatory enteropathy is hypothesized to involve the variable interplay of 4 key components; genetic susceptibility, environmental risk factor, intestinal dysbiosis, and altered GI mucosal immune response [32].

Diet can have many beneficial effects on the GI tract, including on the intestinal microbiota, mucosal immune response, GI permeability and motility, mucosal healing, and gene expression [4]. Therefore, humans with inflammatory bowel disease (IBD) can attain remission with dietary treatment alone [33,34]. It is also hypothesized that diet may act as a significant environmental risk factor in some dogs and cats with chronic inflammatory enteropathy, and therefore removal of this trigger may also help to resolve the GI signs.

Dogs and cats with GI food allergy can present with similar signs as those with FRE, making the clinical distinction between the 2 conditions difficult. However, because studies have shown that intestinal histopathology pretreatment and posttreatment with a successful diet trial in dogs with FRE does not change [6,35], this suggests that the pathogenesis of FRE and food allergy is different. Nevertheless, because the differentiation of FRE from GI food allergy in dogs and cats is not definitively possible at this time, studies assessing diet in animals with chronic inflammatory enteropathy may have included cases with GI food allergy or intolerance. Therefore, dietary strategies recommended or used for GI food allergy may also be applicable for some dogs and cats with suspected FRE. Further studies are needed to help distinguish between FRE, GI food allergy, and GI food intolerance in dogs and cats to help guide optimal dietary management for each condition.

Because the cause of FRE in dogs and cats is unknown, the different dietary strategies discussed in the following paragraphs should be trialed to determine the most effective and before this condition is definitively ruled out. Although owners may find it frustrating to trial different dietary strategies, studies have shown that most dogs and cats with FRE respond quickly, within 1 to 2 weeks, suggesting that these diets do not need to be fed longer term to determine their clinical response [6,36–38].

Commercial therapeutic GI diets can be effective for control of idiopathic chronic GI signs in cats [39,40]. Because these diets have increased digestibility, less protein may present intact to the immune system, which may be dysregulated in chronic inflammatory enteropathy. Conversely, for dogs with chronic inflammatory enteropathy, one study showed that although a therapeutic GI diet was able to induce remission, these dogs were less likely to remain asymptomatic at subsequent rechecks when compared with dogs managed with a hydrolyzed diet [41]. Therefore, further studies comparing therapeutic GI diets with hydrolyzed diets are needed in both dogs and cats to determine the subset of animals with chronic inflammatory enteropathy that are most likely to respond to these diets.

Therapeutic hydrolyzed diets have been shown to be effective in the management of chronic inflammatory enteropathy in both dogs and cats [31,36,41–44], with some studies reporting a positive response in two-third of animals [41,42,45]. Hydrolyzed diets may use the following dietary strategies, which could be beneficial for chronic inflammatory enteropathy in dogs and cats:

- *Hydrolyzed protein:* may help to correct the dysregulated mucosal immune response.
- *Increased digestibility:* as chronic enteropathy may compromise the digestion and absorption of nutrients, diets with high digestibility may be beneficial.
- *Lower fat content:* may be beneficial for some animals with GI disease, due to increased gastric transit and reduced passage of fat into the colon.
- *Soy and/or omega 3 fatty acids:* these ingredients are known to be immunomodulatory.

- *Vegetarian formula*: a study in humans showed that a semivegetarian diet was highly effective for maintaining remission in patients with IBD [46].
- *Gluten-free formula*: a gluten-free diet has been shown to improve clinical symptoms in humans with IBD [47].

Nearly 50% of cats and 60% of dogs with chronic GI signs responded to a novel protein diet [38,48]. One study showed no difference in response rate between hydrolyzed and limited ingredient novel protein diets for dogs with chronic enteropathy [31]. Because some therapeutic limited-ingredient novel protein diets have higher total dietary fiber, these formulas may be additionally beneficial for those cases with large intestinal signs, especially if a highly digestible diet did not help to improve the GI signs. As one study showed the presence of other common food antigens in over-the-counter novel protein diets, these diets should be avoided for the management of chronic inflammatory enteropathy [29].

The following handful of studies has demonstrated the effectiveness of high-fiber diets in dogs and cats with chronic large intestinal signs:

- One retrospective study showed that treatment with a commercial therapeutic highly digestible diet supplemented with soluble fiber resulted in a very good to excellent response in most dogs with chronic idiopathic large bowel diarrhea [49].
- One study with 19 dogs with chronic colitis that had failed a low-fat diet responded to a fiber-supplemented diet, and maintenance could be achieved without the concurrent need for other medications [50].
- One study assessing the effects of chondroitin sulfate and several prebiotics including resistant starch, beta-glucan, and mannooligosaccharides in 27 dogs with IBD showed that the histologic score of dogs that received the supplement together with a hydrolyzed diet decreased by 1.53-fold [51].
- One study documented that the combination of a high-fiber diet and a probiotic mixture in 30 dogs with chronic colitis that were unresponsive to various dietary and pharmacologic interventions was able to induce remission of clinical signs in a mean of 8.5 days [52].
- One study demonstrated positive response to diets high in fiber or supplemented with fiber in cats with colitis [53].

Low-fat diets may be beneficial for GI disease, because dogs and cats with GI disease may experience reduced fat digestion and absorption in the small intestine, which may cause increased passage of fat into the colon, potentially resulting in dysbiosis and secretory diarrhea [11,12]. Therefore, trialing a low-fat diet may be effective in these cases. However, dietary fat did not seem to affect the outcome of cats with chronic diarrhea [54], therefore dietary fat may be less of a concern in cats with chronic inflammatory enteropathy. High-fat diets may also increase the mRNA expression of the innate immune receptors, nucleotide oligomerization domain (NOD) 2, and toll-like receptor (TLR) 5 in rodent models of IBD [10]. Nucleotide oligomerization domain 2 and TLR 5 have been implicated in the pathogenesis of canine chronic enteropathy [55–59]. Therefore, those dogs with a dysregulated intestinal mucosal immune response due to these receptors may benefit from a low-fat diet; however, studies are needed to definitively assess this. Low-fat diets may also be beneficial for those dogs with chronic inflammatory enteropathy leading to secondary lymphangiectasia (please see Intestinal Lymphangiectasia section for more details).

Certain emulsifiers and preservatives can have negative effects on the intestinal microbiota and GI mucosal immune system in rodent gene knockout models of IBD [60–62]. Therefore, some canine and feline chronic inflammatory enteropathy cases, due to their underlying genetic susceptibility, may not be able to tolerate commercial foods, due to these additives, and may need a home-prepared diet for resolution of their GI signs. Home-prepared diets must be formulated under the guidance of a board-certified veterinary nutritionist to ensure they are complete and balanced for long-term feeding.

Unfortunately, only a handful of studies have assessed the efficacy of probiotics in canine chronic enteropathy:

- Two studies assessed the effect of a synbiotic containing *E faecium* in dogs with FRE and failed to show a difference in clinical efficacy, histology scores, expression of intestinal genes, and fecal microbiota richness and density compared with the placebo group [63,64].
- Two studies assessing the effect of VSL#3/Visbiome showed an increase in regulatory T-cell markers and upregulated expression of tight junction proteins in dogs with chronic enteropathy compared with standard treatment [65,66].
- One study showed that *Saccharomyces boulardii* significantly improved clinical activity index, stool frequency and consistency, and BCS in dogs with chronic enteropathy compared with placebo [67].

A slow transition to the new diet should be performed over 7 to 10 days, after which time the diet should be fed exclusively, to allow assessment of the chosen dietary strategy. Most dogs and cats with FRE can be transitioned back to their original diet without showing signs of relapse. In one study, 21% of dogs and in another study, 29% of cats with GI signs relapsed following challenge [6,38]. These cases may have been food allergic, although at this time it is not possible to distinguish food allergy, intolerance, or FRE.

Intestinal lymphangiectasia

Intestinal lymphangiectasia (IL) may be primary or secondary. The main therapeutic strategies for IL include:
- Treatment of the underlying cause if identified.
- Decreased dietary fat intake to decrease chylomicron production, which decreases lymph flow and pressure, and therefore may prevent lacteal dilation, rupture, and leakage.
- Decreased dietary intake of long-chain triglycerides (LCT), which may have proinflammatory effects and therefore, may cause lipogranulomas.
- Glucocorticoids may be used in IL to reduce intestinal inflammation. However, 1 small retrospective study in Yorkshire terriers with IL showed that some dogs could respond satisfactorily in the short-term to a low-fat diet alone [68]. Another study documented that dietary fat restriction could be used as an effective treatment in dogs with IL that were unresponsive to prednisolone or experienced a relapse with dose reduction [69].
- Medium-chain triglycerides (MCT) are used in humans with IL, because they are directly absorbed into the portal vein. However, in dogs MCT are still absorbed into the lymphatic system and therefore may not help to reduce lymph flow [70]. Nevertheless, in an animal model of ileitis, MCT were shown to modulate intestinal inflammation and cause less damage than LCT [71], and therefore their use may help to reduce inflammation in canine IL.

Despite, there being no consensus for the definition of low fat, veterinary nutritionists generally consider less than 20% fat on a metabolizable energy basis to be suitably low. The following commercial therapeutic diets are available that meet this criterion: Royal Canin Veterinary Diet Canine GI Low Fat, Hill's Prescription Diet Canine i/d Low Fat, and Purina Pro Plan Veterinary Diets EN Gastroenteric Low Fat Canine. If an ultra-low-fat diet is required (considered to be <15% fat on a metabolizable energy basis) then consultation with a board-certified veterinary nutritionist is recommended for formulation of a balanced home-prepared diet.

The low-fat diet should be introduced slowly over 7 to 10 days. If a commercial therapeutic low-fat diet does not help to improve GI signs or serum biochemical parameters, then a balanced home-prepared diet formulated by a board-certified veterinary nutritionist to reduce dietary fat further should be considered.

Feline constipation

Constipation is a common clinical problem in cats, in which it may lead to obstipation, necessitating medical intervention. Dietary recommendations vary depending on the extent of colonic motility remaining:
- Feline obstipation:
  - The motility patterns of the large intestine are completely absent, and therefore, a commercial therapeutic GI diet with high digestibility and therefore low residue and high caloric density should be fed to markedly reduce fecal output.
  - Diets with increased fiber content and supplements containing fiber should be avoided in these cats, because they may worsen their GI signs, because all colonic motility has been abolished in these cats.
  - Cats with obstipation should have cleansing enemas, with or without mechanical removal of impacted feces before dietary changes are introduced.
- Feline constipation:
  - Where some level of colonic motility is suspected to remain, insoluble or a mix of insoluble and soluble fiber may help to improve the GI signs.
  - Insoluble fibers provide fecal bulk, which helps to improve colonic motility by causing distension of the colon.
  - Soluble fibers are generally fermentable in the large intestine resulting in the production of short-chain fatty acids, which have several beneficial effects on the colonocytes and colonic motility, as well as increasing fecal water content [72].
  - Cats with constipation should be well hydrated before a high-fiber diet is initiated.

Psyllium is a soluble fiber with low fermentability but is able to form a gel when mixed with water. One uncontrolled trial in cats with constipation showed that a commercial psyllium-enriched dry diet was able to improve stool quality and clinical outcome in more than 80% cats within a week of starting the diet [73].

Feeding multiple small meals throughout the day should be encouraged, because this may help to improve colonic motility and reduce the amount of ingesta entering the colon at each feeding. A tailored weight loss program should be considered for over-weight and obese cats. Ensuring adequate hydration following discharge from the hospital is also important.

PRESENT RELEVANCE AND FUTURE AVENUES TO CONSIDER OR TO INVESTIGATE

Nutrition plays an important role in the management of various canine and feline GI diseases. An understanding of the different dietary strategies available for these different diseases will help to ensure that the most appropriate diet is selected. However, trial and error may be needed to ensure optimization for each disease in the individual animal. Future studies should focus on additional dietary strategies that may be efficacious for the different GI diseases and defining which specific subpopulations within these different conditions are most likely to benefit from these.

SUMMARY/DISCUSSION

- Nutritional assessment is considered the fifth vital sign, after the assessment of temperature, pulse, respiration, and pain.
- Nutritional assessment allows determination of the animal's nutritional status, which helps to identify malnutrition, as well as allow for monitoring of any changes to this status.
- Nutritional assessment involves assessment of the animal, diet, feeding strategy, environment, and re-assessment and monitoring once the chosen dietary strategy has been implemented.
- Nutrition has many direct beneficial effects on the GI tract and is therefore important in the management of various canine and feline GI diseases.
- Nutritional management of acute gastroenteritis in dogs and cats includes consideration of the effects of digestibility, fat, and fiber of the diet, as well as the use of probiotics.
- The diagnosis and management of food allergy or food hypersensitivity in dogs and cats can be achieved with the use of a commercial therapeutic hydrolyzed diet, commercial therapeutic limited-ingredient novel protein diet, or a complete and balanced limited-ingredient novel protein home-prepared diet, formulated by a board-certified veterinary nutritionist.
- Nutritional management of FRE in dogs and cats involves trial and error to determine the most effective dietary strategy. The following category of diets is commonly used for the management of this condition: commercial therapeutic GI diets, commercial therapeutic hydrolyzed diets, commercial therapeutic limited-ingredient novel protein diets, and complete and balanced home-prepared diets. Selection of differing amounts of dietary fat and fiber within these categories of diets can be trialed to determine the most efficacious for the individual animal.

- The main dietary strategy for IL involves decreased fat, because this helps to decrease chylomicron production, which decreases lymph flow and pressure, and therefore may prevent lacteal dilation, rupture, and leakage. Decreased dietary intake of long-chain triglycerides is also important, due to their proinflammatory effects, which may cause lipogranulomas.

- Dietary management is crucial in the treatment of feline constipation, with different recommendations depending on the level of colonic motility remaining. For those cats presenting with constipation that still have some level of colonic motility remaining, insoluble or a mix of insoluble and soluble fiber is recommended. In cats presenting with obstipation, a highly digestible, low-residue diet with a high caloric density is recommended to markedly reduce fecal output.

CLINICS CARE POINTS

- *Nutritional assessment:* Nutritional assessment of dogs and cats with GI disease is paramount to identify if intervention is needed. Adequate nutritional support can preserve lean body mass, reverse the maladaptive metabolic response to injury, maintain organ function, and decrease morbidity.

- *Acute gastroenteritis:* Food should be offered as soon as possible to dogs and cats with acute gastroenteritis, once they have been appropriately stabilized and rehydrated.

- *Adverse reaction to food:* Not all dogs and cats with suspected food allergy or food hypersensitivity will respond to a hydrolyzed diet. Therefore, a commercial therapeutic or home-prepared limited-ingredient novel protein diet should be trialed before definitively ruling out this condition.

- *FRE:* Studies have shown that most dogs and cats with FRE respond quickly to diet, within 1 to 2 weeks, suggesting that these diets do not need to be fed longer term to determine their clinical response.

- *IL:* Dietary fat restriction or further restriction should be considered in those cases of IL that are unresponsive to prednisolone or experience a relapse with dose reduction.
- *Feline constipation:* Determining if a cat is constipated versus obstipated is important, because the 2 conditions have different dietary fiber recommendations.

REFERENCES

[1] Members WNAGTF, Freeman L, Becvarova I, et al. WSAVA Nutritional Assessment Guidelines. J Small Anim Pract 2011;52:385–96.

[2] Schulman RC, Mechanick JI. Metabolic and nutrition support in the chronic critical illness syndrome. Respir Care 2012;57:958–77 [discussion: 977–8].

[3] Baldwin K, Bartges J, Buffington T, et al. AAHA nutritional assessment guidelines for dogs and cats. J Am Anim Hosp Assoc 2010;46:285–96.

[4] Kathrani A. Dietary and Nutritional Approaches to the Management of Chronic Enteropathy in Dogs and Cats. Vet Clin North Am Small Anim Pract 2021;51:123–36.

[5] Jergens AE, Crandell JM, Evans R, et al. A clinical index for disease activity in cats with chronic enteropathy. J Vet Intern Med 2010;24:1027–33.

[6] Allenspach K, Wieland B, Grone A, et al. Chronic enteropathies in dogs: evaluation of risk factors for negative outcome. J Vet Intern Med 2007;21:700–8.

[7] Crane SW. Nutritional aspects of wound healing. Semin Vet Med Surg Small Anim 1989;4:263–7.

[8] Zentek J, Meyer H. Normal handling of diets–are all dogs created equal? J Small Anim Pract 1995;36:354–9.

[9] Laflamme DP. Nutrition for aging cats and dogs and the importance of body condition. Vet Clin North Am Small Anim Pract 2005;35:713–42.

[10] Martinez-Medina M, Denizot J, Dreux N, et al. Western diet induces dysbiosis with increased E coli in CEA-BAC10 mice, alters host barrier function favouring AIEC colonisation. Gut 2014;63:116–24.

[11] Ramakrishna BS, Mathan M, Mathan VI. Alteration of colonic absorption by long-chain unsaturated fatty acids. Influence of hydroxylation and degree of unsaturation. Scand J Gastroenterol 1994;29:54–8.

[12] Devkota S, Wang Y, Musch MW, et al. Dietary-fat-induced taurocholic acid promotes pathobiont expansion and colitis in Il10-/- mice. Nature 2012;487:104–8.

[13] Jones JM. CODEX-aligned dietary fiber definitions help to bridge the 'fiber gap. Nutr J 2014;13:34.

[14] Furusawa Y, Obata Y, Fukuda S, et al. Commensal microbe-derived butyrate induces the differentiation of colonic regulatory T cells. Nature 2013;504:446–50.

[15] Wang H, Shi P, Zuo L, et al. Dietary Non-digestible Polysaccharides Ameliorate Intestinal Epithelial Barrier Dysfunction in IL-10 Knockout Mice. J Crohns Colitis 2016;10:1076–86.

[16] Herstad HK, Nesheim BB, L'Abee-Lund T, et al. Effects of a probiotic intervention in acute canine gastroenteritis–a controlled clinical trial. J Small Anim Pract 2010;51:34–8.

[17] Gomez-Gallego C, Junnila J, Mannikko S, et al. A canine-specific probiotic product in treating acute or intermittent diarrhea in dogs: A double-blind placebo-controlled efficacy study. Vet Microbiol 2016;197:122–8.

[18] Kelley RL, Minikhiem D, Kiely B, et al. Clinical benefits of probiotic canine-derived Bifidobacterium animalis strain AHC7 in dogs with acute idiopathic diarrhea. Vet Ther 2009;10:121–30.

[19] Delucchi L, Fraga M, Zunino P. Effect of the probiotic Lactobacillus murinus LbP2 on clinical parameters of dogs with distemper-associated diarrhea. Can J Vet Res 2017;81:118–21.

[20] Ziese AL, Suchodolski JS, Hartmann K, et al. Effect of probiotic treatment on the clinical course, intestinal microbiome, and toxigenic Clostridium perfringens in dogs with acute hemorrhagic diarrhea. PLoS One 2018;13: e0204691.

[21] Nixon SL, Rose L, Muller AT. Efficacy of an orally administered anti-diarrheal probiotic paste (Pro-Kolin Advanced) in dogs with acute diarrhea: A randomized, placebo-controlled, double-blinded clinical study. J Vet Intern Med 2019;33:1286–94.

[22] Bybee SN, Scorza AV, Lappin MR. Effect of the probiotic Enterococcus faecium SF68 on presence of diarrhea in cats and dogs housed in an animal shelter. J Vet Intern Med 2011;25:856–60.

[23] Will K, Nolte I, Zentek J. Early enteral nutrition in young dogs suffering from haemorrhagic gastroenteritis. J Vet Med A Physiol Pathol Clin Med 2005;52:371–6.

[24] Chan DL, Freeman LM. Nutrition in critical illness. Vet Clin North Am Small Anim Pract 2006;36:1225–41, v-vi.

[25] Pasqui F, Poli C, Colecchia A, et al. Adverse Food Reaction and Functional Gastrointestinal Disorders: Role of the Dietetic Approach. J Gastrointestin Liver Dis 2015; 24:319–27.

[26] Mueller RS, Olivry T. Critically appraised topic on adverse food reactions of companion animals (4): can we diagnose adverse food reactions in dogs and cats with in vivo or in vitro tests? BMC Vet Res 2017;13:275.

[27] Cave NJ. Hydrolysed protein diets for dogs and cats. Vet Clin North Am Small Anim Pract 2006;36:1251–68, vi.

[28] Jackson HA, Jackson MW, Coblentz L, et al. Evaluation of the clinical and allergen specific serum immunoglobulin E responses to oral challenge with cornstarch, corn, soy and a soy hydrolysate diet in dogs with spontaneous food allergy. Vet Dermatol 2003;14:181–7.

[29] Raditic DM, Remillard RL, Tater KC. ELISA testing for common food antigens in four dry dog foods used in dietary elimination trials. J Anim Physiol Anim Nutr (Berl) 2011;95:90–7.

[30] Gaschen FP, Merchant SR. Adverse food reactions in dogs and cats. Vet Clin North Am Small Anim Pract 2011;41: 361–79.

[31] Allenspach K, Culverwell C, Chan D. Long-term outcome in dogs with chronic enteropathies: 203 cases. Vet Rec 2016;178:368.

[32] de Souza HSP, Fiocchi C, Iliopoulos D. The IBD interactome: an integrated view of aetiology, pathogenesis and therapy. Nat Rev Gastroenterol Hepatol 2017;14:739–49.

[33] Borrelli O, Cordischi L, Cirulli M, et al. Polymeric diet alone versus corticosteroids in the treatment of active pediatric Crohn's disease: a randomized controlled open-label trial. Clin Gastroenterol Hepatol 2006;4. 744–53.

[34] Heuschkel RB, Menache CC, Megerian JT, et al. Enteral nutrition and corticosteroids in the treatment of acute Crohn's disease in children. J Pediatr Gastroenterol Nutr 2000;31:8–15.

[35] Schreiner NM, Gaschen F, Grone A, et al. Clinical signs, histology, and CD3-positive cells before and after treatment of dogs with chronic enteropathies. J Vet Intern Med/Am Coll Vet Intern Med 2008;22:1079–83.

[36] Walker D, Knuchel-Takano A, McCutchan A, et al. A comprehensive pathological survey of duodenal biopsies from dogs with diet-responsive chronic enteropathy. J Vet Intern Med 2013;27:862–74.

[37] Schmitz S, Glanemann B, Garden OA, et al. A prospective, randomized, blinded, placebo-controlled pilot study on the effect of Enterococcus faecium on clinical activity and intestinal gene expression in canine food-responsive chronic enteropathy. J Vet Intern Med 2015;29:533–43.

[38] Guilford WG, Jones BR, Markwell PJ, et al. Food sensitivity in cats with chronic idiopathic gastrointestinal problems. J Vet Intern Med 2001;15:7–13.

[39] Perea SC, Marks SL, Daristotle L, et al. Evaluation of Two Dry Commercial Therapeutic Diets for the Management of Feline Chronic Gastroenteropathy. Front Vet Sci 2017;4:69.

[40] Laflamme DP, Xu H, Cupp CJ, et al. Evaluation of canned therapeutic diets for the management of cats with naturally occurring chronic diarrhea. J Feline Med Surg 2012;14:669–77.

[41] Mandigers PJ, Biourge V, van den Ingh TS, et al. A randomized, open-label, positively-controlled field trial of a hydrolysed protein diet in dogs with chronic small bowel enteropathy. J Vet Intern Med 2010;24: 1350–7.

[42] Marks SL, Laflamme DP, McAloose D. Dietary trial using a commercial hypoallergenic diet containing hydrolysed protein for dogs with inflammatory bowel disease. Vet Ther 2002;3:109–18.

[43] Mandigers PJ, Biourge V, German AJ. Efficacy of a commercial hydrolysate diet in eight cats suffering from inflammatory bowel disease or adverse reaction to food. Tijdschr Diergeneeskd 2010;135:668–72.

[44] Wang S, Martins R, Sullivan MC, et al. Diet-induced remission in chronic enteropathy is associated with altered microbial community structure and synthesis of secondary bile acids. Microbiome 2019;7:126.

[45] Kathrani A, Church DB, Brodbelt DC, et al. The use of hydrolysed diets for vomiting and/or diarrhoea in cats in primary veterinary practice. J Small Anim Pract 2020; 61:723–31.

[46] Chiba M, Abe T, Tsuda H, et al. Lifestyle-related disease in Crohn's disease: relapse prevention by a semi-vegetarian diet. World J Gastroenterol 2010;16: 2484–95.

[47] Herfarth HH, Martin CF, Sandler RS, et al. Prevalence of a gluten-free diet and improvement of clinical symptoms in patients with inflammatory bowel diseases. Inflamm Bowel Dis 2014;20:1194–7.

[48] Luckschander N, Allenspach K, Hall J, et al. Perinuclear antineutrophilic cytoplasmic antibody and response to treatment in diarrheic dogs with food responsive disease or inflammatory bowel disease. J Vet Intern Med 2006; 20:221–7.

[49] Leib MS. Treatment of chronic idiopathic large-bowel diarrhea in dogs with a highly digestible diet and soluble fiber: a retrospective review of 37 cases. J Vet Intern Med 2000;14:27–32.

[50] Lecoindre P, Gaschen FP. Chronic idiopathic large bowel diarrhea in the dog. Vet Clin North Am Small Anim Pract 2011;41:447–56.

[51] Segarra S, Martinez-Subiela S, Cerda-Cuellar M, et al. Oral chondroitin sulfate and prebiotics for the treatment of canine Inflammatory Bowel Disease: a randomized, controlled clinical trial. BMC Vet Res 2016;12:49.

[52] Rossi G, Cerquetella M, Gavazza A, et al. Rapid Resolution of Large Bowel Diarrhea after the Administration of a Combination of a High-Fiber Diet and a Probiotic Mixture in 30 Dogs. Vet Sci 2020;7.

[53] Dennis JS, Kruger JM, Mullaney TP. Lymphocytic/plasmacytic colitis in cats: 14 cases (1985-1990). J Am Vet Med Assoc 1993;202:313–8.

[54] Laflamme DP, Xu H, Long GM. Effect of diets differing in fat content on chronic diarrhea in cats. J Vet Intern Med 2011;25:230–5.

[55] Kathrani A, Lee H, White C, et al. Association between nucleotide oligomerisation domain two (Nod2) gene polymorphisms and canine inflammatory bowel disease. Vet Immunol Immunopathol 2014;161:32–41.

[56] Kathrani A, House A, Catchpole B, et al. Polymorphisms in the TLR4 and TLR5 gene are significantly associated with inflammatory bowel disease in German shepherd dogs. PLoS One 2010;5:e15740.

[57] Kathrani A, Holder A, Catchpole B, et al. TLR5 risk-associated haplotype for canine inflammatory bowel disease confers hyper-responsiveness to flagellin. PLoS One 2012;7:e30117.

[58] Swerdlow MP, Kennedy DR, Kennedy JS, et al. Expression and function of TLR2, TLR4, and Nod2 in primary canine colonic epithelial cells. Vet Immunol Immunopathol 2006;114:313–9.

[59] Allenspach K, House A, Smith K, et al. Evaluation of mucosal bacteria and histopathology, clinical disease activity and expression of Toll-like receptors in German

shepherd dogs with chronic enteropathies. Vet Microbiol 2010;146:326–35.

[60] Chassaing B, Koren O, Goodrich JK, et al. Dietary emulsifiers impact the mouse gut microbiota promoting colitis and metabolic syndrome. Nature 2015;519:92–6.

[61] Shang Q, Sun W, Shan X, et al. Carrageenan-induced colitis is associated with decreased population of anti-inflammatory bacterium, Akkermansia muciniphila, in the gut microbiota of C57BL/6J mice. Toxicol Lett 2017;279:87–95.

[62] Watt J, Marcus R. Carrageenan-induced ulceration of the large intestine in the guinea pig. Gut 1971;12:164–71.

[63] Schmitz S, Henrich M, Neiger R, et al. Stimulation of duodenal biopsies and whole blood from dogs with food-responsive chronic enteropathy and healthy dogs with Toll-like receptor ligands and probiotic Enterococcus faecium. Scand J Immunol 2014;80:85–94.

[64] Pilla R, Guard BC, Steiner JM, et al. Administration of a Synbiotic Containing Enterococcus faecium Does Not Significantly Alter Fecal Microbiota Richness or Diversity in Dogs With and Without Food-Responsive Chronic Enteropathy. Front Vet Sci 2019;6:277.

[65] Rossi G, Pengo G, Caldin M, et al. Comparison of microbiological, histological, and immunomodulatory parameters in response to treatment with either combination therapy with prednisone and metronidazole or probiotic VSL#3 strains in dogs with idiopathic inflammatory bowel disease. PLoS One 2014;9:e94699.

[66] White R, Atherly T, Guard B, et al. Randomized, controlled trial evaluating the effect of multi-strain probiotic on the mucosal microbiota in canine idiopathic inflammatory bowel disease. Gut Microbes 2017;8:451–66.

[67] D'Angelo S, Fracassi F, Bresciani F, et al. Effect of Saccharomyces boulardii in dog with chronic enteropathies: double-blinded, placebo-controlled study. Vet Rec 2018;182:258.

[68] Rudinsky AJ, Howard JP, Bishop MA, et al. Dietary management of presumptive protein-losing enteropathy in Yorkshire terriers. J small Anim Pract 2017;58:103–8.

[69] Okanishi H, Yoshioka R, Kagawa Y, et al. The clinical efficacy of dietary fat restriction in treatment of dogs with intestinal lymphangiectasia. J Vet Intern Med 2014;28:809–17.

[70] Jensen GL, McGarvey N, Taraszewski R, et al. Lymphatic absorption of enterally fed structured triacylglycerol vs physical mix in a canine model. Am J Clin Nutr 1994;60:518–24.

[71] Tsujikawa T, Ohta N, Nakamura T, et al. Medium-chain triglycerides modulate ileitis induced by trinitrobenzene sulfonic acid. J Gastroenterol Hepatol 1999;14:1166–72.

[72] Jha R, Fouhse JM, Tiwari UP, et al. Dietary Fiber and Intestinal Health of Monogastric Animals. Front Vet Sci 2019;6:48.

[73] Freiche V, Houston D, Weese H, et al. Uncontrolled study assessing the impact of a psyllium-enriched extruded dry diet on faecal consistency in cats with constipation. J Feline Med Surg 2011;13:903–11.

Advances in Small Animal Care 3 (2022) 121–131

ADVANCES IN SMALL ANIMAL CARE

Challenges in Differentiating Chronic Enteropathy from Low-Grade Gastrointestinal T-cell Lymphoma in Cats

Julien Dandrieux, BSc, Dr med vet, PhD, DACVIM(SAIM)[a,*], Valérie Freiche, Dr med vet, PhD, DESV-IM[b]

[a]U-Vet, Faculty of Veterinary and Agricultural Sciences, University of Melbourne, 250 Princes Highway, Werribee, Victoria 3030, Australia;
[b]Ecole Nationale Vétérinaire d'Alfort, CHUVA, Unité de Médecine Interne, Maisons-Alfort, F-94700, France

---

KEYWORDS

- Feline • Inflammatory bowel disease • Low-grade intestinal T-cell lymphoma • Histology
- Immunohistochemistry • PCR for antigen receptor rearrangements

KEY POINTS

- Low-grade gastrointestinal T-cell lymphoma (LGITL) and chronic enteropathy (CE) cannot be differentiated by clinical signs, physical examination findings, or diagnostic imaging.
- LGITL has a favorable prognosis with oral chemotherapy (chlorambucil).
- Gold-standard for diagnosis is based on histology findings, including immunohistochemical analysis.
- Clonal rearrangement is present in most LGITL cases but clonality alone (reported in some healthy elderly cats) does not allow discrimination between CE and LGITL.
- There is no supporting evidence that cats with LGITL treated with prednisolone alone will not respond to chlorambucil later. However, prior administration of prednisolone may delay the establishment of a final diagnosis.

INTRODUCTION

Chronic gastrointestinal (GI) signs are common in middle age to older cats and can include presenting complaints of vomiting, diarrhea, hypo-/anorexia, and weight loss [1]. Work-up of these unspecific problems involves ruling out extraintestinal disease (eg, chronic kidney disease, hyperthyroidism, hepatopathies) and intestinal parasitic infection. In their absence, chronic enteropathy (CE) or other GI infiltrative process (lymphoma) is often suspected, and the next step is to empirically rule out food-responsive enteropathy (FRE). Abdominal ultrasound should be considered before or after a diet trial to further assess the abdominal organs of interest; that is, the gastro-intestinal tract

and any indication of involvement of the abdominal lymph nodes, as well as presence of comorbidities in the pancreas, liver, and other abdominal organs, because they can often be seen in elderly cats.

In the absence of response to an elimination diet and exclusion of extra-GI disease, the 2 remaining differential diagnoses are an inflammatory process requiring the use of immunosuppressant treatment (immunosuppressant-responsive enteropathy, immunosuppressant-responsive enteropathy (IRE), also called steroid-responsive enteropathy or idiopathic inflammatory bowel disease) or low-grade gastrointestinal T-cell lymphoma (LGITL). Other lymphoma subtypes described in cats include intermediate-/high-grade alimentary

---

Funded by: CAUL.

*Corresponding author, *E-mail addresses:* julien.dandrieux@unimelb.edu.au; jdandrieux@gmail.com

lymphoma (I/HGAL), and large granular lymphoma (LGL). However, their clinical presentation and abdominal ultrasound features are far less ambiguous when attempting to differentiate from IRE (eg, presence of significant mesenteric lymphadenopathy).

Generally, the GI tract is the most common location for lymphoma in cats, especially in a referral population [2]. There is a steady increase of GI lymphoma prevalence in cats since the 1990s [2], which has been reported in several studies both in Europe and North America [3–5].

Although laboratory testing and diagnostic imaging findings can be useful to rule out other causes, they do not clearly differentiate between IRE and LGITL. For this reason, a combination of histology, immunohistochemistry (IHC), and polymerase chain reaction (PCR) for antigen receptor rearrangements (PARRs) are currently utilized to reach a final diagnosis [6]. However, the 2 diseases are likely to be a *continuum*, with progression from an inflammatory process to a neoplastic one, and remain challenging to conclusively differentiate.

Some clinically relevant questions covered in this article include:

- How best to differentiate IRE from LGITL? What are the limitations of the current methods?
- What is the risk of treating with prednisolone alone, if my patient has LGITL rather than IRE? Could it delay the final diagnosis? Can I cause resistance to treatment?
- What is the risk of CE progression to a large cell lymphoma?
- How do I treat LGITL, what do I need to tell the client?

SIGNIFICANCE

As outline above, the clinician is often faced with the dilemma to differentiate between an inflammatory process (FRE, IRE) versus a neoplastic process (LGITL or other types of lymphoma). GI lymphoma is characterized by a clonal expansion of lymphocytes and is by far the most frequent digestive tract neoplasia in cats. The gut-associated lymphoid tissue is the primary site of neoplastic cell proliferation. Lymphoma in cats has previously been classified by anatomical location, cell size, and immunophenotype (Table 1). Several studies previously highlighted an increase in prevalence over time reported in North America and in Europe [2,4,7]. The following types of lymphoma have been described in cats:

- Low-grade alimentary lymphoma or LGITL
- I/HGAL
- LGL.

Among lymphomas, LGITL is an indolent disease and is the most common, affecting elderly cats. Its incidence has significantly increased during the 2 past decades representing 60% to 75% of GI lymphomas [3,8–11]. Table 2 summarizes some of the differences among LGITL, I/HGAL, and LGL. LGITL originate typically from T-cells (CD3$^+$, CD56$^-$, pSTAT3$^-$, pSTAT5$^+$, KI67 = 30% in the lamina propria), I/HGAL from B-cell or T-cell (CD79a$^+$ or CD3$^+$) and LGL from cytotoxic T-cell (CD3$^+$/CD8$^+$/CD79a$^-$) or natural killer (NK) cells (CD8$^+$/CD79a$^-$). Both I/HGAL and LGL are more likely to cause intestinal masses or significant enlargement of the lymph nodes. For this reason, a combination of abdominal ultrasound and fine-needle aspirates of the abnormal organs will often be diagnostic, with an increased proportion of intermediate to large lymphocytes on cytology with or without granulation. Because the diagnostic is usually achieved with imaging and cytology, these 2 types of lymphoma will not be further discussed.

In contrast, LGITL is defined by variable infiltration of the intestinal mucosa by a monomorphic population of small lymphocytes, mostly involving the epithelium but also the lamina propria and potentially the submucosa and the muscularis. On abdominal ultrasound, the wall layering is usually preserved, and a mild-to-moderate lymphadenopathy can be present. These findings are very similar to what is expected from cats with IRE [3]. Lymph node cytology is unrewarding because most lymphocytes are expected to be small, and the differentiation between LGITL or other types of CE is not possible.

LGITL was first compared with monomorphic epitheliotropic T-cell lymphoma (MEITL, previously named enteropathy-associated T-cell lymphoma, enteropathy-associated T-cell lymphoma (EATL), type 2) in people [8]. However, MEITL differs in several ways to LGITL and most notably by having a very aggressive clinical course. More recently, LGITL has attracted attention as a transitional model for a rarer T-cell GI lymphoma in people with an indolent clinical course, called indolent T-cell lymphoproliferative disorder of the GI tract (GI-TLPD), which was added to the World Health Organization (WHO) classification of lymphoid neoplasms in 2016 [12,13]. Similarly to what has been described in people with GI-TLPD, LGITL in cats is characterized by a monomorphic infiltrate of small lymphocytes in the lamina propria, and shows an indolent clinical course [14]. Epitheliotropism is strong in cats and variable in people. Most neoplastic lymphocytes are CD3$^+$ CD56$^-$ pSTAT3$^-$ in both species [14]. All feline lymphomas were also pSTAT5$^+$, whereas this is not

TABLE 1
General Classification of Lymphoma in Cats

Location[a]	Cell Size	Immunophenotype
Gastrointestinal	Small	T cell
Nasal	Intermediate	B cell
Mediastinal	Large	
Peripheral nodal		
Renal		

[a] These are the most common location for lymphoma in cats. Gastrointestinal lymphoma is by far the most common presentation.

always the case in people. Interestingly, a mutation of STAT5 (STAT5BN642H) described in people has also recently been detected in 29% of cats with LGITL [15]. Hence, LGITL is an interesting transitional model that seems to be closely related to GI-TLPD.

Several parameters have been studied as markers to differentiate cats with IRE from cats with LGITL, including signalment, clinical signs, laboratory tests, and diagnostic imaging. Overall, there are no clinical parameters that can definitely differentiate IRE from LGITL. Although clinical signs were significantly longer in cats with LGITL in one study, there is marked overlap between both groups limiting its use for differentiation between the 2 [16]. Hypocobalaminemia is more frequently seen with LGITL than in IRE [16]. In any case, if present, cobalamin supplementation is recommended.

The Role of Diagnostic Imaging

Abdominal ultrasonography is a key step in the workup of cats with suspected CE or lymphoma to rule out organomegaly, intestinal masses, and/or peritoneal effusion and to assess for comorbidities. Fine-needle aspirates should be obtained in cases with organomegaly, or masses, or abnormal ultrasonographic appearance to rule out aggressive forms of lymphoma or other neoplasia (such as carcinoma or mast cell tumor). Any free fluid should be analyzed (protein content, cell count, cytology) to rule in/out other possible diagnoses.

Other features that can be detected on ultrasound include diffuse or focal thickening of the intestinal wall, as well as loss of normal wall layering. Ultrasonographic distinction between diffuse neoplastic infiltration and inflammatory disease is not possible: both entities show a diffuse thickening of the muscular layer [16,17]. Diagnostic cut-offs values for intestinal wall thickness are not clearly defined for either IRE or LGITL. The ratio of mucosa muscularis width to submucosal width can be of interest, with measurements of 0.5 and greater considered abnormal [17]. Regional lymph nodes (mainly jejunal/mesenteric and ileo-colic) may frequently appear rounded, hypoechoic, and enlarged in both inflammatory infiltrations and LGITL. In a recent prospective study, a range of altered ultrasonographic findings suggestive of jejunal lymphadenopathy (eg, increased lymph node thickness, rounded shape and hyperechoic perinodal fat, hypoechogenicity) were more commonly seen in cats with LGITL than in cats with IRE [16]. Similarly, the presence of abdominal effusion (although in small volume) was more often seen in cats with LGITL than IRE. However, these features can also be seen in cats with IRE and for this reason cannot be used for definitive diagnosis.

In conclusion, ultrasonography is helpful to rule out aggressive cancers but does not allow definitive differentiation of IRE from LGITL. Furthermore, normal ultrasonographic examination does not exclude underlying IRE or LGITL [18]. Thus, histological analysis is mandatory to establish a definitive diagnosis,

TABLE 2
Comparison of the 3 Main Types of Lymphoma Described in Cats

Characteristics	LGITL	I/HGAL	LGL
Clinical presentation	Indolent	Acute	Acute
Immunophenotype	CD3$^+$/CD56$^-$/STAT5$^+$	CD79a$^+$ or CD3$^+$	CD3$^+$/CD8$^+$/CD79a$^-$ or CD3$^-$/CD79a$^-$
Cell size	Small	Intermediate-large	Intermediate-large
Prognosis	Good	Poor	Bad

Abbreviations: I/HGAL, Intermediate-/high-grade alimentary lymphoma; LGITL, low-grade intestinal T-cell lymphoma; LGL, large granular lymphoma.

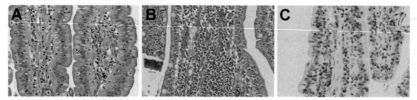

FIG. 1 Comparison of the histology of the small intestinal mucosal villi in a normal cat (**A**) and a cat with low-grade gastrointestinal T-cell lymphoma (**B**). Note the monomorphic population of small lymphocytes, which expand the villus lamina propria and extend into the epithelial layer in the cat with lymphoma. These cells are confirmed to be T-lymphocytes with immunohistochemistry (primary Ab CD3) (**C**). Objective 40×. (*Courtesy of* Richard Ploeg, BVSc, DACVP, Melbourne, AU.)

except in cases where fine needle aspirate (FNA) of abnormal organs have confirmed other neoplasia.

Tissue Sampling

Biopsy collection and histopathologic examination of multiple intestinal tissue biopsies are mandatory to differentiate IRE from LGITL. That said, the best sampling technique (endoscopic mucosal pinch biopsies vs full-thickness biopsies obtained via coeliotomy) remains debatable. Adequate quality of representative GI biopsies is paramount to reach a diagnosis, which can be more difficult to achieve with endoscopic techniques, and various other pros and cons for each technique need to be considered on a case-by-case basis:

• GI endoscopy

GI endoscopy is a minimally invasive technique. It allows a direct visualization of the gastric, duodenal, proximal jejunal, colonic, and, in some cases, distal ileal mucosa (depending on the size of the cat and the endoscope used). At least 6 to 10 good quality biopsies per site are ideally needed to reach a final diagnosis, and macroscopic visualization is not reliable to predict the histopathologic features [19]. To promote a standardized interpretation of inflammatory changes in the GI mucosa of dogs and cats, the World Small Animal Veterinary Association (WSAVA) GI Standardization Group guidelines have been published [20,21]. However, in LGITL, some lesions can emerge within the jejunal mucosa, which is not routinely reached with endoscopy [22].

• Exploratory coeliotomy

Exploratory coeliotomy is more invasive than endoscopy but it allows direct inspection of the GI tract. Full-thickness biopsies can be obtained from both the GI tract and any other affected organs (pancreas, liver, spleen, and lymph nodes) as indicated. Even if the risk of dehiscence postsampling has been reported, the incidence is low, and the procedure is generally safe. During surgery, thorough palpation of the GI tract can be helpful to identify local areas of intestinal

thickening. Jejunal or ileal biopsies can be more easily performed compared with endoscopy but the number of samples is usually smaller.

Histology, Immunohistochemistry, and Polymerase Chain Reaction for Antigen Receptor Rearrangement

The current gold standard to establish a diagnosis of IRE or LGITL is based on a thorough histologic and immunohistochemical analysis of GI biopsies (Fig. 1).

• *Histology criteria to differentiate IRE from LGITL*

   In a recent study, following the 2016 revision of the WHO classification of lymphoid neoplasms, several histologic criteria were suggested to distinguish IRE from LGITL more accurately [22]. It has been suggested that a separate assessment of the lamina propria and the epithelium could limit interobserver discrepancies and improve the diagnostic accuracy of IRE versus LGITL.

   ○ Epitheliotropism (homing of neoplastic T-cells to the mucosal epithelium) is stronger in LGITL cases compared with IRE, and *lymphocyte monomorphism* is typical of LGITL. Although LGITL can exhibit polymorphism, polymorphism is more pronounced in IRE.

   ○ Lamina propria cellularity is marked in LGITL. Other features seen more commonly in cats with LGITL than IRE include the presence of villous atrophy or fusion.

   ○ An apical-to-basal gradient has recently been reported in LGITL cases.

   ○ Other features suggestive of LGITL include lymphocytic cryptitis and lymphoid plaques and nests.

   ○ In full-thickness biopsies, LGITL is occasionally characterized by a transmural infiltration (muscularis, serosa) that is not seen in IRE.

• IHC

In addition to standard histological examination, IHC is an essential complementary molecular technique, which can help in differentiating IRE from LGITL. CD3 antibodies are used to detect T-lymphocytes, CD20 and CD79 antibodies for B-lymphocytes, and CD 57 antibodies for NK cells. LGITL is of T-cell phenotype in more than 90% of cases, and hence predominantly CD3$^+$.

Another marker, Ki67, is used to assess cell proliferation. Ki67 activity increases during cell division and decreases after each mitosis. In a recent prospective study, Ki67 expression in lamina propria lymphocytes and intraepithelial lymphocytes was significantly increased in LGITL cases compared with IRE cases.

As expected, in IRE, a polymorphic disease, CD3 expression is low, whereas CD20 is higher than in LGITL. Ki67 expression is low [22].

In 2 recent studies, pSTAT5 has been shown to be expressed in LGITL cases [15,22]. These data may suggest that the STAT5 pathway has a key role in indolent feline LGITL.

A new model of lymphomagenesis has thus emerged and suggests a continuum between inflammatory enteropathy toward low-grade T-cell intestinal lymphoma. In this model, the immunohistochemical study has highlighted the JAK/STAT pathway activation, leading to pSTAT5 expression.

- Clonality testing (PARR)

Clonality testing is a diagnostic tool based on PCR amplification of the immunoglobulin heavy chain genes for B-cells and the CDR3 region of the T-cell receptor gamma gene for T-cells [23]. This test is also called PARR, and it demonstrates clonally expanded lymphocyte populations in the submitted samples. PARR can be performed on DNA extracted from formalin-fixed tissue slides by multiplex PCR or from fresh frozen GI biopsy samples. However, PARR should never replace IHC investigations because it cannot determine lymphocyte phenotype and tissue localization. As previously mentioned, most LGITL exhibit monoclonality. However, in a recent study, a high number of IRE cases also displayed monoclonality, whereas others showed monoclonality on a polyclonal background [22,24]. PARR clonality on its own can hence not be used to differentiate CE from LGITL. It has been hypothesized that clonal IRE could result either from emerging neoplastic clonal cells on a previously purely polyclonal (inflammatory) background (part of the suspected *continuum* from inflammation to cancer) or from a strong antigenic stimulation in feline GI inflammation [22].

In conclusion, a combination of histological and immunophenotypic findings ± PARR should remain the gold-standard criteria to differentiate IRE from LGITL to avoid the risks of a misdiagnosis. Reclassification of equivocal cases from IRE to LGITL or vice versa might be necessary based on findings of these diagnostic tools but should not be exclusively based on PARR test results.

Present Relevance and Future Avenues to Consider or to Investigate

What are the limitations of the current methods?

The main limitations of our current methods to diagnose LGITL are that there is an overlap between cats with IRE and LGITL, with the need for multiple tests as outline above.

The disease can be multifocal, and the biopsies might not be representative of the true lesions. Additionally, clonality has been described in healthy elderly cats, which can lead to a wrong diagnosis, if not used in conjunction with histology and IHC. For these reasons, there is LGITL, which is likely missed as a diagnosis in some cats while wrongly diagnosed in others. This can lead to inappropriate use of chemotherapy with risk both for the pet and the owner.

There are currently no biomarkers that have been identified to separate the 2 diseases. Newer methods, such as assessment of the fecal microbiome and untargeted metabolomic, have been recently studied to compare healthy cats with cats with IRE or LGITL [25,26]. Although differences are present between healthy and sick cats, there were no differences in the fecal microbiome between cats with IRE and cats with LGITL, and only limited differences in the metabolome.

The same group has recently assessed the use of histology-guided mass spectrometry on duodenal biopsies between cats with IRE and LGITL with very promising results [6]. However, this method is currently not commercially available and further studies are required to confirm these preliminary findings. If confirmed and more widely available, histology-guided mass spectrometry has the potential to become an excellent tool for diagnosis cats with LGITL, although the need of noninvasive diagnostic would remain.

What is the risk of treating with prednisolone alone, if my patient has low-grade gastrointestinal T-cell lymphoma rather than IRE? Can we cause resistance to treatment?

One question that is frequently debated is the relevance of differentiating IRE from LGITL. Some clinicians advocate to treat empirically rather than obtaining biopsies in cats after ruling out other differentials. The principal argument is that the differentiation between the 2 entities remains difficult with our current diagnostic tools. For this reason, one strategy is to treat with prednisolone and, if the cats are not responding satisfactorily, then to add chlorambucil.

An argument against this approach is that the prognosis for LGITL, although good with chlorambucil treatment, is worse than for CE. In the opinion of the authors, for some clients, this information is invaluable and helps guiding how they want to treat their cats. The final diagnosis is required for their decision-making. Another limitation is that reaching a final diagnosis of LGITL might be harder in cat treated with prednisolone before obtaining biopsies.

Another consideration is to that treatment with steroids as a single agent might affect later treatment with chemotherapeutic drugs, so-called corticosteroid-induced resistance, but evidence to support clinical relevance is currently lacking.

One ex vivo study has attempted to assess this using 2 feline lymphoma cell lines (1 B cell and 1 T cell) [27]. A reduction in the cytotoxicity of both doxorubicin and vincristine was noted after pretreatment with steroids. Additionally, there was an increase in transcription of proteins with the potential of causing multidrug resistance. Limitations of this study includes that both lines were from large-cell lymphomas and the effect of prednisolone pretreatment on resistance to an alkylating agent, such as chlorambucil, was not assessed.

In vivo, some feline studies have reported no effect of pretreatment with steroids on the efficacy of chemotherapy, whereas another reported a reduction in the median survival time (MST) in cats achieving complete remission [28–30]. However, the relevance of these studies is very limited for the treatment of LGITL because they included only 3 cats treated with chlorambucil. In one study, where cats with LGITL received treatment with prednisolone and chlorambucil, the treatment was discontinued after a year, due to disease remission (n = 18) or for diverse other reasons [31]. A rescue protocol with the same treatment was attempted in 9 cats, and overall remission rates were similar after the after the rescue protocol compared with the first treatment.

What is the risk of progression to a large cell lymphoma?

A small but significant number of cats (6%–14% depending on the study) will develop another neoplasia after the diagnosis of LGITL [31–33]. The most frequent neoplasia is I/HGAL in different locations (intestinal, renal, splenic, hepatic) and carcinomas (intestinal or extraintestinal). In the largest study, 12/121 cats (10%) with LGITL developed I/HGAL, and 9 of these received a rescue chemotherapy protocol [32]. The duration from LGITL diagnosis to development of I/HGAL was several months to years (548 ± 378 days). The cats were reassessed either after developing clinical signs, on detection of a mass on physical examination, or development of azotemia. Anemia and hypoalbuminemia were noted more frequently at relapse. MST after initiation of the rescue protocol was 25 days (2–183 days). In addition, the authors identified 3.7% of cats in the same studies that were diagnosed with simultaneously LGITL and I/HGAL, which is similar to percentages reported in an earlier study (3.3%), further supporting the notion of a *continuum* between diseases [8].

How do I treat low-grade gastrointestinal T-cell lymphoma, what do I need to tell the client?

Treatment of low-grade gastrointestinal T-cell lymphoma. General treatment of cats with CE has been reviewed recently, and the reader should refer to this article for more information [1]. Apart from standard treatments (diet, prednisolone), modulation of the microbiome is also under investigation as a therapeutic option, namely antibiotics, probiotics, or fecal microbiota transplants but there is currently limited evidence on the clinical utility of these treatment of CE in cats.

A combination of chlorambucil and prednisolone is the chemotherapy protocol of choice for cats diagnosed with LGITL and is also used for cats with poorly or nonresponsive CE.

The authors consider a dose of 1 to 2 mg/kg q24 h prednisolone as a starting dose. Similar to dogs, common adverse effects of glucocorticoids include polyuria, polydipsia, and polyphagia but cats have comparatively fewer side effects than dogs at an equivalent dosage. However, cats can also develop acute congestive heart failure and diabetes mellitus secondary to insulin resistance. Diabetes mellitus was reported in 9.7% of cats treated with a dose of prednisolone greater than 1.9 mg/kg/d in one study, with the majority of cats developing the disease within 3 months of starting therapy [34]. Although the use of budesonide has been described off-label, there is currently not enough evidence to recommend its use instead of prednisolone in cats.

Once remission is achieved (defined as resolution of clinical signs and biochemical and ultrasonographic changes if present), a consideration is to reduce the

TABLE 3
Commonly Used Drugs in Cats Diagnosed with LGAL

Name	Dosage	Adverse Effects Reported in Cats[a]	Interactions, Other Considerations	Monitoring
Prednisolone	1–2 mg/kg q24 h	**Polyuria, polydipsia, and polyphagia. Steroid hepatopathy** Onset of diabetes mellitus. Onset of congestive heart failure. Secondary infections		Clinical response (body weight, BCS, fecal scoring) Baseline same as for chlorambucil (see below). Spot glucose and urinalysis, if onset of diabetes mellitus is suspected
Budesonide	0.5–1 mg/cat q24 h		Not sufficient evidence-based data to support its use currently	
Chlorambucil • Metabolized in the liver • Excreted in the urine	1.5–4 mg/m² PO q24 h (interval is adjusted in small cats to account for the tablet size, typically 2 mg PO q48–72 h) 15 mg/m² PO q24 h for 4 d q3weeks or 20 mg/m² PO q2weeks	**Anemia, leukopenia, thrombocytopenia Vomiting, diarrhea** Neurotoxicity Fanconi syndrome	Use gloves and do not split or crush the tablets Increased risk of myelosuppression if used with additional myelosuppressive agents	• Baseline CBC, chemistry, urinalysis including UPC • Repeat CBC after 1 mo, thereafter q2-3 mo • Biochemistry and urinalysis including UPC q3 months

Abbreviations: BCS, Body condition score; CBC, Complete blood LGAL, low grade alimentarly lymphoma; UPC, Urine protein:creatinine ratio.
  [a] More frequent adverse effects are bolded.

prednisolone dosage over the following months to a dosage of 0.5 to 1 mg/kg per Os (PO) q24 h to reduce the risk of adverse effects over time.

Treatment with chlorambucil as either continuous (2 mg/cat PO q48–72 h) or pulse dosing (every 2 or 3 weeks) has been described (Table 3 for dosages) [33,35,36]. Continuous treatment can be better tolerated in cats developing GI signs with high dose of chlorambucil but pulse dosing has the potential benefit of reduced exposure for the owner and less handling of the cat [37]. This strategy is used by some clinicians for treatment in the hospital setting for cats difficult to handle.

One study reported adverse effects in approximately one-third of cats (19/56) treated with prednisolone and chlorambucil [31].

- Myelosuppression was the most common adverse effect (n = 11). Anemia, leukopenia, and thrombocytopenia usually developed within the first 2 weeks of treatment and resolved in the same time frame after chlorambucil discontinuation. Marked

thrombocytopenia developed occasionally months after starting treatment and took months to resolve (see Table 3 for monitoring).

- GI adverse effects (inappetence, vomiting, and diarrhea) and hepatotoxicity were reported on 7 occasions, and while usually being mild and self-limiting, reduction of chlorambucil dose or discontinuation (in particular for hepatotoxicity) was required. In the author's experience, transitioning from a pulse protocol to continuous treatment can be useful in some cats developing vomiting with pulse therapy. Chlorambucil was withdrawn in 5/6 cats with hepatotoxicity and alanine transferase (ALT) improved in all cats in an average of 76 days (6–228 days). The severity of hepatotoxicity described in other case reports is more variable but the contribution of an underlying disease process was not always excluded [31].
- Reversible neurologic signs (agitation, facial twitching, myoclonus, and tonic-clonic seizures) were reported in 1 cat following a drug overdose [38].

BOX 1
List of Considerations for the Owners Before Treating Their Cats with Chlorambucil

- The following people should not be involved with drug administration or cleaning of any cat excreta:
  - Women who are trying to conceive, pregnant, or lactating.
  - Young children.
  - In any doubt, the owners should consult with their personal doctor before treating their cat.
- Follow the posology recommended by your veterinarian.
- Prevent direct skin contact with the drug. Use chemotherapy-rated gloves to handle, do not crush the tablets, wash your hands after handling.
- The drug is excreted in the saliva, urine, feces, or vomit.
  - The pet should not urinate or defecate, where children play or community areas.
  - The litter tray should be cleaned once a day using disposable gloves. Use disposable plastic bags in the litter box.
  - Keep the cat inside during the period of excretion (2 days after treatment) and ideally in a controlled environment (eg, one room that is easy to clean, if any spills occur).
  - If the cat has an accident in the house (urination, defecation, or vomiting):
    - Use disposable gloves and absorptive disposable towels. Rinse with dilute bleach once gross contamination is removed. Avoid cleaning with high-pressure sprays. Double bag all wastes before disposal. Dispose of it like chemical waste.
  - Avoid stroking your cat. Wash your hands after close contact (the coat is contaminated by saliva).
  - Any soft items, such as bedding or towels, should be washed twice. Keep separate from other laundry and ideally bleach.
- Keep the chlorambucil in its original package and outside the reach of kids or pets. Do not store near medications for humans or food.
- Bring the leftovers of the chlorambucil to your veterinarian.

- Acquired Fanconi syndrome was reported in 4 cats within 2 to 26 months of starting chlorambucil treatment [39]. Improvement or resolution occurred in 3/4 cats within 3 months of discontinuing treatment.

Monitoring During Treatment of Low-Grade Gastrointestinal T-Cell Lymphoma

There is no strict consensus on the frequency of laboratory monitoring for potential chlorambucil-induced adverse effects. The authors' recommendation is to obtain baseline hematology, biochemistry, and urinalysis. For continuous dosing, repeat hematology should be considered 1 month after starting treatment and every 2 to 3 months thereafter. For pulse treatment, hematology should be repeated 1 week after the treatment. Treatment should be discontinued if platelets are lower than 75,000/μL or there is other significant evidence of myelosuppression. As outlined above, marked thrombocytopenia can develop months after starting treatment and for this reason, on-going monitoring is recommended.

Biochemistry and urinalysis (glucosuria in case of Fanconi syndrome or new onset of diabetes mellitus) should be considered after 1 month, and if normal every 3 months thereafter.

It is recommended to measure vitamin B12 concentration at the time of diagnosis because hypocobalaminemia is a common finding in cats with LGITL. Two parenteral protocols with either hydroxocobalamin or cyanocobalamin have been prospectively evaluated [40,41]. The former resulted in normalization of vitamin B12 concentration and methylmalonic acid concentration (consistent with cellular replenishment). A successful oral cobalamin supplementation protocol with 0.25 mg cyanocobalamin tablets PO q24 h for 1 to 3 months in cats with LGITL has also been described [42].

Chlorambucil Handling and Safety

Guidelines on the use of cytotoxic drugs in veterinary medicine are available from the European College of Veterinary Medicine (https://www.ecvim-ca.org/images/downloads/guidelines/Guidelines_ECVIM_Hazards_Cytotoxic_drugs_2nd_version_July_2007.pdf) and as a Consensus Statement by the American College of Veterinary Medicine [37]. The reader is referred to these documents for in depth information and any local legal requirements on handling and disposing of cytotoxic drugs.

The discussion is limited to chlorambucil, which is the most common chemotherapeutic use to treat LGITL, and discussion with an oncologist is recommended, if alternative protocols are considered.

Chlorambucil is classified in Group 1 (drug which is carcinogenic) by the Agency for Research on Cancer. The duration of excretion of chlorambucil in cats has not been studied; for this reason, guidelines are based on research in people. Excretion of chlorambucil is expected in urine, feces, saliva, and vomitus. The period of risk after administration of chlorambucil is 2 days (human data).

Chlorambucil is a nitrogen mustard derivative that is metabolized in the liver to its active metabolite and further metabolized in the liver to other inactive metabolites that are excreted in the urine and feces. The cytotoxic effect is noncell cycle specific by alkylation of DNA strands. Chlorambucil has also teratogenic effects, which is relevant for the veterinary staff handling the drug and the owners. For these reasons, chlorambucil should be avoided in immunosuppressed owners, in pregnancies, and care should be taken with young kids. Owners should be given written discharge instructions and a list of routine recommendations for owners is listed in Box 1. Staff handling animals treated with chlorambucil should be specifically trained. The reader should refer to the American College of Veterinary Internal Medicine (ACVIM) guidelines for further information on care of cats in the clinic.

The handling of chlorambucil and monitoring plan for adverse effects as listed above are best given as written notes to the owner.

SUMMARY/DISCUSSION

Both IRE and LGITL are frequently diagnosed in cats with chronic gastrointestinal signs.

Thorough work-up is required to rule out other diseases, whereas sampling of intestinal tissue is required to reach a definitive diagnosis. The diagnosis remains challenging, and there is a likely *continuum* between IRE and LGITL, as well as potentially between LGITL and other types of GI lymphoma or cancer.

Although the prognosis for cats with LGITL is worse than cats with IRE, MST is typically more than 2 years with combined chlorambucil and prednisolone treatment, which is superior to MSTs of other types of intestinal lymphoma.

Because chlorambucil is a chemotherapy drug, clear instructions on handling, disposal, and side effects are required for owners treating their pet with this drug.

CLINICS CARE POINTS

- Definitive diagnosis of low-grade gastrointestinal T-cell lymphoma (LGITL) requires intestinal biopsies and a combination of histology, immunohistochemistry, +/− polymerase chain reaction for antigen receptor rearrangement testing.
- The treatment of choice for LGITL is a combination of chlorambucil and prednisolone with a median survival time of years.
- Chlorambucil is a chemotherapy drug, and owners need a clear understanding of the implications. It might, hence, not be an option for individual cases where young children or women who are conceiving, pregnant, or lactating could come into contact with the drug or the cat's excreta.
- Diabetes mellitus can develop in any cat receiving high doses of glucocorticoids; hence monitoring for the development of typical signs such as polyuria (PU)/polydipsia (PD) and weight loss should trigger a recheck.
- Thrombocytopenia can develop months after the initiation of treatment with chlorambucil, and for this reason, platelet counts should be monitored regularly long-term.

SUMMARY

CE and LGITL can be difficult to differentiate one from another but different laboratory methods using paraffin-fixed biopsies (for histopathology, IHC, and PARR) can be helpful. Although a staged treatment starting with steroids and adding chlorambucil in the absence of response can be used, determining from the outset if an LGITL is present can be helpful for prognosis and to increase confidence that aggressive treatment is indicated.

DISCLOSURE

J. Dandrieux: Panel member for IDEXX. Funding: ATMO(R) and CannPal(TM). Grants: ACVIM Resident Research Grant and Canine Research Foundation. V. Freiche: Funding: Royal Canin.

REFERENCES

[1] Marsilio S. Feline chronic enteropathy. J Small Anim Pract 2021;62(6):409–19.

[2] Louwerens M, London CA, Pedersen NC, et al. Feline lymphoma in the post—feline leukemia virus era. J Vet Intern Med 2005;19(3):329–35.

[3] Norsworthy GD, Estep JS, Hollinger C, et al. Prevalence and underlying causes of histologic abnormalities in cats suspected to have chronic small bowel disease: 300 cases (2008-2013). J Am Vet Med Assoc 2015;247: 629–35.

[4] Manuali E, Forte C, Vichi G, et al. Tumours in European Shorthair cats: a retrospective study of 680 cases. J Feline Med Surg 2020;22(12):1095–102.

[5] Rissetto K, Villamil JA, Selting KA, et al. Recent trends in feline intestinal neoplasia: an epidemiologic study of 1,129 cases in the veterinary medical database from 1964 to 2004. J Am Anim Hosp Assoc 2011;47(1): 28–36.

[6] Marsilio S, Newman SJ, Estep JS, et al. Differentiation of lymphocytic-plasmacytic enteropathy and small cell lymphoma in cats using histology-guided mass spectrometry. J Vet Intern Med 2020;34(2):669–77.

[7] Meichner K, Kruse DB, Hirschberger J, et al. Changes in prevalence of progressive feline leukaemia virus infection in cats with lymphoma in Germany. Vet Rec 2012; 171(14):348.

[8] Moore PF, Rodriguez-Bertos A, Kass PH. Feline gastrointestinal lymphoma: mucosal architecture, immunophenotype, and molecular clonality. Vet Pathol 2012;49: 658–68.

[9] Chino J, Fujino Y, Kobayashi T, et al. Cytomorphological and immunological classification of feline lymphomas: clinicopathological features of 76 Cases. J Vet Med Sci 2013;75(6):701–7.

[10] Swanson CM, Smedley RC, Saavedra PV, et al. Expression of the Bcl-2 apoptotic marker in cats diagnosed with inflammatory bowel disease and gastrointestinal lymphoma. J Feline Med Surg 2012;14(10):741–5.

[11] Kiupel M, Smedley RC, Pfent C, et al. Diagnostic algorithm to differentiate lymphoma from inflammation in feline small intestinal biopsy samples. Vet Pathol 2011; 48:212–22.

[12] Swerdlow SH, Campo E, Pileri SA, et al. The 2016 revision of the World Health Organization classification of lymphoid neoplasms. Blood 2016;127(20):2375–90.

[13] Wolfesberger B, Fuchs-Baumgartinger A, Greß V, et al. World Health Organisation classification of lymphoid tumours in veterinary and human medicine: a comparative evaluation of gastrointestinal lymphomas in 61 cats. J Comp Pathol 2018;159:1–10.

[14] Freiche V, Cordonnier N, Paulin MV, et al. Feline low-grade intestinal T cell lymphoma: a unique natural model of human indolent T cell lymphoproliferative disorder of the gastrointestinal tract. Lab Invest 2021; 101(6):794–804.

[15] Kieslinger M, Swoboda A, Kramer N, et al. A Recurrent STAT5BN642H driver mutation in feline alimentary t cell lymphoma. Cancers (Basel) 2021;13(20):5238.

[16] Freiche V, Fages J, Paulin MV, et al. Clinical, laboratory and ultrasonographic findings differentiating low-grade intestinal T-cell lymphoma from lymphoplasmacytic enteritis in cats. J Vet Intern Med 2021;35(6):2685–96.

[17] Daniaux LA, Laurenson MP, Marks SL, et al. Ultrasonographic thickening of the muscularis propria in feline small intestinal small cell T-cell lymphoma and inflammatory bowel disease. J Feline Med Surg 2014;16(2): 89–98.

[18] Jugan MC, August JR. Serum cobalamin concentrations and small intestinal ultrasound changes in 75 cats with clinical signs of gastrointestinal disease: a retrospective study. J Feline Med Surg 2017;19:48–56.

[19] Willard MD, Mansell J, Fosgate GT, et al. Effect of sample quality on the sensitivity of endoscopic biopsy for detecting gastric and duodenal lesions in dogs and cats. J Vet Intern Med 2008;22:1084–9.

[20] Day MJ, Bilzer T, Mansell J, et al. Histopathological standards for the diagnosis of gastrointestinal inflammation in endoscopic biopsy samples from the dog and cat: a report from the World Small Animal Veterinary Association Gastrointestinal Standardization Group. J Comp Pathol 2008;138(Suppl 1):S1–43.

[21] Washabau RJ, Day MJ, Willard MD, et al. Endoscopic, biopsy, and histopathologic guidelines for the evaluation of gastrointestinal inflammation in companion animals. J Vet Intern Med 2010;24:10–26.

[22] Freiche V, Paulin MV, Cordonnier N, et al. Histopathologic, phenotypic, and molecular criteria to discriminate low-grade intestinal T-cell lymphoma in cats from lymphoplasmacytic enteritis. J Vet Intern Med 2021;35(6): 2673–84.

[23] Moore PF, Woo JC, Vernau W, et al. Characterization of feline T cell receptor gamma (TCRG) variable region genes for the molecular diagnosis of feline intestinal T cell lymphoma. Vet Immunol Immunopathol 2005; 106(3–4):167–78.

[24] Marsilio S, Ackermann MR, Lidbury JA, et al. Results of histopathology, immunohistochemistry, and molecular clonality testing of small intestinal biopsy specimens from clinically healthy client-owned cats. J Vet Intern Med 2019;33(2):551–8.

[25] Marsilio S, Pilla R, Sarawichitr B, et al. Characterization of the fecal microbiome in cats with inflammatory bowel disease or alimentary small cell lymphoma. Sci Rep 2019;9.

[26] Marsilio S, Chow B, Hill SL, et al. Untargeted metabolomic analysis in cats with naturally occurring inflammatory bowel disease and alimentary small cell lymphoma. Sci Rep 2021;11(1):9198.

[27] Hlavaty J, Ertl R, Mekuria TA, et al. Effect of prednisolone pre-treatment on cat lymphoma cell sensitivity towards chemotherapeutic drugs. Res Vet Sci 2021;138:178–87.

[28] Fabrizio F, Calam AE, Dobson JM, et al. Feline mediastinal lymphoma: a retrospective study of signalment, retroviral status, response to chemotherapy and prognostic indicators. J Feline Med Surg 2014;16(8):637–44.

[29] Taylor SS, Goodfellow MR, Browne WJ, et al. Feline extranodal lymphoma: response to chemotherapy and survival in 110 cats. J Small Anim Pract 2009;50(11):584–92.

[30] Wolfesberger B, Skor O, Hammer SE, et al. Does categorisation of lymphoma subtypes according to the World Health Organization classification predict clinical outcome in cats? J Feline Med Surg 2017;19(8):897–906.

[31] Pope KV, Tun AE, McNeill CJ, et al. Outcome and toxicity assessment of feline small cell lymphoma: 56 cases (2000–2010). Vet Med Sci 2015;1(2):51–62.

[32] Wright KZ, Hohenhaus AE, Verrilli AM, et al. Feline large-cell lymphoma following previous treatment for small-cell gastrointestinal lymphoma: incidence, clinical signs, clinicopathologic data, treatment of a secondary malignancy, response and survival. J Feline Med Surg 2019;21(4):353–62.

[33] Stein TJ, Pellin M, Steinberg H, et al. Treatment of feline gastrointestinal small-cell lymphoma with chlorambucil and glucocorticoids. J Am Anim Hosp Assoc 2010;46:413–7.

[34] Nerhagen S, Moberg HL, Boge GS, et al. Prednisolone-induced diabetes mellitus in the cat: a historical cohort. J Feline Med Surg 2020. https://doi.org/10.1177/1098612X20943522.

[35] Kiselow MA, Rassnick KM, McDonough SP, et al. Outcome of cats with low-grade lymphocytic lymphoma: 41 cases (1995-2005). J Am Vet Med Assoc 2008;232:405–10.

[36] Lingard AE, Briscoe K, Beatty JA, et al. Low-Grade alimentary lymphoma: clinicopathological findings and response to treatment in 17 cases. J Feline Med Surg 2009;11(8):692–700.

[37] Smith AN, Klahn S, Phillips B, et al. ACVIM small animal consensus statement on safe use of cytotoxic chemotherapeutics in veterinary practice. J Vet Intern Med 2018;32(3):904–13.

[38] Benitah N, de Lorimier LP, Gaspar M, et al. Chlorambucil-induced myoclonus in a cat with lymphoma. J Am Anim Hosp Assoc 2003;39(3):283–7.

[39] Reinert NC, Feldman DG. Acquired Fanconi syndrome in four cats treated with chlorambucil. J Feline Med Surg 2016;18(12):1034–40.

[40] Kempf J, Hersberger M, Melliger RH, et al. Effects of 6 weeks of parenteral cobalamin supplementation on clinical and biochemical variables in cats with gastrointestinal disease. J Vet Intern Med 2017;31(6):1664–72.

[41] Kook PH, Melliger RH, Hersberger M. Efficacy of intramuscular hydroxocobalamin supplementation in cats with cobalamin deficiency and gastrointestinal disease. J Vet Intern Med 2020;34(5):1872–8.

[42] Toresson L, Steiner JM, Olmedal G, et al. Oral cobalamin supplementation in cats with hypocobalaminaemia: a retrospective study. J Feline Med Surg 2017;19(12):1302–6.

Advances in Small Animal Care 3 (2022) 133–143

ADVANCES IN SMALL ANIMAL CARE

Update on Acute Hemorrhagic Diarrhea Syndrome in Dogs

Kathrin Busch, DVM, Dr med vet, DECVIM-CA[a], Stefan Unterer, DVM, Dr med vet, Dr habil, DECVIM-CA[b],*

[a]Clinic of Small Animal Medicine, Centre for Clinical Veterinary Medicine, Ludwig-Maximilians-University, Munich, Germany; [b]Clinic for Small Animal Internal Medicine, Vetsuisse Faculty, University of Zurich, Zurich, Switzerland

KEYWORDS
- Hemorrhagic gastroenteritis • Gastrointestinal bleeding • *Clostridium perfringens* • Pore-forming toxin • NetF
- Chronic enteropathy

KEY POINTS

- Acute hemorrhagic diarrhea syndrome (AHDS) of dogs is characterized by a sudden onset of severe bloody diarrhea associated with a dramatic loss of fluid into the intestinal lumen.
- A normal-to-increased packed cell volume helps to differentiate AHDS from true GI bleeding, in which anemia is usually observed.
- Whereas a positive PCR for NetF encoding *Clostridium perfringens* strains is suggestive for AHDS, neither a fecal culture for *C perfringens* nor a fecal ELISA test for *C perfringens* enterotoxin nor a fecal PCR for *C perfringens* α toxin gene are diagnostic.
- Rapid volume replacement through a large-bore IV catheter is the mainstay of treatment. Antibiotics are usually not necessary because translocation of bacteria through the damaged intestinal mucosa can usually be compensated for by the dog.
- Most dogs recover, but the mortality rate is high if untreated. Only 10% to 15% of dogs have repeat occurrences of AHDS, but 28% of dogs develop chronic or chronic recurrent signs of GI disease later in life.

INTRODUCTION

Hemorrhagic diarrhea is much more commonly observed in dogs in comparison with cats and humans, and the gut is considered as the main shock organ in this species [1]. Numerous causes for acute hemorrhagic diarrhea (AHD) exist and hemorrhagic diarrhea is not a diagnosis per se, because it only reflects the severity of intestinal mucosal damage. The two most important causes of AHD are canine parvovirus infection and acute hemorrhagic diarrhea syndrome (AHDS). Dogs with canine parvovirus infection are typically young, and have a low hematocrit and/or total protein and albumin levels. Any disease causing intestinal destruction associated with significant fluid loss into the intestinal lumen can clinically resemble AHDS, but this syndrome has unique clinical features that help distinguish it from other conditions (Box 1). Clostridial overgrowth and the associated release of clostridial toxins seem to be responsible for epithelial cell injury and the rapid movement of large amounts of fluid and electrolytes into the gut lumen (Fig. 1). AHDS is not only an acute life-threatening gastrointestinal (GI) disorder, but a significant number of dogs develop long-term consequences. A recently published, retrospective, longitudinal study reported that about 30% of dogs with AHDS develop chronic diarrhea later in life,

*Corresponding author, *E-mail address:* stefan.unterer@uzh.ch

https://doi.org/10.1016/j.yasa.2022.06.003
2666-450X/22/

> **BOX 1**
> **Unique Clinical Features of AHDS**
>
> - Vomiting as first clinical sign in 80% of cases
> - Sudden onset of severe bloody diarrhea
> - Significant loss of fluid into the intestinal lumen
> - Blood loss is usually minor in proportion to fluid loss
> - Rapid clinical improvement with adequate fluid therapy
> - Not transmissible to other dogs or species

supporting the theory that severe intestinal mucosal damage and associated barrier dysfunction might trigger chronic GI diseases [2].

PATHOGENESIS

A primary pathogenic role of *Clostridium perfringens* in dogs with AHDS was first suspected in the late 1980s, when the first cases with peracute hemorrhagic enteritis and necropsy examinations were reported. Gram-positive bacilli adherent to the necrotic epithelial surfaces of the intestinal tract were found, and large numbers of *C perfringens* (published at the time with the former name *Clostridium welchii*) were cultured from the intestinal content [3]. Interpretation of those findings was difficult, because *C perfringens* is part of the normal colonic flora and clostridial overgrowth is a possible postmortem sequela. However, a prospective study that included 10 dogs with AHD confirmed this hypothesis. Endoscopy was performed within the first 12 hours of presentation in all dogs and clostridial

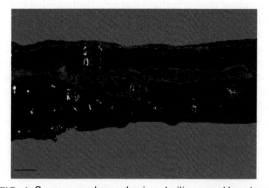

FIG. 1 Severe necrohemorrhagic enteritis caused by a type A *Clostridium perfringens* strain in a dog with AHDS. In the intestinal lumen "raspberry jam" characteristic stool is observed.

strains identified as *C perfringens* by culture and mass spectrometry using matrix-assisted laser desorption/ionization-time of flight were detected on the surface of the small intestinal mucosa by immunohistochemistry (Fig. 2) [4]. *C perfringens* is rarely cultured from the small intestine and clostridial-type bacteria are not visible with routine histology in healthy dogs or dogs with intestinal disorders, such as chronic enteropathies and canine parvovirus infection. In 5 of 10 dogs with AHDS clostridial strains could be cultured from biopsy samples of the duodenum and each of the five genotyped isolates encoded the pore-forming toxin NetF, which is a β-pore-forming toxin that belongs to the leucocidin/hemolysin superfamily [4]. In vitro experiments showed that the NetF toxin is able to form pores in susceptible cells leading to plasma membrane destruction and subsequent osmotic cell lysis. In an experimental study, a NetF insertional inactivation mutant of *C perfringens* was created, and this strain was no longer toxic for an equine ovarian cell line. Additionally, antiserum against NetF toxin neutralized the cytotoxicity of wild-type NetF-producing *C perfringens* type A strains isolated from a dog with AHD [5]. All of these findings suggest that NetF is likely to be the major virulence factor in *C perfringens* strains responsible for canine AHDS. Although NetF-encoding *C perfringens* strains are not present in every dog with AHDS, several studies showed a higher prevalence of *C perfringens* encoding the *netF* gene in fecal samples from dogs with AHDS compared with healthy dogs and dogs with other intestinal diseases. For example, in dogs with parvovirus infection, which show similar intestinal lesions to dogs with AHDS, no *C perfringens* strains encoding *netF* could be detected [6]. It can hence be concluded that the overgrowth of clostridial strains is not only a secondary consequence to a primary insult of the intestinal tract, as has been speculated previously. In addition to the pore-forming toxins, *C perfringens* produces numerous extracellular enzymes and minor toxins, such as collagenase (κ-toxin), neuraminidase, caseinase (λ-toxin), deoxyribonuclease (η-toxin), hyaluronidase (μ-toxin), and urease, which might be released during the bacterial proliferation phase and additionally contribute to the damage of the intestinal mucosa. *C perfringens* enterotoxin (CPE) is a cytotoxic (causing tissue damage) enterotoxin, and its production and release are associated with sporulation. However, CPE cannot consistently be detected in the feces of dogs with AHDS, and is therefore not considered to be the primary toxin causing mucosal lesions and hemorrhagic diarrhea. In contrast to CPE encoding strains, which are

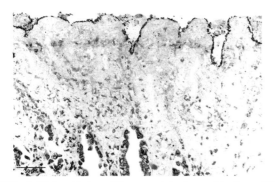

FIG. 2 Histopathology (Giemsa, original magnification ×20) of a dog with AHDS. Extensive necrosis of the superficial colonic mucosa, which demonstrates a complete loss of the mucus layer. Note the plump, rod-shaped bacteria directly attached to surface of the colon. Destruction of the intestinal lining and of the mucus layer represent two main features of intestinal barrier dysfunction.

histopathologic features in dogs with AHDS. Lesions with the highest histologic scores were detectable in the colon, whereas proximal parts of the small intestines had lower scores, and the gastric mucosa was not affected [4]. It can therefore be speculated that clostridial overgrowth and toxin release starts in the large intestine and subsequently affects the small intestine. In cases with a lethal outcome, the observation of *C perfringens* on the surface of the gastric mucosa has also been described, but this most likely represents severe, rare forms of AHDS. Based on in vivo endoscopy and histology findings from dogs with AHDS, the stomach is typically not affected, and therefore the most commonly used name "hemorrhagic gastroenteritis" seems inadequate and should be replaced by the more precise description "acute hemorrhagic diarrhea syndrome" [8].

permanently present in the feces of some dogs after recovering from AHDS and in healthy dogs, *netF* drops lower than the detection limit of the polymerase chain reaction (PCR) assay within 7 days following presentation with AHDS in all dogs (Fig. 3) [7]. No specific cause inciting clostridial proliferation and toxin release, such as food poisoning, has been identified to date. Thus, it is likely that different causes are responsible for the abrupt clostridial overgrowth and clinical consequence, which is AHDS.

A necrotizing and neutrophilic inflammation often affecting the entire gut, but with individual severity in different areas, represents the characteristic

SIGNALMENT, CLINICAL, AND CLINICOPATHOLOGIC ABNORMALITIES

AHDS is often reported in small breed dogs, such as Miniature Schnauzer, Cavalier King Charles Spaniel, Dachshund, Chihuahua, Yorkshire Terrier, Maltese, Miniature Pinschers, and small mix breeds [9,10]. However, in one study Labrador Retrievers were the most prevalent breed in a dog population presenting with AHDS, so large breed dogs must also be considered predisposed [11]. The incidence of AHDS was higher in middle-aged dogs with a median of 5 years, compared with the general hospital population, which had a median of 10 years, as described in a study including 108 cases of dogs with AHDS [9]. A sex predilection has not been documented.

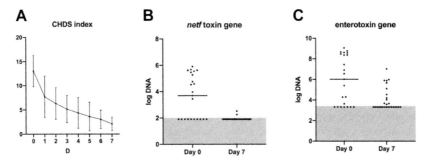

FIG. 3 Clinical course, abundance of *Clostridium perfringens* encoding enterotoxin, and NetF toxin in dogs with AHDS. Characteristic clinical course of dogs with uncomplicated AHDS based on the acute hemorrhagic diarrhea index (**A**). Associated with the rapid clinical improvement of this self-limiting syndrome is the reduction of *C perfringens* strains encoding for the NetF toxin to such a degree that after 7 days these strains can usually not be detected by a sensitive PCR assay in any dog (**B**). Abundance of clostridial strains encoding for enterotoxin also declines, but a significant number of dogs stay positive for these toxigenic strains (**C**). CHDS, canine haemorrhagic diarrhoea severity index.

AHDS dogs characteristically present with an acute to peracute history of GI signs of less than 24 hours duration [9]. Chronic enteropathies may predispose to AHDS, because a significant number of dog owners describe the presence of chronic intestinal signs before the onset of AHD (personal communication Skotnitzki). Vomiting is observed as the first clinical sign in about half of the dogs with AHDS, and 80% of dog owners describe hematemesis. It is noteworthy that some dogs with severe AHD at presentation do not have any or few bowel movements on Days 2 and 3 after presentation, because of an empty GI tract and reduced intestinal motility secondary to the acute intestinal inflammation. Soft stools are present until Day 10, because the severely damaged intestinal mucosa might need time to completely recover [12].

Depending on the severity of dehydration at presentation, lethargy, weakness, tachycardia, prolonged capillary refill time, and weak pulses may be detected. The most consistent physical examination finding is tachycardia, which is a compensatory mechanism because of the hypovolemia or a stress response caused by abdominal discomfort and nausea [9]. Although dogs with AHDS typically have a significant loss of fluid through the intestinal tract, skin turgor may appear normal in many cases because of the peracute onset and the lag time in compartmental fluid shifts. It is important to know that dogs with AHDS consistently have low to low-normal rectal temperature. Pyrexia is an unusual clinical presentation in dogs with AHDS and should raise concerns for the presence of another infectious agent (eg, *Salmonella* spp), translocation of bacteria from the GI tract to the systemic circulation (septicemia), or a strong inflammatory reaction involving other organs (eg, pancreatitis) [9,11]. Despite the severe lesions in the intestinal tract of dogs with AHDS, significant abdominal pain is usually not present on physical examination.

Although substantial lesions are present in the entire intestinal tract of dogs with AHDS and hematemesis and/or AHD are observed, blood loss is usually minor in proportion to fluid loss [4]. As a result, dogs with AHDS characteristically have an increased packed cell volume at presentation, with a median packed cell volume of 57% and a range of 33% to 76% described in one study [9]. A packed cell volume in the normal and greater than the normal range is helpful to differentiate this form of hemorrhagic enteritis from true GI bleeding, in which anemia is usually present. The presence of anemia at presentation in a dog with hemorrhagic diarrhea is always indicative of a true intestinal bleed (eg, hemostatic disorders, ulceration, intestinal neoplasia).

C perfringens is an enterotoxigenic pathogen that causes significant necrosis of the intestinal mucosa but is not invasive. Translocation of bacteria through the damaged intestinal mucosa can usually be compensated for despite the significant loss of the epithelial integrity [13]. Leukogram changes, which reflect systemic bacterial infection or septicemia/sepsis, such as significant neutrophilia ($>25 \times 10^{12}/L$) or neutropenia and a severely increased number of band neutrophils ($>2.5 \times 10^{12}/L$), is not observed in dogs with an uncomplicated form of AHDS. A mild left shift is seen in about 50% of dogs, which most likely reflects the increased demand of neutrophils for the first-line defense at the surface of the destroyed intestinal mucosa [9]. Presence of an inflammatory leukogram characterized by a significant elevation of mature neutrophils and/or banded neutrophils in contrast to a stress leukogram in any dog with AHD should always prompt a search for other causes of AHD or suspicion of another enteropathogenic, enteroinvasive bacterial infection.

Neutropenia should also raise the suspicion of canine parvovirus infection, especially if the dog is young and/or inadequately vaccinated [14]. Severe GI tract hemorrhage is also described in dogs with hypoadrenocorticism [15,16]. Therefore, a basal serum cortisol concentration is generally useful in every dog with unexplained hemorrhagic diarrhea to rule out hypoadrenocorticism, but is mandatory in dogs with history of recurrent episodes of acute diarrhea, depression, and weakness and with the absence of a stress leukogram, lymphocytosis, and eosinophilia or characteristic electrolyte changes (eg, hyperkalemia, hyponatremia).

Although few dogs have low serum albumin concentration at presentation, some dogs show a significant hypoalbuminemia after fluid resuscitation. Albumin levels should especially be monitored in dogs that have a decreased or low-normal level initially and in dogs with peripheral edema and body cavity effusions because they might require colloid osmotic support with fresh frozen plasma (small breed dogs) or albumin solutions (large breed dogs). Azotemia is only rarely observed in dogs with AHDS despite the presence of severe dehydration. Therefore, it is important to determine urine specific gravity before fluid administration to differentiate between prerenal and renal azotemia if present. Alkaline phosphatase activity is usually normal in dogs with AHDS, whereas alanine aminotransferase activity is increased in about 20% of the cases. This is most likely secondary hepatocellular damage caused by decreased hepatic perfusion during hypovolemia. Because dogs with primary acute liver failure can also present with AHD, it is important to attempt differentiating primary liver disease from reactive hepatopathy by reevaluating alanine aminotransferase, total bilirubin, and serum bile acids 3 to 5 days after rehydration. Alanine aminotransferase usually drops by about 50% and total bilirubin and serum bile acids normalize in secondary hepatopathies, such as AHDS (personal observation Unterer). Serum lactate elevation reflects the severity of hypovolemia and reduced peripheral perfusion and is hence an unspecific finding [9].

RECENT DISCOVERIES

In August and November 2019 an outbreak of AHD was observed in dogs living in the Oslo region of Norway. Hundreds of dogs were affected, and many dogs died across Norway. At the beginning of the outbreak a presumptive diagnosis of idiopathic AHDS had been made because no underlying cause could be identified. However, three arguments speak against an AHDS diagnosis: (1) AHDS is a syndrome affecting individual dogs and is not a transmissible disease, as suspected/documented in Oslo; (2) AHDS has a low mortality rate and this is in contrast to the high number of fatal cases during the outbreak; and (3) one major finding was the positive fecal culture results of *Providencia alcalifaciens* with 100% sequence identity in different affected dogs. *P alcalifaciens* is a gram-negative bacterium, which was not a part of the normal dog fecal microbiota in the time before the outbreak. It was concluded from this study that the increased abundance of *P alcalifaciens* in dogs with AHD relative to healthy dogs might explain the unexpectedly high numbers of dogs suffering from a severe form of AHDS during this outbreak. Transmission of *P alcalifaciens* may have triggered the concurrent outgrowths of *C perfringens* in a dysbiotic background microbiota [17]. However, a recent unpublished observational case-control study shows that *P alcalifaciens* can also be found in dogs with acute nonhemorrhagic diarrhea and that these dogs are not more severely affected, needing more aggressive treatment or having a worse prognosis than dogs with acute nonhemorrhagic diarrhea in which this pathogen was not isolated (personal communication Dr S. Salavati). Hence, the pathologic significance of *P alcalifaciens* remains unclear.

A recently published study showed a 28% prevalence of chronic GI signs in dogs with a previous episode of AHDS, which was significantly higher compared with an age and breed matched control group with a prevalence of 14% [2]. It is speculated that because of destruction of the epithelial mucosal barrier an increased number of food antigens and bacteria can pass the intestinal barrier and influence the immune system. A subset of dogs with a high AHDS-index (>9) have significantly increased intestinal permeability, as assessed by iohexol [18]. In these dogs, small proteins and allergens crossing the epithelial barrier might trigger a breakdown of oral tolerance to specific food components [19].

It is also known that the physiologic composition and diversity of the intestinal bacterial communities is essential to prevent the development of allergic and immune-mediated diseases [20]. Thus, dysbiosis typically characterized by a significant clostridial overgrowth associated with reduced abundances of *Blautia*, *Turicibacter*, *Faecalibacterium*, and *Streptococcus* spp in dogs with AHDS might represent an additional factor for the increased risk for long-term consequences of acute enteritis [21].

DIAGNOSTIC STRATEGY AND MONITORING

A diagnosis can reliably be made based on GI biopsies when *C perfringens* is observed on the necrotic surface, because *C perfringens* attached to the intestinal mucosal is not seen [4,8] in either healthy dogs or in dogs with any other GI disease. However, because of the potential risk for the patient, financial expense, and lack of therapeutic consequence, a gastroduodenoscopy and colonoscopy are not recommended for the diagnosis of AHDS. Instead, noninvasive tests are preferred, but unfortunately, they all have limitations.

Fecal culture positive for *Clostridium* spp is not diagnostic for AHDS, because many clostridial strains are found in feces of healthy dogs [22]. Most fecal PCRs for clostridial toxin genes, such as CPE or α-toxin, are not helpful for the diagnosis of AHDS. Detecting CPE protein in feces based on enzyme-linked immunosorbent assay also does not confirm the diagnosis, because only up to 30% of dogs with AHDS, but also 14% of healthy dogs, can test positive according to one report [23]. Other tests, such as increases in fecal inflammatory or "leakage" markers (eg, calprotectin, S100A12, α1-proteinase inhibitor), reflect intestinal damage, but these parameters are not specific for AHDS and are unhelpful to guide treatment or prognosis [24].

A positive PCR for *C perfringens* type A strains, which encode for the pore-forming toxin NetF, supports the diagnosis of AHDS [6]. However, because fecal NetF toxin expression decreases rapidly, dogs presenting late in the course of the disease can test negative [7]. Hence, in many dogs, diagnosis of AHDS is still based on clinical observations and exclusion of other known causes of AHD.

Taking a thorough history is essential to rule out the ingestion of toxins or drugs that might cause mucosal irritation, or a previous event that may have caused intestinal damage (eg, severe hypotension or heat stroke). Fecal examinations, including flotation and giardia antigen enzyme-linked immunosorbent assay, should be used to identify parasites, which although rarely solely responsible for such severe GI signs, may contribute to the clinical course. Hemoconcentration is a typical finding in AHDS, which is characterized by GI fluid loss rather than true GI bleeding. A routine serum biochemistry profile is necessary to exclude hepatic and renal disease. Baseline cortisol level should be performed as a standard screening test to rule out hypoadrenocorticism, followed by further endocrine testing if baseline cortisol concentration is less than 2 μg/dL (<55 nmol/L), even if typical electrolyte changes (hyperkalemia, hyponatremia) are not present. Diagnostic imaging, especially abdominal ultrasound, can identify other abnormalities, such as acute pancreatitis or intestinal obstruction (eg, foreign body, intussusception). A recent study showed correlation of C-reactive protein concentrations with the severity of the AHDS on the day of admission, but could not predict the duration of hospitalization or mortality [11]. Additional tests might need to be performed depending on the clinical course, especially if the patient does not significantly improve with fluid therapy or develops pyrexia (Fig. 4).

The AHDS index (Table 1) is a useful tool to assess clinical disease activity and to monitor the clinical course (discussed later) [9,11].

TREATMENT AND CLINICAL COURSE

Severe dehydration caused by vomiting, anorexia, and diarrhea generally requires intravenous (IV) fluid replacement therapy. The peracute and severe onset of the disease, and the frequent presence of paralytic ileus, which can sequester large fluid volumes, may lead to an underestimation of actual fluid loss or requirements. Therefore, frequent reevaluation (every 2–6 hours) of clinical parameters and adjustments of fluid therapy are essential.

Rapid volume replacement with balanced electrolyte solutions by giving a shock bolus as fast as 30 mL/kg over 10 minutes, repeated up to three times, might be needed, followed by continuous replacement of ongoing losses if there is no risk of fluid overload (eg, compromised cardiac function). Usually, patients improve quickly with aggressive fluid resuscitation, which should be continued and adapted until the dog

is able to match losses with voluntary oral intake. This usually takes 2 to 3 days and electrolytes should be measured regularly (every 12–24 hours) during that time.

Some patients suffer from severe protein loss because of gut barrier destruction, which may lead to a reduced intravascular oncotic pressure and subsequent edema and/or ascites. Therefore, serum albumin should be measured initially and after rehydration. In patients with severe hypoalbuminemia (<18 g/L) administration of synthetic colloids, albumin, or plasma should be considered.

In addition, symptomatic treatment comprised of antiemetics (eg, maropitant, 1 mg/kg once a day IV or subcutaneously [SC]; metoclopramide, 0.2–0.5 mg/kg three times a day IV, SC, or orally) and pain medication (eg, metamizole, 30–50 mg/kg three times a day IV, SC, or orally; buprenorphine, 5–20 μg/kg IV or SC) should be administered as needed. Nonsteroidal anti-inflammatory drugs are not recommended because of their propensity to cause further GI injury. The administration of omeprazole is also not indicated in AHDS, because these dogs characteristically do not have gastric bleeding and indeed may even be contraindicated because proton pump inhibitors are suspected to further affect the integrity of the intestinal tight junction complex and might represent an additional factor responsible for intestinal dysbiosis [25].

The general treatment recommendations in several textbooks for AHD include the administration of antimicrobials. The likely rational behind this is that either primary intestinal infection with enteropathogens is difficult to diagnose or the assumption of a compromised intestinal barrier, which is a major risk factor for translocation of commensal bacteria and subsequent septicemia. Approximately half of dogs with AHDS are classified as having systemic inflammatory response syndrome at presentation, based on the criteria defined by de Laforcade and colleagues (2003) [26] and Hauptman and others (1997) [27]. Although most of these abnormalities might be driven by hypovolemia alone, a prospective study conducted by one of the authors showed that the incidence of detectable true bacteremia in dogs with AHDS is low (11%) and not different from healthy control dogs (14%) [13]. The likely conclusion from these observations is that even though bacterial translocation might still occur during AHDS, septicemia is often prevented by effective elimination of bacteria and their toxins from the portal circulation by the liver. We hence presume that risk of septicemia and sepsis is low in dogs with AHDS as long as portal vasculature and hepatic function are

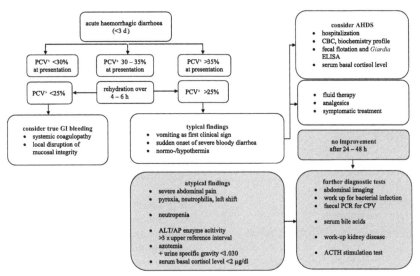

FIG. 4 Summary of the approach to diagnose AHDS and to identify possible complications. ACTH, corticotropin; ALT, alanine aminotransferase; AP, alkaline phosphatase; CBC, complete blood count; CPV, canine parvovirus; ELISA, enzyme-linked immunosorbent assay; PCV, packed cell volume. [a]PCV reference range: 35% to 58%.

not compromised, and patients are otherwise immuno-competent. In addition to this, two independent studies (one an unpublished doctoral thesis) have evaluated the benefit of antibiotics in dogs with AHDS. When using amoxicillin/clavulanic acid in a prospective, placebo-controlled, blinded setup in dogs with AHDS without systemic inflammatory response syndrome, the clinical course (as measured by AHD activity index) and outcome (duration of hospitalization, survival) was not different between the placebo and treatment groups [12]. It was concluded that in dogs with aseptic AHDS, antibiotics may not be necessary as part of treatment [12]. Another study evaluated whether the combination of metronidazole plus amoxicillin-clavulanate is superior to the monoantibiotic therapy with amoxicillin-clavulanate, where again, there was no significant difference in hospitalization time between treatment groups, nor in daily clinical scores. Hence the addition of metronidazole does not confer a clinical benefit when treating even severe cases of hemorrhagic diarrhea in dogs [28]. Based on the available evidence, routine administration of antibiotics is thus not

TABLE 1
Criteria for Assessment of the Canine AHDS Activity Index

Parameter	0	1	2	3
Activity reduction	Not reduced	Mildly	Moderately	Severely reduced
Appetite reduction	Not reduced	Mildly	Moderately	Severely reduced
Vomiting (times/d)	0	1	2–3	>3
Fecal consistency	Normal	Slightly soft	Very soft	Watery diarrhea
Defecation (n/d)	1	2–3	4–5	>5
Dehydration (%)	0	<5	5–10	>10
Total AHDS score	*0–3*	*4–5*	*6–8*	*9 or greater*
Clinical significance of disease	Clinically insignificant	Mild AHDS	Moderate AHDS	Severe AHDS

AHD index is calculated as the sum of the scoring of all the parameters listed in the table. Each parameter is scored from 0–3 on any individual treatment day, and the sum of scores (maximum 18) yield a total cumulative score.

TABLE 2
Indications for Broad-Spectrum Antibiotics in Dogs with Intestinal Disorders

History	
• Immunocompromised patients (eg, hyperadrenocorticism, immunosuppressive treatment, portosystemic shunt)	
Physical examination finding at presentation	
• Hyperthermia (°F/°C)	>103.1/39.5
Physical examination findings after rehydration and pain management	
• Tachycardia (beats/min)	>140 (small breed dogs) >120 (large breed dogs)
• Tachypnea (breaths/min)	>40
• Hypothermia	
• Hypotension	
Hematologic and serum biochemical changes	
• Neutrophilia (cells/µL)	>20,000
• Neutropenia (cells/µL)	<3000
• Band neutrophils (cells/µL)	>2500
• Hypoglycemia (mmol/L)	<3.5

recommended. Not only does routine usage of antibiotics not have a benefit, it can have detrimental effects on the intestinal microbiota, sustaining dysbiosis and promoting the development of multi-resistant bacteria [29,30]. Data from human medicine suggest that dysbiosis induced by antimicrobials is associated with an increased risk for developing asthma, postinfectious irritable bowel disease, and chronic enteropathies such as Crohn disease [31–35]. However, because recognizing septic events and infections with enteropathogens at presentation is challenging, especially when dogs show clinical signs of hypovolemia, close monitoring and assessment of the clinical response to adequate fluid therapy is mandatory in these cases.

Because about one-third of dogs with AHDS develop chronic GI sings, antibiotic-induced dysbiosis might represent one important factor in triggering chronicity. Thus, antibiotics should be used judiciously and be restricted to patients with clinical signs of sepsis, additional immunocompromise, or a reduced capacity to

eliminate bacteria from the portal blood (eg, portosystemic shunt, significant loss of liver function) (Table 2).

In addition to aggressive fluid and symptomatic therapy, early enteral nutrition with a highly digestible diet is important in dogs with AHD, because it promotes enterocyte proliferation and improves intestinal barrier integrity [36,37]. Adding dietary fiber might be useful because it functions as an important substrate for potentially beneficial microbes in the large intestine, and acts as an energy source for colonocytes. In addition, dietary polysaccharides might have a direct impact on the colonic mucus layer, which is important for barrier function and thus prevention of bacteria translocation [38–40]. It has been suggested that restricting the diet to one protein source or even feeding a hydrolyzed diet in the acute phase of diarrhea might help to avoid sensitizing the immune system to a variety of antigens, but there is little evidence for this.

Probiotics have so far not shown to reduce the time of clinical recovery, but a high dose of a probiotic mixture (eg, Slab51 bacterial blend) might be useful to accelerate the normalization of the intestinal microbiota and to displace toxigenic *C perfringens* strains. Bacteria considered as beneficial, such as *Blautia* spp and *Faecalibacterium*, had significantly higher abundance on Day 7 in dogs with AHDS treated with a probiotic compared with placebo. Probiotics might also have a positive long-term impact on the intestinal microbiota, because enterotoxin genes were significantly lower in dogs with AHDS receiving a Slab51 probiotic blend compared with a placebo group after 3 weeks of supplementation [7].

Fecal microbiota transplantation (FMT) is an important treatment modality in people with *Clostridium difficile* infections (CDI). Similar to canine AHDS, CDI is characterized by an overgrowth of clostridial strains and bacterial toxin release causing mucosal lesions. One important difference is the comparatively milder clinical course of AHDS and rapid clinical improvement even of many severe cases with symptomatic treatment only. This is in contrast to human CDI, which can cause significant morbidity, requires aggressive antibiotic treatment, and antibiotic resistance and recurrence even after appropriate antibiotic treatment are common. Therefore, it is not unexpected that although FMT is a successful treatment of primary or recurrent CDI in people, FMT in dogs with AHDS did not have a significant effect on hospitalization times or clinical signs compared with the control treatment group [41–43]. However, the same study showed promising trends of accelerated normalization of the fecal microbiota composition and richness in dogs with AHDS after receiving a single FMT rectally. Rapid improvement of gut homeostasis may have a positive long-term impact on intestinal health in these dogs, but this still needs to be evaluated.

SUMMARY

Several investigations have provided new insight into the pathogenesis and role of bacteria in AHDS. Based on current information, it is assumed that NetF-toxin is likely a major bacterial virulence factor driving this syndrome [5,6]. The trigger for transient clostridial overgrowth is not known and it is possible that AHDS is initiated by different causes (eg, motility changes, nutritional factors, food poisoning) or represents a multifactorial disorder. The peracute loss of intestinal mucosal integrity in AHDS frequently results in a dramatic fluid shift into the intestinal lumen, which requires aggressive treatment. Although response to IV fluid therapy and symptomatic treatments is usually rapid, some dogs might need prolonged fluid and colloid support because of protein loss, whereas antibiotics are rarely needed or beneficial. Development of pyrexia should raise suspicion for an additional underlying disease. Clinicians are advised to be mindful of overzealous antibiotic use in this condition, because of their detrimental effects on the intestinal microbiota, which could possibly predispose to GI problems later in life. AHDS can have long-term impacts in a significant number of dogs [2], mainly an increased risk for chronic GI disorders [2,44–48], which can develop in up to 30% of dogs following an episode of AHDS [19]. Although probiotics and FMT have not been shown to have a positive effect on clinical severity, hospitalization times, or overall outcome in AHDS, they could be important adjunctive treatments that reestablish the defunct microbiota. Future research should hence focus on establishing strategies to prevent chronicity, such as modulation of the intestinal microbiota (eg, FMT, probiotics) or therapeutic agents improving intestinal integrity.

CLINICS CARE POINTS

- In any dog with acute hemorrhagic diarrhea a packed cell volume has to be performed to differentiate between true GI bleeding and hemorrhagic enteritis.
- In young and inadequately vaccinated dogs with acute hemorrhagic diarrhea testing for canine parvovirus infection is mandatory.

- When dogs with acute hemorrhagic diarrhea have a history of episodes with lethargy or vague and nonspecific clinical problems, check a serum basal cortisol level to rule out hypoadrenocorticism.
- When albumin levels are already low initially at the time of presentation do not forget to reassess this parameter after fluid resuscitation to identify those dogs that may require colloids, plasma, or albumin solutions.
- If there is evidence of hypovolemia, such as lethargy, weakness, tachycardia, prolonged capillary refill time, and weak pulse pressure, a rapid volume replacement through a large-bore IV catheter is required.
- Do not administer antibiotics routinely, but in dogs with AHDS and signs of systemic infection, immunosuppression, and reduced liver function, and in dogs inadequately responding to symptomatic therapy, antibiotic treatment might be indicated/necessary.

DISCLOSURE

The authors mentioned the study Ziese AL, Suchodolski JS, Hartmann K, et al. Effect of probiotic treatment on the clinical course, intestinal microbiome, and toxigenic Clostridium perfringens in dogs with acute hemorrhagic diarrhea. *PLoS One* 2018;13:e0204691. Anna Lena Ziese was working with us and in this study the probiotic (trade name Vivomixx) was provided by the company MENDES S.A. (Via Giacometti, 1, 6900 Lugano Switzerland). Anna Lena Ziese received travel support from MENDES S.A. to travel to an international conference. However, this support does not influence the data of this review article. In addition to this disclosure, the authors have nothing to disclose.

REFERENCES

[1] Hackett TB. Gastrointestinal complications of critical illness in small animals. Vet Clin North Am Small Anim Pract 2011;41(4):759–66, vi.

[2] Skotnitzki E, Suchodolski JS, Busch K, et al. Frequency of signs of chronic gastrointestinal disease in dogs after an episode of acute hemorrhagic diarrhea. J Vet Intern Med 2022;36(1):59–65.

[3] Prescott JF, Johnson JA, Patterson JM, et al. Haemorrhagic gastroenteritis in the dog associated with *Clostridium welchii*. Vet Rec 1978;103(6):116–7.

[4] Leipig-Rudolph M, Busch K, Prescott JF, et al. Intestinal lesions in dogs with acute hemorrhagic diarrhea syndrome associated with netF-positive *Clostridium perfringens* type A. J Vet Diagn Invest 2018;30(4):495–503.

[5] Mehdizadeh Gohari I, Parreira VR, Nowell VJ, et al. A novel pore-forming toxin in type A Clostridium perfringens is associated with both fatal canine hemorrhagic gastroenteritis and fatal foal necrotizing enterocolitis. PLoS One 2015;10(4):e0122684.

[6] Sindern N, Suchodolski JS, Leutenegger CM, et al. Prevalence of Clostridium perfringens netE and netF toxin genes in the feces of dogs with acute hemorrhagic diarrhea syndrome. J Vet Intern Med 2019;33(1):100–5.

[7] Ziese AL, Suchodolski JS, Hartmann K, et al. Effect of probiotic treatment on the clinical course, intestinal microbiome, and toxigenic Clostridium perfringens in dogs with acute hemorrhagic diarrhea. PLoS One 2018; 13(9):e0204691.

[8] Unterer S, Busch K, Leipig M, et al. Endoscopically visualized lesions, histologic findings, and bacterial invasion in the gastrointestinal mucosa of dogs with acute hemorrhagic diarrhea syndrome. J Vet Intern Med 2014;28(1): 52–8.

[9] Mortier F, Strohmeyer K, Hartmann K, et al. Acute haemorrhagic diarrhoea syndrome in dogs: 108 cases. Vet Rec 2015;176(24):627.

[10] Allen-Deal A, Lewis D. Prevalence of Clostridium perfringens alpha toxin and enterotoxin in the faeces of dogs with acute haemorrhagic diarrhoea syndrome. J Small Anim Pract 2021;62(5):373–8.

[11] Dupont N, Jessen LR, Moberg F, et al. A retrospective study of 237 dogs hospitalized with suspected acute hemorrhagic diarrhea syndrome: disease severity, treatment, and outcome. J Vet Intern Med 2021;35(2): 867–77.

[12] Unterer S, Strohmeyer K, Kruse BD, et al. Treatment of aseptic dogs with hemorrhagic gastroenteritis with amoxicillin/clavulanic acid: a prospective blinded study. J Vet Intern Med 2011;25(5):973–9.

[13] Unterer S, Lechner E, Mueller RS, et al. Prospective study of bacteraemia in acute haemorrhagic diarrhoea syndrome in dogs. Vet Rec 2015;176(12):309.

[14] Schnelle AN, Barger AM. Neutropenia in dogs and cats: causes and consequences. Vet Clin North Am Small Anim Pract 2012;42(1):111–22.

[15] Busch K, Wehner A, Dorsch R, et al. [Acute haemorrhagic diarrhoea as a presenting sign in a dog with primary hypoadrenocorticism]. Tierarztl Prax Ausg K Kleintiere Heimtiere 2014;42(5):326–30, Akuter blutiger Durchfall als Vorstellungsgrund bei einem Hund mit primärem Hypoadrenokortizismus.

[16] Medinger TL, Williams DA, Bruyette DS. Severe gastrointestinal tract hemorrhage in three dogs with hypoadrenocorticism. J Am Vet Med Assoc 1993;202(11):1869–72.

[17] Herstad KMV, Trosvik P, Haaland AH, et al. Changes in the fecal microbiota in dogs with acute hemorrhagic diarrhea during an outbreak in Norway. J Vet Intern Med 2021. https://doi.org/10.1111/jvim.16201.

[18] Reisinger A SH, Ishii P, Suchodolski J, Unterer S, Steiner J, Lidbury JA, Hartmann K, Busch K. Iohexol as marker of intestinal barrier dysfunction in dogs with acute

hemorrhagic diarrhea syndrome. presented at: ACVIM Forum; 2022; June 23-25 in Austin, Texas.

[19] Wesemann DR, Nagler CR. The microbiome, timing, and barrier function in the context of allergic disease. Immunity 2016;44(4):728–38.

[20] Plunkett CH, Nagler CR. The influence of the microbiome on allergic sensitization to food. J Immunol 2017;198(2):581–9.

[21] Suchodolski JS, Markel ME, Garcia-Mazcorro JF, et al. The fecal microbiome in dogs with acute diarrhea and idiopathic inflammatory bowel disease. PLoS One 2012;7(12):e51907.

[22] Marks SL, Rankin SC, Byrne BA, et al. Enteropathogenic bacteria in dogs and cats: diagnosis, epidemiology, treatment, and control. J Vet Intern Med 2011;25(6): 1195–208.

[23] Busch K, Suchodolski JS, Kuhner KA, et al. Clostridium perfringens enterotoxin and Clostridium difficile toxin A/B do not play a role in acute haemorrhagic diarrhoea syndrome in dogs. Vet Rec 2015;176(10):253.

[24] Heilmann RM, Guard MM, Steiner JM, et al. Fecal markers of inflammation, protein loss, and microbial changes in dogs with the acute hemorrhagic diarrhea syndrome (AHDS). J Vet Emerg Crit Care (San Antonio) 2017;27(5):586–9.

[25] Konig J, Wells J, Cani PD, et al. Human intestinal barrier function in health and disease. Clin Transl Gastroenterol 2016;7(10):e196.

[26] de Laforcade AM, Freeman LM, Shaw SP, et al. Hemostatic changes in dogs with naturally occurring sepsis. J Vet Intern Med 2003;17(5):674–9.

[27] Hauptman JG, Walshaw R, Olivier NB. Evaluation of the sensitivity and specificity of diagnostic criteria for sepsis in dogs. Vet Surg 1997;26(5):393–7.

[28] Ortiz V, Klein L, Channell S, et al. Evaluating the effect of metronidazole plus amoxicillin-clavulanate versus amoxicillin-clavulanate alone in canine haemorrhagic diarrhoea: a randomised controlled trial in primary care practice. J Small Anim Pract 2018;59(7):398–403.

[29] Werner M, Suchodolski JS, Straubinger RK, et al. Effect of amoxicillin-clavulanic acid on clinical scores, intestinal microbiome, and amoxicillin-resistant Escherichia coli in dogs with uncomplicated acute diarrhea. J Vet Intern Med 2020;34(3):1166–76.

[30] Torres-Henderson C, Summers S, Suchodolski J, et al. Effect of Enterococcus faecium strain SF68 on gastrointestinal signs and fecal microbiome in cats administered amoxicillin-clavulanate. Top Companion Anim Med 2017; 32(3):104–8.

[31] Kummeling I, Stelma FF, Dagnelie PC, et al. Early life exposure to antibiotics and the subsequent development of eczema, wheeze, and allergic sensitization in the first 2 years of life: the KOALA Birth Cohort Study. Pediatrics 2007;119(1):e225–31.

[32] Metsala J, Lundqvist A, Virta LJ, et al. Prenatal and postnatal exposure to antibiotics and risk of asthma in childhood. Clin Exp Allergy 2015;45(1):137–45.

[33] Klem F, Wadhwa A, Prokop LJ, et al. Prevalence, risk factors, and outcomes of irritable bowel syndrome after infectious enteritis: a systematic review and meta-analysis. Gastroenterology 2017;152(5):1042–54.e1.

[34] Umamaheswari B, Biswal N, Adhisivam B, et al. Persistent diarrhea: risk factors and outcome. Indian J Pediatr 2010;77(8):885–8.

[35] Ungaro R, Bernstein CN, Gearry R, et al. Antibiotics associated with increased risk of new-onset Crohn's disease but not ulcerative colitis: a meta-analysis. Am J Gastroenterol 2014;109(11):1728–38.

[36] Will K, Nolte I, Zentek J. Early enteral nutrition in young dogs suffering from haemorrhagic gastroenteritis. J Vet Med A Physiol Pathol Clin Med 2005;52(7):371–6.

[37] Mohr AJ, Leisewitz AL, Jacobson LS, et al. Effect of early enteral nutrition on intestinal permeability, intestinal protein loss, and outcome in dogs with severe parvoviral enteritis. J Vet Intern Med 2003;17(6):791–8.

[38] Desai MS, Seekatz AM, Koropatkin NM, et al. A dietary fiber-deprived gut microbiota degrades the colonic mucus barrier and enhances pathogen susceptibility. Cell 2016;167(5):1339–53.e21.

[39] Li N, Zheng B, Cai HF, et al. Cost-effectiveness analysis of oral probiotics for the prevention of Clostridium difficile-associated diarrhoea in children and adolescents. J Hosp Infect 2018;99(4):469–74.

[40] Vernocchi P, Del Chierico F, Fiocchi AG, et al. Understanding probiotics' role in allergic children: the clue of gut microbiota profiling. Curr Opin Allergy Clin Immunol 2015;15(5):495–503.

[41] Gal A, Barko PC, Biggs PJ, et al. One dog's waste is another dog's wealth: a pilot study of fecal microbiota transplantation in dogs with acute hemorrhagic diarrhea syndrome. PLoS One 2021;16(4):e0250344.

[42] Keithlin J, Sargeant J, Thomas MK, et al. Systematic review and meta-analysis of the proportion of Campylobacter cases that develop chronic sequelae. BMC Public Health 2014;14:1203.

[43] Ajene AN, Fischer Walker CL, Black RE. Enteric pathogens and reactive arthritis: a systematic review of Campylobacter, Salmonella and Shigella-associated reactive arthritis. J Health Popul Nutr 2013;31(3):299–307.

[44] Kilian E, Suchodolski JS, Hartmann K, et al. Long-term effects of canine parvovirus infection in dogs. PLoS One 2018;13(3):e0192198.

[45] Sato-Takada K, Flemming AM, Voordouw MJ, et al. Parvovirus enteritis and other risk factors associated with persistent gastrointestinal signs in dogs later in life: a retrospective cohort study. BMC Vet Res 2022;18(1):96.

[46] Francino MP. Antibiotics and the human gut microbiome: dysbioses and accumulation of resistances. Front Microbiol 2015;6:1543.

[47] Stefka AT, Feehley T, Tripathi P, et al. Commensal bacteria protect against food allergen sensitization. Proc Natl Acad Sci U S A 2014;111(36):13145–50.

[48] Zheng D, Liwinski T, Elinav E. Interaction between microbiota and immunity in health and disease. Cell Res 2020;30(6):492–506.

SECTION IV: INFECTIOUS DISEASE

Advances in Small Animal Care 3 (2022) 145–159

ADVANCES IN SMALL ANIMAL CARE

Feline Immunodeficiency Virus

Current Knowledge and Future Directions

Paweł M. Bęczkowski, DVM, PhD, Dip. ECVIM-CA, MRCVS[a],*,
Julia A. Beatty, BVetMed, PhD, FANZCVS (Feline med), GradCertEd (Higher Ed), FRCVS, GAICD[a,b]

[a]Department of Veterinary Clinical Sciences, Jockey Club College of Veterinary Medicine and Life Sciences, City University of Hong Kong, Tat Chee Avenue, Kowloon, Hong Kong; [b]Centre for Animal Health and Welfare, Jockey Club College of Veterinary Medicine and Life Sciences, City University of Hong Kong, Tat Chee Avenue, Kowloon, Hong Kong

---

KEYWORDS

- Retrovirus • Lentivirus • Immunodeficiency • Viral diversity • Receptor usage • CD134 • CXCR4 • Vaccine

KEY POINTS

- Clinical outcomes in FIV-infected cats are variable and poorly defined. The immunodeficiency that accompanies infection can, and often does, remain subclinical.
- FIV infection is lifelong. Serology is the first-line diagnostic test to identify infected cats. PCR is available for confirmation if required.
- Viral, host, and environmental factors that influence prognosis in individual FIV-infected cats are unclear. Reliable surrogate markers to predict clinical progression are not available.
- Key to the management of FIV-infected cats is preventive health care and early detection and investigation of clinical problems.
- A commercial FIV vaccine is available in only a few regions including Australia, New Zealand, and Japan. Interference with diagnostic testing by the commercial FIV vaccine is largely resolved, but vaccine efficacy in the field remains questionable. FIV vaccination is classified as noncore by WSAVA Vaccination Guidelines Group.

INTRODUCTION

Overview

Feline immunodeficiency virus (FIV) is a ubiquitous pathogen of domestic cats. Transmission occurs primarily via biting during territorial fights and results in persistent lifelong infection. Although progressive decline of CD4+T cells is a hallmark of FIV infection, clinical manifestations in naturally infected cats are often inapparent. Many infected cats have treatable medical problems that are common in cats irrespective of their retroviral status. In those cats that do develop immunodeficiency-associated diseases, it is often difficult to assign clinical relevance to their FIV status. The initial diagnosis is based on detection of circulating antibodies to the viral capsid protein p24. Although different strains of FIV circulate among wild Felidae and Hyaenidae, the virus presents no known zoonotic risk.

Background

FIV was first isolated from cats in 1986 during the height of the human immunodefiency virus (HIV)-AIDS pandemic in the Western world, at a time when licensed HIV treatments were not yet available. This historical context provides insight into the intensity of the research effort that has been focused on FIV. FIV causes

---

The authors have no conflicts of interest to declare that are relevant to the content of this article.

*Corresponding author, E-mail address: pbeczkow@cityu.edu.hk

https://doi.org/10.1016/j.yasa.2022.05.007
2666-450X/22/

immunodeficiency in infected cats that closely resembles that seen in human HIV infection. Hence experimental infection of cats with FIV was widely adopted as a model to develop an HIV vaccine. This research program provided new tools to investigate the feline immune response, which benefited our understanding greatly. A commercial FIV vaccine became available 2 decades ago, but this vaccine has limited availability and its efficacy in the field is poor.

In the 35 years since the discovery of FIV, it has become apparent that the immunodeficiency that accompanies natural infection is often subclinical, contrasting starkly with the predictable decline to terminal AIDS in untreated HIV-infected patients. Perhaps the area in greatest need of research is the outcomes associated with natural FIV infection. Which cats progress and why? Which features of the infecting virus, the individual cat, or the environment contribute to clinical outcome? Can we predict the outcome in an individual cat? Are we recognizing subtle or unexpected consequences of FIV infection?

THE VIRUS
Discovery and Origins
- FIV was discovered in Petaluma, California, USA in 1986 in group-housed cats displaying signs suggesting an underlying immunodeficiency [1].
- FIV originated among wild felids in Africa between 5 and 2.5 million years ago, disseminated through the Panthera lineage and ancestors of the African lion, then globally among New World cats as species-specific strains [2].
  - FIV-Fca (the FIV strain infecting domestic cats, *Felis catus)*, as inferred by comparative genomic analyses, has a more recent evolutionary origin, having been in coexistence with its host for much shorter period than FIV strains infecting wild cats (eg, FIV-Pca, FIV-Ppa).
- FIV is genetically more closely related to ungulate retroviruses (equine infectious anemia virus, bovine immunodeficiency virus, caprine arthritis and encephalitis virus), but resembles primate lentiviruses in its ability to cause a clinical immunodeficiency [1].

Virion Structure and Genomic Organization
- FIV belongs to the family Retroviridae, subfamily Orthoretrovirinae, genus *Lentivirus.*
- The FIV virion is an enveloped, spherical particle that contains 2 copies of a positive-stranded RNA within the viral core (Fig. 1).

- The genome contains approximately 9400 nucleotides comprising 3 major genes: *gag, pol,* and *env* [3] (Fig. 2).
  - Additional accessory and regulatory genes (*vif, orf-A,* and *rev*) have a role in viral replication, trafficking of viral RNA from the nucleus to cytosol, virus release, and defense against host restriction factors.
- The envelope bears heavily glycosylated proteins (Env) that interact with cellular receptor for the virus. Mutations within the *env* gene facilitate immune evasion [4].

Viral Diversity on the Population Level
- FIV-Fca forms a phylogenetically diverse group of viruses distributed among domestic cats worldwide [2]. Based on sequence diversity of a highly variable V3-V5 region of *env,* FIV is classified into 5 subtypes (clades), A to E [5]. Diversity can reach 26% between isolates and likely reflects independent viral coevolution in different geographic areas (Fig. 3).
- Clinical significance of specific subtypes has not been determined in natural infections. There is no convincing evidence that one subtype is more pathogenic than the other.
- Genetic diversity is generated by point mutations, introduced by an error-prone reverse transcriptase (RT) and recombination between viral variants [6,7].
  - Recombination can occur between viral variants of the same or different subtypes. Recombination is facilitated by the (1) presence of 2 RNA molecules within each virion and (2) the ability of RT to switch between the 2 RNA genomes during provirus formation.
  - Concurrent infection of the host with different strains of the virus may lead to the emergence of novel variants with altered properties such as pathogenicity or infectivity.

Intrahost Viral Diversity and Intrahost Evolution
- FIV exists within the host as closely related variants referred to as viral quasi-species that collectively contribute to the characteristics of the viral population [8].
- The intrahost diversity and rate of intrahost evolution of FIV *env* is relatively low when compared with that of HIV [7].
- When contrasted with pathogenic and rapidly evolving human HIV counterparts, and compared with less pathogenic bovine immunodeficiency virus (BIV), which exhibits little sequence variation [9],

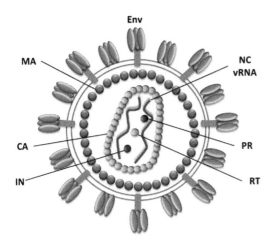

FIG. 1 Schematic representation of FIV virion. The virion is a spherical particle of approximately 120 nm in diameter. The virion contains 2 copies of single-stranded, positive-sense viral RNA (vRNA) surrounded by the nucleocapsid (NC), p24 capsid (CA), matrix (MA), and heavily glycosylated envelope glycoprotein (Env). Reverse transcriptase (RT), integrase (IN), and protease (PR) enzymes are responsible for DNA synthesis from viral RNA, integration of proviral DNA into the DNA of the host cell, and cleavage of precursor protein products, respectively.

the relative genetic stability of FIV likely reflects a long period of coexistence between the virus and the host; this may contribute to lower pathogenicity and explain why many FIV-infected cats do not progress to the terminal-stage disease [7].

EPIDEMIOLOGY
Prevalence
- FIV is distributed globally with a seroprevalence ranging between less than 2.5 and greater than 14% [10].
- Risk factors for FIV seropositivity are presented in Table 1.

- Average age at the time of diagnosis is 6 years, with male cats being almost 5 times more likely to be seropositive than females [11].

Transmission
- Horizontal transmission via inoculation of virus in saliva or blood during aggressive territorial fights is predominant [12].
- Vertical, perinatal, and postnatal queen to kitten transmission is rarely documented, unless the queen becomes infected during pregnancy [13].
  - Perinatal infection of 1 kitten does not imply infection of the whole litter.
- Virus can be isolated from semen, but natural sexual transmission of FIV has not been documented [14].
- Transmission of FIV among naturally infected cats cohabiting in stable households is infrequent [15].
- Cats used as blood donors must be free from FIV infection because iatrogenic transmission by this route is inevitable [16].

PATHOGENESIS
Cell Tropism
- Infection commences with binding of the viral Env to the viral receptor on susceptible cells.
  - FIV preferentially targets CD4+ T cells, CD4+CD25 regulatory T cells, macrophages, monocytes, neuroglia, CD8+ T cells, and B cells.
  - The virus uses feline CD134 as its primary receptor [17] and CXCR4 as a coreceptor [18].
  - CD134 is expressed on feline CD4+ T lymphocytes consistent with progressive depletion of CD4+ lymphocytes during disease progression [17].
  - Structurally, the extracellular domain of CD134 is composed of 3 cysteine-rich domains (CRD-1, CRD-2, and CRD-3) (Fig. 4).
  - Understanding the structure of CD134 is important in deciphering the nature of virus-host interaction, because different strains of FIV have

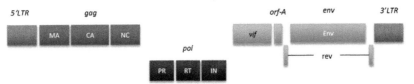

FIG. 2 Genomic organization of FIV (simplified). The genome consists of 3 major genes: (1) *gag*, which encodes core proteins: matrix (MA), capsid (CA, p24), and nucleocapsid (NC); (2) *pol*, which encodes key enzymes: integrase (IN), protease (PR), and reverse transcriptase (RT); and (3) *env*, which encodes envelope glycoprotein (Env), one regulatory (*rev*), and 2 accessory genes (*vif, orf-a*). The genes are bordered by long terminal repeats (LTRs) within the provirus.

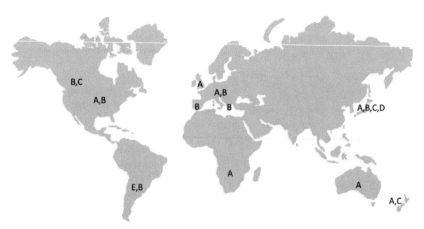

FIG. 3 Global distribution of FIV subtypes. Subtype A is most prevalent in the Australia, United Kingdom, South Africa, the west coast of the United States, and some parts of Japan. Subtype B has been identified in cats in southern Europe, Brazil, Canada, the United States, and Japan. Subtype C has been isolated in New Zealand and Canada. Subtypes D and E have been described only in Japan and Argentina.

different affinity for the primary entry receptor [19] (see Fig. 4).

○ Some strains of the virus (often referred as "early" variants), require stringent interaction with determinants on both cysteine-rich domains (CRD-1 and CRD-2) of CD134 to achieve productive infection [20]. In contrast, "late" variants can infect susceptible cells via interaction with a first cysteine-rich domain (CRD-1) alone [20].

○ Data from experimental [20] and natural infections [21] reveal that the virus changes the way it interacts with its primary receptor during the course of disease, similar to the receptor switch observed during progression of HIV infection [22].

○ In naturally infected cats, CRD-2-dependent viral variants dominate in early infection, and evolve toward CRD-2 independence during disease progression (late infection) [21].

○ Emergence of "late," CRD-2 independent viral variants segregates with declining clinical status and onset of immunodeficiency [21,23].

Correlates of Immune Protection

FIV infection elicits a robust innate immune response, followed by cell-mediated and humoral adaptive responses. However, sterilizing immunity is not achieved and persistent infection is established. Subsequent progressive depletion of CD4+ lymphocytes and paradoxic global immune activation and immune suppression leads to immune dysfunction [24].

• Cell-mediated immunity is governed by cytotoxic CD8+ T lymphocytes (CTLs). This immunity develops within weeks postexposure and is responsible for the subsequent decline in plasma viral load seen during the "asymptomatic" stage of infection [25,26].

○ The antiviral activity of CD8+ T cells is mediated through (a) noncytotoxic, non-antigen-specific CD8+ T cells [26] and (b) major histocompatibility complex (MHC) class I-restricted CTLs [27].

■ Nonspecific CD8+ T cells appear approximately 1 week postexposure and target the virus via contact-dependent or contact-independent noncytotoxic mechanisms.

TABLE 1
Risk Factors for Feline Immunodeficiency Virus Infection

	High-Risk	Low-Risk
Age	Adult	Young
Sex	Male	Female
Neuter status	Entire	Neutered
Environment	Outdoor	Indoor
Breed	Mixed breed	Pure breed
Health status	Sick	Healthy

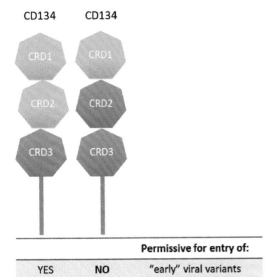

		Permissive for entry of:
YES	NO	"early" viral variants
YES	YES	"late" viral variants

FIG. 4 Schematic representation of the structure of CD134 primary cellular receptor for FIV. CD134 consists of 3 cysteine-rich domains (CRDs) 1 to 3. Some FIV variants (referred as "early"), require stringent interaction with determinants on both cysteine-rich domains (CRD-1 and CRD-2) of CD134 to achieve productive infection, whereas others (referred as "late") are able to infect susceptible cells via interaction with a first cysteine-rich domain (CRD-1) alone. During progression of natural infection, FIV changes the way it interacts with CD134. Emergence of "late" CRD-2-independent variants coincides with decreasing numbers of CD4+ T cells and declining clinical status [21,23].

- Typical MHC class I-restricted CD8+ T cells are primed against specific viral proteins (Gag, Pol, and Env) and are detectable as early as 2 weeks postexposure.
  ○ CD8+ T-cell numbers increase throughout infection and decline only at the terminal stage [24].
- Humoral, B-cell-mediated immunity elicited against Gag and Env viral proteins, and manifested by increased IgG immunoglobulin plasma levels, is detectable within 2 to 4 weeks postinfection [28,29].
  ○ Additional immunity is provided by virus neutralizing antibodies (VNAbs), which, although detectable within 30 days postinfection, take several months to fully develop [30].
    ■ VNAbs' interaction with epitopes on the Env interferes with, or blocks, cellular entry of the virus, thus preventing the infection (antibody-mediated viral neutralization).

- Autoantibodies against the primary receptor for FIV, CD134, provide additional protection against the virus in some infected cats [31].
- Although presence of VNAbs can be beneficial, or at least neutral, antibody-dependent enhancement has also been documented [32].
- Intrinsic immunity represented by cellular-based antiviral restriction factors provides additional protection that controls almost every stage of retroviral life cycle. Intrinsic retroviral restriction factors encoded by the feline genome include APOBEC3G [33] and Tetherin/BST-2 proteins [34].
  ○ APOBEC3G (apolipoprotein B messenger RNA [mRNA]-editing enzyme catalytic polypeptide-like 3 G) operates during reverse transcription causing accumulation of guanosine to adenosine substitutions in a positive-strand viral DNA, subsequent accumulation of premature stop codons and inhibition of viral replication by hypermutation, and degradation of viral genomic material.
  ○ Feline Tetherin/BST-2 retains the FIV virion on the cell surface preventing its release, but not the cell-to-cell spread of the virus.

Despite vigorous responses, innate, intrinsic, and adaptive immunity fail to clear the virus, and FIV infection eventually leads to variable degrees of immune dysfunction. Although depletion of CD4+ T cells plays an important role, long-standing immune activation and impaired regenerative capacity of the bone marrow progenitor cells seems to be equally important in development of immunodeficiency.

The Course of Feline Immunodeficiency Virus Infection and Clinical Signs

Infected cats are often normal on clinical examination, and it can be difficult to assign the significance of retroviral status to presenting clinical signs. Nevertheless, it is plausible to attribute FIV's role in cases with refractory infections, which fail to respond to standard and prolonged therapies. The disease course is characterized by 3 distinct stages [35] (Fig. 5):

- Acute, primary stage, which is defined by a rapid viral replication and subsequent viremia. The virus replicates in CD4+ T cells, macrophages, and dendritic cells. Plasma viral load peaks at 8 to 12 weeks postinfection.
  ○ Transient nonspecific clinical signs such as lethargy, inappetence, and pyrexia may be detected. Generalized lymphadenopathy and

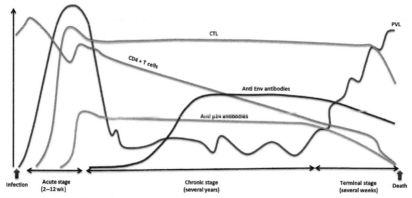

FIG. 5 Clinical course of FIV infection. Following infection, there is an acute stage, which is characterized by peak viral replication. Pyrexia, lymphadenopathy, and other nonspecific clinical signs may coincide. The subsequent robust immune response suppresses viral replication, and infected cats enter the chronic stage of infection. Sometimes referred as "asymptomatic" this stage is accompanied by a sustained cytotoxic T lymphocyte response (CTL), emergence of neutralizing antibodies, suppressed plasma viral load (PVL), and a progressive depletion of CD4+ T cells. It is unknown why some cats remain well in this stage of infection, whereas others progress to profound immunodeficiency and eventually succumb. Env, envelope glycoprotein; p24, viral capsid protein.

neutropenia may occur and persist for several months [12].

○ Rapid depletion of CD4+ T cells and subsequent excessive production of CD8+ T cells results in an inversion of the CD4:CD8 ratio, which is often lifelong.

○ The immune response curtails viral replication but fails to clear virus.

• Silent, subclinical stage with mild or inapparent clinical signs.

○ Plasma viral loads are suppressed.

○ CD4+ T lymphocyte numbers, after an initial rebound, continue to decline progressively.

○ Combination of immunosuppression and immune hyperactivation contributes to FIV-induced immune dysregulation, which variably affects individual cats. Transient nonspecific clinical signs include hyporexia, lethargy, intermittent pyrexia, and lymphadenopathy.

○ Feline chronic gingivostomatitis, which has a complex and multifactorial cause, is frequently seen in infected cats [36,37] (Fig. 6).

○ Declining numbers of CD4+ T cells, and subsequent decreased production of cytokines such as interferon (IFN)-γ, interleukin (IL)-2, IL-10, and IL-12 contribute to impaired immunity and opportunistic infections [38]; more pronounced clinical signs associated with pathogens as documented for *Toxoplasma gondi* [39], and *Listeria*

monocytogenes [40]; and indirect predisposition for neoplasia [41].

○ Owing to incompletely understood reasons, some infected cats remain in this phase for life, whereas others progress to the terminal stage of disease [38].

• Terminal stage is characterized by progressive immune depletion, subsequent escape of the virus from the immune surveillance, and onset of clinical signs compatible with a profound

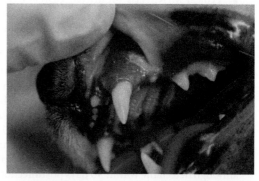

FIG. 6 Feline chronic gingivostomatitis (FCGS). Although not causal, FIV may contribute to the severity of FCGS with infected cats having significant differences in their oral microbiota when compared with uninfected ones [37]. (*Courtesy of* Matthew Oxford, BVM&S GPCert (SAS) MRCVS, Winchester, Hampshire, UK.)

immunodeficiency. Persistent neutropenia is frequently documented [42,43], and increases the risk of atypical and refractory bacterial, viral, fungal, and parasitic infections. Some cats develop neoplasia and neurologic disease.

o Weight loss, resembling HIV-associated "wasting syndrome," is frequently observed [44]. The underlying cause is multifactorial with altered hypermetabolism, cytokine effects, and hyporexia being quoted as the main contributors.

o Concurrent infections include bacterial pyodermas, demodicosis, disseminated cowpox, cryptococcosis, mycobacteriosis, and lungworm [28,45–47]. These infections tend to be more severe and more difficult to treat than in immunocompetent cats.

o Neuropathogenesis is attributed to actions of monocytes and macrophages, which carry the virus across the blood-brain barrier resulting in progressive encephalitis. Stereotypic behavioral and circadian rhythm changes, aggression, tremors, and delayed pupillary light reflexes have all been attributed to FIV-induced neuropathogenesis [48].

o Nephropathy and presence of proteinuria, but not renal azotemia, have been reported [49]. Potential underlying mechanisms include glomerular deposition of viral-antibody immune complexes, direct viral infection of renal epithelial cells, and thrombotic microangiopathy.

o FIV-associated impairment of the antineoplastic immune control capacity and its consequences are the most likely reason why infected cats are 5 to 6 times more likely to develop lymphoma when compared with their FIV-negative counterparts [41].

■ Chronic hyperstimulation of the B-cell compartment is another mechanism rendering cells more prone to neoplastic transformation [50].

■ Furthermore, FIV-induced immune dysregulation may reveal oncogenic potential of other viruses. Any role for recently discovered *Felis catus* gammaherpesvirus 1 in lymphomagenesis in FIV-infected cats remains to be established [51–53].

PROGNOSIS

In contrast to HIV infection, surrogate markers to monitor disease progression or response to treatment are not well established for FIV infection. Although many infected cats achieve similar life spans to their uninfected counterparts [42,43,54], it remains unknown why some cats progress to the terminal-stage disease, whereas others remain asymptomatic.

• In a study examining the long-term outcome of natural retroviral infections, the survival rate for FIV-infected cats at 6 years postdiagnosis was 65%, compared with 90% for uninfected control cats [54]. The decision on euthanasia around the time of diagnosis of FIV infection is one of the main reasons for reported decreased survival of infected cats. In the same study, after exclusions of cats that were euthanized or died within 100 days postdiagnosis, the survival rate for FIV-infected cats at 3 and 6 years was 94% and 80%, respectively, when compared with controls [54].

• There is no justification for euthanasia of healthy cats based on their FIV status.

• CD4:CD8 ratio, a well-established surrogate marker to monitor progression of HIV infection, is not of diagnostic value because no correlation between inversion of CD4:CD8 and disease progression in FIV-infected cats has been found [55,56].

• The plasma viral load is suggested to be a promising prognostic marker [57], but its potential clinical utility remains to be established.

DETECTION AND DIAGNOSIS

The retroviral status of every feline patient should, ideally, be known to improve their individual health care and to prevent spread of the virus to other cats [58]. FIV infection can be diagnosed by (1) serology, followed by (2) polymerase chain reaction (PCR).

• Serologic, point-of-care (POC) screening tests using lateral flow immunochromatography or bidirectional-flow enzyme-linked immunosorbent assay (ELISA) technologies, and laboratory-based ELISA assays that detect antibodies against nucleocapsid, p24 capsid, or Env viral proteins can be reliably used for diagnosis in most cases and are the diagnostic tests of choice [58].

o Although antibodies to the virus can be detected approximately 2 to 4 weeks postexperimental infection [28], in most cases seroconversion occurs within 60 days postexposure [59].

o Maternal-derived antibodies (MDAs) from FIV-infected or vaccinated queens can persist for up to 5 months and could be responsible for false-positive serology results in young kittens [60].

In such cases, cats should be retested after 6 months of age.

- ○ Fel-O-Vax FIV (Boehringer Ingelheim Pty Limited, NSW, Australia) vaccine-induced antibodies can confound the serologic diagnosis and differentiation between infected, vaccinated, and vaccinated and infected cats [61].
  - In cats with prior FIV vaccination history, it is important to select the serologic test that can distinguish between natural infection and vaccine-induced antibodies.
  - The SNAP Combo FeLV Ag/FIV Ab Test (IDEXX Laboratories, Inc, Westbrook, ME, USA) is highly sensitive and specific but does not differentiate between the antibodies induced by natural infection and those induced by the vaccination.
  - Anigen Rapid FIV Ab/FeLV Ag Test Kit (Bionote, Inc, Hwaseong-si, South Korea) and WITNESS FeLV-FIV Test Kit (Zoetis, Inc, Florham Park, NJ, USA) seem to differentiate FIV-infected cats from annually vaccinated cats with 100% specificity [62]. However, caution is still needed in interpretation of those 2 POC test results in cats with a recent history of primary vaccination (3 doses, 2–4 weeks apart). Some immunized cats can potentially return false-positive results up to 22 weeks after receiving the final dose of primary vaccination [62].
- • Additional serologic assays include Western blot and immunofluorescent antibody assay. These assays are technically demanding, potentially less sensitive, and more challenging to interpret than ELISA assays [63].
- • Molecular PCR tests detect integrated DNA provirus or plasma viral RNA.
  - ○ PCR is not recommended as a screening test, but as an adjunct to serology in doubtful situations. PCR can be useful in determination of true FIV status in
    - seropositive cats that have been vaccinated against FIV,
    - seropositive kittens, where presence of anti-FIV MDAs is suspected, and
    - seronegative cats that may have been recently infected but where not enough time has lapsed for seroconversion to occur.
  - ○ Variable performance of FIV PCR tests has been reported [64]. The overall sensitivity has been estimated 5% to 15% lower than that of serologic assays [65].

- ■ Lower sensitivity can be attributed to inability of the primers to detect all field isolates, poor sample quality, and low viral and provirus load [66].

MANAGEMENT OF INFECTED CATS
Environment and Housing Conditions
Predicting the outcome for individual FIV-infected cats is challenging because the relationship between FIV infection and various clinical presentations is unclear.

- • There are several studies that demonstrated that FIV infection does not adversely affect the longevity of infected cats [42,43,67].
- • Housing conditions, appropriate nutrition, and husbandry are crucial to maintain FIV-infected cats in good health [44].
  - ○ Stable, indoor households, are most suitable. Low-density housing not only seems to reduce the risk of disease progression but also lowers the risk of transmission to other cats.
  - ○ Overcrowded shelter conditions, environmental stress, and exposure to infectious agents can have a significant negative impact on FIV-infected cats leading to onset of the terminal-stage disease.
  - ○ Cats should be fed complete, balanced diets matched for the age and nutritional needs imposed by concurrent medical conditions. Raw diets are discouraged to avoid exposure to food-borne infectious diseases.
  - ○ Neutering is crucial in reducing roaming and aggressive behaviors.

HEALTH CARE
Preventive Health Care
FIV-infected cats should ideally undergo a thorough routine clinical examination every 6 to 12 months.

- • Hematology, biochemistry, and full urine analysis should be performed annually [58] and any problems investigated.
- • Routine, ectoparasite and endoparasite prophylaxis, including heartworm control, is crucial.
- • Recommendation for vaccination of immunocompromised cats has been clarified by the most recent ABCD guidelines [68].
  - ○ Booster vaccinations for previously vaccinated FIV-infected cats that live indoors are not recommended.

○ Outdoor cats that are at risk of exposure to infectious diseases should be considered for vaccination, ideally with inactivated formulations classified as "core" vaccines.

- Where surgery is indicated in FIV-infected cats, perioperative antibiotics should be reserved for cats with persistent neutropenia, or those at moderate to high risk of bacterial contamination of the surgical site [69].
- Infected cats should not be hospitalized in isolation wards to minimize their risk of exposure to communicable infectious diseases.
- Given very low environmental persistence, there is a minimal risk of hospital-acquired virus transmission as long as standard biosecurity protocols are followed.

Supportive Treatment

FIV-infected cats often have treatable diseases. As such, their medical problems need to be approached and investigated with this mindset, but a higher consideration is given for differentials concerning ectoparasites and endoparasites, unusual opportunistic infections, and neoplasia.

- The response of FIV-infected cats to medical therapy is often similar to that of negative cats, but more aggressive or a longer course of treatment is sometimes needed. Antibiotic choice, when indicated, needs to be guided by culture and susceptibility results [69].
- Treatment with griseofulvin has been associated with myelosuppression and severe neutropenia [70] in FIV-infected cats.
- Use of glucocorticoids seems counterintuitive, because they have the potential to exacerbate the lentiviral infection. However, their judicious use in some circumstances for treatment of immune-mediated conditions can be beneficial [71].
- Cats diagnosed with lymphoma seem to respond to multiagent chemotherapy in a similar way as retrovirus-negative cats [72]. Cytotoxic treatments should therefore not be discouraged, but patients need to be more closely monitored for chemotherapy-induced myelosuppression.
- Treatment of FIV-associated neutropenia has been attempted with a recombinant human G-CSF (granulocyte colony-stimulation factor) [73]. Although associated with a short-term positive response, G-CSF tends to promote viral replication and enhancement of infection [74]. The safe use of G-CSF is further impeded by development of antibodies to human G-CSF, which could cross-react with endogenous feline G-CSF to cause refractory agranulocytosis [73].

- Although studies in FIV-infected cats are lacking, anemia can be treated with darbepoetin [75], which is less antigenic than previously recommended erythropoietin [74].
- Insulinlike growth factor I (rHuIGF-1) has been shown to stimulate thymic function, and increase the number of circulating T lymphocytes in juvenile experimentally infected cats [76], but there are no studies assessing its efficacy in naturally acquired infections.

Immunomodulatory and Specific Antiviral Therapies

Clear clinical guidelines as when to start immunomodulatory and specific antiretroviral treatments are not available for cats. However, in patients whose health status is clearly adversely affected by FIV infection, and where recurrent infections are persistent despite aggressive conventional therapies, it is reasonable to consider these treatment options. The expectations and potential benefits of antiviral therapies need to be carefully balanced against the risk as well as monetary considerations.

- Interferon therapy has both immunomodulatory and antiviral effects [77–79]. Although in vivo data documenting treatment benefit are limited, IFNs can be considered for some infected cats.
  ○ Recombinant human interferon-α (rHuIFN-α) has been shown to have antiviral activity against FIV *in vitro*. [80] rHuIFN-α can be administered as subcutaneous (SC) injection at 10^4 to 10^6 U/kg every 24 hours. However, within 3 to 7 weeks, treated cats develop anti-human IFN antibodies, rendering rHuIFN-α ineffective [81].
  ○ Recombinant feline interferon-ω (rFeIFN-ω, Virbagen Omega, Virbac) is not antigenic, and prolonged therapy is not associated with any major side effects [82]. rFeIFN-ω can be given at 10^6 U/kg SC every 24 hours on 5 consecutive days for 3 series starting on days 0, 14, and 60. An alternative protocol also exists where rFeIFN-ω is administered orally at 10^5U/cat every 24 hours for 90 consecutive days [83]. Although IFN-ω suppresses FIV replication *in vitro*, [80] its efficacy *in vivo* is much more variable; some studies reported an improvement of clinical scores and laboratory parameters, whereas others failed to demonstrate a clear benefit [80,83,84].

- Antiviral therapies consist of an impressive arsenal of drugs specifically designed for treatment of HIV infection. Although most are either noneffective or toxic for cats, 2 groups: 1) nucleoside analogue reverse transcriptase inhibitors (NARTIs) and 2) receptor antagonists, can be considered for off-license treatment of some infected cats.
  - Zidovudine (3'-azido-2',3'-dideoxythymidine, AZT) has been studied as a potential therapeutic for FIV infection [85–87].
    - Zidovudine, a NARTI, inhibits viral replication *in vitro* and *in vivo*, with resultant decrease in plasma viral load and improvement of clinical status. The recommended dosage is at 5 to 10 mg/kg every 12 hours orally or SC.
    - Zidovudine can lead to myelosuppression. Nonregenerative anemia is one of the most common side effects. Complete blood cell count should be therefore monitored initially every week, and if no concerns are identified during the first month of treatment, once monthly thereafter. In cats that have developed drug-induced anemia, discontinuation of treatment results in a prompt improvement of hematocrit values.
    - Other limiting side effects include gastrointestinal disturbances and anorexia.
    - Although some cats can tolerate treatment beyond 2 years, resistance to zidovudine can develop as early as 6 months after initiation of treatment [88].
  - Receptor antagonists bind to either the cell surface receptor or the virus itself, thus inhibiting the virus receptor interaction and virus entry. Of receptor antagonists identified for HIV, only bicyclams have been investigated as a potential treatment of cats.
    - Plerixafor (1,1'-(1,4-phenylenbismethylene)-bis(1,4,8,11-tetraazacyclotetradecane)-octachlo-ride dehydrate, AMD3100) is a selective CXCR4 antagonist, which is licensed as a stem cell activator for human patients undergoing bone marrow transplant. Plerixafor has been studied *in vitro* and *in vivo* in FIV-infected cats. Based on a study of 40 cats, treatment at 0.5 mg/kg every 12 hours SC for 6 weeks was associated with decreased viral loads and improvement in clinical parameters with no apparent side effects [89].

Chimeric antigen receptor-modified T cells (CAR-T) therapies have been studied extensively, particularly over the last decade, as treatment options for various hemato-oncological diseases [90] and as a cure for HIV-infected humans [91]. The potential of CAR-T to target the virus within latently infected cells, otherwise inaccessible to antiretroviral drugs, offers a promising therapeutic option not only for HIV-infected humans but also for FIV-infected cats and merits further investigation in this species. In summary, when compared with HIV infection where specific, widely available, and relatively safe antiviral therapies can almost completely inhibit viral replication, conclusions on the efficacy and safety of antiretroviral drugs and specific treatment recommendations for FIV infection are more difficult to make. Well-designed, long-term treatment trials, including assessment of novel CAR-T therapies, in naturally infected cats are needed to address this knowledge gap.

VACCINATION

Since its discovery FIV served as a valuable animal model in pursuit of a safe and efficacious lentiviral vaccine. This global research effort culminated in the release of the first commercial FIV vaccine in 2002. The vaccine was licensed in the United States based on 80% efficacy against homologous and heterologous challenge [92]. Twenty years later, multiple studies that examined its efficacy under experimental and field conditions suggest that full protection remains elusive.

Although not what we have hoped for, lessons learned along the way, briefly reviewed in the following points, will inform development of a new generation of vaccines.

- Development of lentiviral vaccine is associated with several major obstacles:
  - Remarkable genetic diversity of the viral *env* gives virus a tremendous populational antigenic plasticity, making it difficult to design one vaccine that would protect against all strains worldwide.
  - Potential superinfection events, error-prone nature of RT, and its propensity for recombination are additional mechanisms indirectly responsible for the enormous plasticity of the virus and resultant immune evasion.
  - The ability of lentiviruses to establish latent infection in nondividing cells, where integrated provirus is inaccessible to the immune system until the cell becomes activated, provides an additional escape mechanism.

○ Vaccine-induced enhancement of infection has been described in multiple studies where prototypic vaccines instead of protecting, render immunized subjects more susceptible to infection [93].

- Multiple studies informed development of a commercial dual subtype inactivated vaccine (Fel-O-Vax FIV).
  ○ The vaccine consists of inactivated FIV Petaluma (clade A) and FIV Shizuoka (clade D)-infected whole cells [92].
  ○ Fel-O-Vax FIV was licensed based on encouraging efficacy data. However, it has been shown that the protection achieved in initial reported studies [94–96] did not extend to experimental challenge with a primary, virulent UK strain of the virus [97]. The vaccine was never licensed in Europe.
  ○ Cats vaccinated against FIV and subsequently diagnosed with infection are reported [98–100]. The efficacy of the vaccine in Australia is estimated at 56% [99].
  ○ The FIV vaccine, which is regarded as "noncore" by the WSAVA, is still available in Australia, New Zealand, and Japan but has been discontinued in North America since 2015.

SUMMARY

Over the last 20 years it has become increasingly evident that the FIV vaccine, which stood behind this unprecedented research effort, is far from being fully efficacious. Lessons learned from the cat helped us to better understand its immune system and the immunodeficiency virus at a level not available for any other feline pathogen. Data gained along the way has influenced our current clinical decision making when approaching FIV-infected patients in a hospital setting. Knowledge of the viral and host factors helps to better understand and substantiate clinical observation that many naturally FIV-infected cats remain healthy and do not progress to terminal disease during their often-normal life spans. Although a safe and fully efficacious lentiviral vaccine is not within our reach yet, the vast knowledge about viral immunology learned from the feline model will inform efforts in the development of next-generation lentiviral vaccines. In the next 20 years, an improved understanding of outcomes in naturally infected cats will assist in designing evidence-based interventions to improve the quality of life of millions of FIV-infected cats worldwide.

CLINICS CARE POINTS

- Interpreting the results of FIV serology requires careful consideration of risk factors identified in patient signalment, history, and physical examination. Repeat serology and/or PCR testing may be indicated for confirmation of FIV infection status.
- FIV subtype, often reported with PCR testing results, has no established clinical relevance at this time.
- FIV-infected cats are likely to have a degree of immune dysfunction, even though this is often not clinically apparent. Regular health checks, preventive medicine, and owner education are important for maintaining optimal health.
- Considering contribution, if any, of FIV infection to current clinical signs in infected cats is key to managing the case.
- Reliable clinical prognostic markers for FIV infection are not available.
- Cats used as blood donors should be established to be free from FIV infection by repeated testing.
- FIV-infected cats should not be hospitalized in isolation wards on the basis of their FIV status alone because at these places potentially immunosuppressed cats are at unnecessary risk.
- There is no justification for euthanasia of healthy cats solely based on their FIV infection status.
- FIV poses no known zoonotic risk.

REFERENCES

[1] Pedersen NC, Ho EW, Brown ML, et al. Isolation of a T-lymphotropic virus from domestic cats with an immunodeficiency-like syndrome. Science 1987;235:790–3.

[2] Pecon-Slattery J, Troyer JL, Johnson WE, et al. Evolution of feline immunodeficiency virus in Felidae: implications for human health and wildlife ecology. Vet Immunol Immunopathol 2008;123:32–44.

[3] Talbott RL, Sparger EE, Lovelace KM, et al. Nucleotide sequence and genomic organization of feline immunodeficiency virus. Proc Natl Acad Sci U S A 1989;86:5743–7.

[4] Willett BJ, McMonagle EL, Logan N, et al. A single site for N-linked glycosylation in the envelope glycoprotein of feline immunodeficiency virus modulates the virus-receptor interaction. Retrovirology 2008;5:77.

[5] ABCD. Feline Immunodeficiency Virus ABCD guidelines on prevention and management. 2017. Available at: http://www.abcdcatsvets.org/feline-immunodeficiency/. Accessed February 2, 2022.

[6] Bęczkowski PM, Hughes J, Biek R, et al. Feline immunodeficiency virus (FIV) *env* recombinants are common in natural infections. Retrovirology 2014;11:80.

[7] Bęczkowski PM, Hughes J, Biek R, et al. Rapid evolution of the *env* gene leader sequence in cats naturally infected with feline immunodeficiency virus. J Gen Virol 2015;96:893–903.

[8] Holland JJ, De La Torre JC, Steinhauer DA. RNA virus populations as quasispecies. Curr Top Microbiol Immunol 1992;176:1–20.

[9] Carpenter S, Vaughn EM, Yang J, et al. Antigenic and genetic stability of bovine immunodeficiency virus during long-term persistence in cattle experimentally infected with the BIVR29 isolate. J Gen Virol 2000;81: 1463–72.

[10] Buch J, Beall M, o'Connor T. Worldwide clinic-based serologic survey of FIV antibody and FeLV antigen in cats. ACVIM Forum Research Abstract Program, J Vet Intern Med. 2017;31:1315.

[11] Levy JK, Scott HM, Lachtara JL, et al. Seroprevalence of feline leukemia virus and feline immunodeficiency virus infection among cats in North America and risk factors for seropositivity. J Am Vet Med Assoc 2006;228: 371–6.

[12] Pedersen NC, Yamamoto JK, Ishida T, et al. Feline immunodeficiency virus infection. Vet Immunol Immunopathol 1989;21:111–29.

[13] O'Neil LL, Burkhard MJO, Hoover EA. Frequent perinatal transmission of feline immunodeficiency virus by chronically infected cats. J Virol 1996;70:2894–901.

[14] Bishop SA, Stokes CR, Gruffydd-Jones TJ, et al. Vaginal and rectal infection of cats with feline immunodeficiency virus. Vet Microbiol 1996;51:217–27.

[15] Litster AL. Transmission of feline immunodeficiency virus (FIV) among cohabiting cats in two cat rescue shelters. The Vet J 2014;201:184–8.

[16] Pennisi MG, Hartmann K, Addie DD, et al. Blood transfusion transfusion in cats ABCD guidelines for minimising risks of infectious iatrogenic complications. J Feline Med Surg 2015;17:588–93.

[17] Shimojima M, Miyazawa T, Ikeda Y, et al. Use of CD134 as a primary receptor by the feline immunodeficiency virus. Science 2004;303:1192–5.

[18] Willett BJ, Hosie MJ, Neil JC, et al. Common mechanism of infection by lentiviruses. Nature 1997;385:587.

[19] Willett BJ, McMonagle EL, Bonci F, et al. Mapping the domains of CD134 as a functional receptor for feline immunodeficiency virus. J Virol 2006;80:7744–7.

[20] Willett BJ, McMonagle EL, Ridha S, et al. Differential utilization of CD134 as a functional receptor by diverse strains of feline immunodeficiency virus. J Virol 2006; 80:3386–94.

[21] Bęczkowski PM, Techakriengkrai N, Logan N, et al. Emergence of CD134 cysteine-rich domain 2 (CRD2)-independent strains of feline immunodeficiency virus (FIV) is associated with disease progression in naturally infected cats. Retrovirology 2014;11:95.

[22] Regoes RR, Bonhoeffer S. The HIV coreceptor switch: a population dynamical perspective. Trends Microbiol 2005;13:269–77.

[23] Hosie MJ, Techakriengkrai N, Bęczkowski PM, et al. The comparative value of feline virology research: can findings from the feline lentiviral vaccine be translated to humans? Vet Sci 2017;4:7.

[24] Ackley CD, Yamamoto JK, Levy N, et al. Immunologic abnormalities in pathogen-free cats experimentally infected with feline immunodeficiency virus. J Virol 1990;64:5652–5.

[25] Beatty JA, Willett BJ, Gault EA, et al. A longitudinal study of feline immunodeficiency virus-specific cytotoxic T lymphocytes in experimentally infected cats, using antigen-specific induction. J Virol 1996;70: 6199–206.

[26] Bucci JG, English RV, Jordan HL, et al. Mucosally transmitted feline immunodeficiency virus induces a CD8+ antiviral response that correlates with reduction of cell-associated virus. J Infect Dis 1998;177:18–25.

[27] Flynn JN, Beatty JA, Cannon CA, et al. Involvement of gag- and env-specific cytotoxic T lymphocytes in protective immunity to feline immunodeficiency virus. AIDS Res Hum Retroviruses 1995;11:1107–13.

[28] Yamamoto JK, Sparger E, Ho EW, et al. Pathogenesis of experimentally induced feline immunodeficiency virus infection in cats. Am J Vet Res 1988;49:1246–58.

[29] Egberink HF, Keldermans CE, Koolen MJ, et al. Humoral immune response to feline immunodeficiency virus in cats with experimentally induced and naturally acquired infections. Am J Vet Res 1992;53:1133–8.

[30] Bęczkowski PM, Logan N, McMonagle E, et al. An investigation of the breadth of neutralizing antibody response in cats naturally infected with feline immunodeficiency virus. The J Gen Virol 2015;96:671–80.

[31] Grant CK, Fink EA, Sundstrom M, et al. Improved health and survival of FIV-infected cats is associated with the presence of autoantibodies to the primary receptor, CD134. Proc Natl Acad Sci U S A 2009;106: 19980–5.

[32] Siebelink KH, Tijhaar E, Huisman RC, et al. Enhancement of feline immunodeficiency virus infection after immunization with envelope glycoprotein subunit vaccines. J Virol 1995;69:3704–11.

[33] McEwan WA, Schaller T, Ylinen LM, et al. Truncation of TRIM5 in the Feliformia Explains the Absence of Retroviral Restriction in Cells of the Domestic Cat. J Virol 2009;83:8270–5.

[34] Dietrich I, McMonagle EL, Petit SJ, et al. Feline tetherin efficiently restricts release of feline immunodeficiency virus but not spreading of infection. J Virol 2011;85: 5840–52.

[35] Hartmann K. Clinical aspects of feline retroviruses: a review. Viruses 2012;4:2684–710.

[36] Lee DB, Verstraete FJM, Arzi B. An Update on Feline Chronic Gingivostomatitis. Vet Clin North Am Small Anim Pract 2020;50:973–82.

[37] Weese SJ, Nichols J, Jalali M, et al. The oral and conjunctival microbiotas in cats with and without feline immunodeficiency virus infection. Vet Res 2015;46:21.

[38] Tompkins MB, Tompkins WA. Lentivirus-induced immune dysregulation. Vet Immunol Immunopathol 2008;123:45–55.

[39] Davidson MG, Rottman JB, English RV, et al. Feline immunodeficiency virus predisposes cats to acute generalized toxoplasmosis. Am J Pathol 1993;143:1486–97.

[40] Dean GA, Bernales JA, Pedersen NC. Effect of feline immunodeficiency virus on cytokine response to Listeria monocytogenes in vivo. Vet Immunol Immunopathol 1998;65:125–38.

[41] Shelton GH, Grant CK, Cotter SM, et al. Feline immunodeficiency virus and feline leukemia virus infections and their relationships to lymphoid malignancies in cats: a retrospective study (1968-1988). J Acquir Immune Defic Syndr 1990;3:623–30.

[42] Liem B, Dhand N, Pepper A, et al. Clinical Findings and Survival in Cats Naturally Infected with Feline Immunodeficiency Virus. J Vet Intern Med 2013;27:798–805.

[43] Gleich S, Hartmann K. Hematology and Serum Biochemistry of Feline Immunodeficiency Virus-Infected and Feline Leukemia Virus-Infected Cats. J Vet Intern Med 2009;23:552–8.

[44] Bęczkowski PM, Litster A, Lin TL, et al. Contrasting clinical outcomes in two cohorts of cats naturally infected with feline immunodeficiency virus (FIV). Vet Microbiol 2015;176:50–60.

[45] Ishida T, Washizu T, Toriyabe K, et al. Feline immunodeficiency virus infection in cats of Japan. J Am Vet Med Assoc 1989;194:221–5.

[46] Barrs VR, Martin P, Nicoll RG, et al. Pulmonary cryptococcosis and Capillaria aerophila infection in an FIV-positive cat. Aust Vet J 2000;78:154–8.

[47] Taffin ER, Casaert S, Claerebout E, et al. Morphological variability of Demodex cati in a feline immunodeficiency virus-positive cat. J Am Vet Med Assoc 2016;249:1308–12.

[48] Meeker RB, Hudson L. Feline Immunodeficiency Virus Neuropathogenesis: A Model for HIV-Induced CNS Inflammation and Neurodegeneration. Vet Sci 2017;4:14.

[49] Baxter KJ, Levy JK, Edinboro CH, et al. Renal disease in cats infected with feline immunodeficiency virus. J Vet Intern Med 2012;26:238–43.

[50] Beatty JA, Callanan JJ, Terry A, et al. Molecular and immunophenotypical characterization of a feline immunodeficiency virus (FIV)-associated lymphoma: a direct role for FIV in B-lymphocyte transformation? J Virol 1998;72:767–71.

[51] Beatty J. Viral causes of feline lymphoma: retroviruses and beyond. Vet J 2014;201:174–80.

[52] McLuckie AJ, Barrs VR, Smith AL, et al. Detection of Felis catus gammaherpesvirus 1 (FcaGHV1) in peripheral blood B- and T-lymphocytes in asymptomatic, naturally-infected domestic cats. Virology 2016;497:211–6.

[53] Troyer RM, Beatty JA, Stutzman-Rodriguez KR, et al. Novel gammaherpesviruses in North American domestic cats, bobcats, and pumas: identification, prevalence, and risk factors. J Virol 2014;88:3914–24.

[54] Levy J., Lorentzen L., Shields J., et al., Long-term outcome of cats with natural FeLV and FIV infection, Proceedings of the 8th International Feline Retrovirus Research Symposium, October 8-11, 2006, Washington, DC, USA.

[55] Hoffmann-Fezer G, Thum J, Ackley C, et al. Decline in CD4+ cell numbers in cats with naturally acquired feline immunodeficiency virus infection. J Virol 1992;66:1484–8.

[56] Walker C, Canfield PJ, Love DN. Analysis of leucocytes and lymphocyte subsets for different clinical stages of naturally acquired feline immunodeficiency virus infection. Vet Immunol Immunopathol 1994;44:1–12.

[57] Goto Y, Nishimura Y, Baba K, et al. Association of plasma viral RNA load with prognosis in cats naturally infected with feline immunodeficiency virus. J Virol 2002;76:10079–83.

[58] Little S, Levy J, Hartmann K, et al. 2020 AAFP Feline Retrovirus Testing and Management Guidelines. J Feline Med Surg 2020;22:5–30.

[59] Barr MC. FIV, FeLV, and FIPV: interpretation and misinterpretation of serological test results. Semin Vet Med Surg (Small Anim) 1996;11:144–53.

[60] MacDonald K, Levy JK, Tucker SJ, et al. Effects of passive transfer of immunity on results of diagnostic tests for antibodies against feline immunodeficiency virus in kittens born to vaccinated queens. J Am Vet Med Assoc 2004;225:1554–7.

[61] Levy JK, Crawford PC, Kusuhara H, et al. Differentiation of feline immunodeficiency virus vaccination, infection, or vaccination and infection in cats. J Vet Intern Med 2008;22:330–4.

[62] Westman M, Yang D, Green J, et al. Antibody Responses in Cats Following Primary and Annual Vaccination against Feline Immunodeficiency Virus (FIV) with an Inactivated Whole-Virus Vaccine (Fel-O-Vax® FIV). Viruses 2021;13:470.

[63] Levy JK, Crawford PC, Slater MR. Effect of vaccination against feline immunodeficiency virus on results of serologic testing in cats. J Am Vet Med Assoc 2004;225:1558–61.

[64] Crawford PC, Slater MR, Levy JK. Accuracy of polymerase chain reaction assays for diagnosis of feline immunodeficiency virus infection in cats. J Am Vet Med Assoc 2005;226:1503–7.

[65] Morton JM, McCoy RJ, Kann RKC, et al. Validation of real-time polymerase chain reaction tests for diagnosing feline immunodeficiency virus infection in domestic cats using Bayesian latent class models. Prev Vet Med 2012;104(1–2):136–48.

[66] Bienzle D, Reggeti F, Wen X, et al. The variability of serological and molecular diagnosis of feline immunodeficiency virus infection. Can Vet J 2004;45: 753–7.

[67] Addie DD, Dennis JM, Toth S, et al. Long-term impact on a closed household of pet cats of natural infection with feline coronavirus, feline leukaemia virus and feline immunodeficiency virus. Vet Rec 2000;146: 419–24.

[68] ABCD. ABCD guidelines on Vaccination of Immunocompromised Cats. 2020. Available at: http://www.abcdcatsvets.org/vaccination-of-immunocompromised-cats/. Accessed February 2, 2022.

[69] Weese JS, Giguère S, Guardabassi L, et al. ACVIM consensus statement on therapeutic antimicrobial use in animals and antimicrobial resistance. J Vet Intern Med 2015;29:487–98.

[70] Shelton GH, Grant CK, Linenberger ML, et al. Severe neutropenia associated with griseofulvin therapy in cats with feline immunodeficiency virus infection. J Vet Intern Med 1990;4:317–9.

[71] Barr MC, Huitron-Resendiz S, Selway DR, et al. Exogenous glucocorticoids alter parameters of early feline immunodeficiency virus infection. J Infect Dis 2000;181: 576–86.

[72] Collette SA, Allstadt SD, Chon EM, et al. Treatment of feline intermediate- to high-grade lymphoma with a modified university of Wisconsin-Madison protocol: 119 cases (2004-2012). Vet Comp Oncol 2016; 14(Suppl 1):136–46.

[73] Phillips K, Arai M, Tanabe T, et al. FIV-infected cats respond to short-term rHuG-CSF treatment which results in anti-G-CSF neutralizing antibody production that inactivates drug activity. Vet Immunol Immunopathol 2005;108:357–71.

[74] Arai M, Darman J, Lewis A, et al. The use of human hematopoietic growth factors (rhGM-CSF and rhEPO) as a supportive therapy for FIV-infected cats. Vet Immunol Immunopathol 2000;77:71–92.

[75] Winzelberg Olson S, Hohenhaus AE. Feline non-regenerative anemia: Diagnostic and treatment recommendations. J Feline Med Surg 2019;21:615–31.

[76] Woo JC, Dean GA, Lavoy A, et al. Investigation of recombinant human insulin-like growth factor type I in thymus regeneration in the acute stage of experimental FIV infection in juvenile cats. AIDS Res Hum Retroviruses 1999;15:1377–88.

[77] Tompkins WA. Immunomodulation and therapeutic effects of the oral use of interferon-alpha: mechanism of action. J Interferon Cytokine Res 1999;19:817–28.

[78] Pedretti E, Passeri B, Amadori M, et al. Low-dose interferon-alpha treatment for feline immunodeficiency virus infection. Vet Immunol Immunopathol 2006;109: 245–54.

[79] Gomez-Lucia E, Collado VM, Miró G, et al. Clinical and Hematological Follow-Up of Long-Term Oral Therapy with Type-I Interferon in Cats Naturally Infected with Feline Leukemia Virus or Feline Immunodeficiency Virus. Animals 2020;10:1464.

[80] Tanabe T, Yamamoto JK. Feline immunodeficiency virus lacks sensitivity to the antiviral activity of feline IFN-gamma. J Interferon Cytokine Res 2001;21: 1039–46.

[81] Zeidner NS, Myles MH, Mathiason-DuBard CK, et al. Alpha interferon (2b) in combination with zidovudine for the treatment of presymptomatic feline leukemia virus-induced immunodeficiency syndrome. Antimicrob Agents Chemother 1990;34:1749–56.

[82] de Mari K, Maynard L, Sanquer A, et al. Therapeutic effects of recombinant feline interferon-omega on feline leukemia virus (FeLV)-infected and FeLV/feline immunodeficiency virus (FIV)-coinfected symptomatic cats. J Vet Intern Med 2004;18:477–82.

[83] Gil S, Leal RO, McGahie D, et al. Oral Recombinant Feline Interferon-Omega as an alternative immune modulation therapy in FIV positive cats: clinical and laboratory evaluation. Res Vet Sci 2014;96:79–85.

[84] Leal RO, Gil S, Duarte A, et al. Evaluation of viremia, proviral load and cytokine profile in naturally feline immunodeficiency virus infected cats treated with two different protocols of recombinant feline interferon omega. Res Vet Sci 2015;99:87–95.

[85] Bisset LR, Lutz H, Böni J, et al. Combined effect of zidovudine (ZDV), lamivudine (3TC) and abacavir (ABC) antiretroviral therapy in suppressing in vitro FIV replication. Antivir Res 2002;53:35–45.

[86] Schwartz AM, McCrackin MA, Schinazi RF, et al. Antiviral efficacy of nine nucleoside reverse transcriptase inhibitors against feline immunodeficiency virus in feline peripheral blood mononuclear cells. Am J Vet Res 2014; 75:273–81.

[87] Smith RA, Remington KM, Lloyd RM Jr, et al. A novel Met-to-Thr mutation in the YMDD motif of reverse transcriptase from feline immunodeficiency virus confers resistance to oxathiolane nucleosides. J Virol 1997;71:2357–62.

[88] Hartmann K. Efficacy of antiviral chemotherapy for retrovirus-infected cats: What does the current literature tell us? J Feline Med Surg 2015;17:925–39.

[89] Hartmann K, Stengel C, Klein D, et al. Efficacy and adverse effects of the antiviral compound plerixafor in feline immunodeficiency virus-infected cats. J Vet Intern Med 2012;26:483–90.

[90] Mochel JP, Ekker SC, Johannes CM, et al. CAR T Cell Immunotherapy in human and veterinary oncology: changing the odds against hematological malignancies. AAPS J 2019;21:50.

[91] Mu W, Carrillo MA, Kitchen SG. Engineering CAR T Cells to target the HIV reservoir. Front Cell Infect Microbiol 2020;10:410.

[92] Uhl EW, Heaton-Jones TG, Pu R, et al. FIV vaccine development and its importance to veterinary and human medicine: a review FIV vaccine 2002 update and review. Vet Immunol Immunopathol 2002;90:113–32.

[93] Huisman W, Martina BE, Rimmelzwaan GF, et al. Vaccine-induced enhancement of viral infections. Vaccine 2009;27:505–12.

[94] Pu RY, Coleman A, Omori M, et al. Dual-subtype FIV vaccine protects cats against in vivo swarms of both homologous and heterologous subtype FIV isolates. AIDS 2001;15:1225–37.

[95] Pu R, Coleman J, Coisman J, et al. Dual-subtype FIV vaccine (Fel-O-Vax FIV) protection against a heterologous subtype B FIV isolate. J Feline Med Surg 2005;7:65–70.

[96] Kusuhara H, Hohdatsu T, Okumura M, et al. Dual-subtype vaccine (Fel-O-Vax FIV) protects cats against contact challenge with heterologous subtype B FIV infected cats. Vet Microbiol 2005;108:155–65.

[97] Dunham SP, Bruce J, MacKay S, et al. Limited efficacy of an inactivated feline immunodeficiency virus vaccine. Vet Rec 2006;158:561–2.

[98] Bęczkowski PM, Harris M, Techakriengkrai N, et al. Neutralising antibody response in domestic cats immunised with a commercial feline immunodeficiency virus (FIV) vaccine. Vaccine 2015;33:977–84.

[99] Westman ME, Malik R, Hall E, et al. The protective rate of the feline immunodeficiency virus vaccine: An Australian field study. Vaccine 2016;34:4752–8.

[100] Stickney A, Ghosh S, Cave NJ, et al. Lack of protection against feline immunodeficiency virus infection among domestic cats in New Zealand vaccinated with the Fel-O-Vax® FIV vaccine. Vet Microbiol 2020;250:108865.

Advances in Small Animal Care 3 (2022) 161–176

ADVANCES IN SMALL ANIMAL CARE

Diagnostic Testing for Infectious Respiratory Tract Disease

Sean E. Hulsebosch, DVM, DACVIM[a], Jennifer C. Chan, DVM[b], Lynelle R. Johnson, DVM, MS, PhD, DACVIM[a],*

[a]Department of Veterinary Medicine and Epidemiology, University of California-Davis, One Garrod Drive, Davis, CA 95616, USA; [b]William R. Pritchard Veterinary Medical Teaching Hospital, University of California-Davis, One Garrod Drive, Davis, CA 95616, USA

KEYWORDS
- Biopsy • Bronchoscopy • Culture • Cytology • Rhinoscopy • Thoracocentesis • Tracheal wash

KEY POINTS
- Primary bacterial infection of the nasal cavity is uncommon, whereas primary airway or lung infections, as well as pleural infections, are commonly encountered.
- Molecular testing for acute or chronic upper respiratory tract disease in the cat is of limited value given the high prevalence of viruses in the feline population and the presence of a latent carrier state.
- Airway cytology and culture are necessary to confirm a diagnosis of bacterial infection and to determine appropriate antimicrobial therapy.
- Pleural infection is typically related to a penetrating injury or foreign body, although geographic location and lifestyle can affect the commonality of these etiologies.
- Pleural infections are typically polymicrobial, and bacteria are visible cytologically in thoracic fluid.

INTRODUCTION TO NASAL DISEASES

- The most common causes of nasal disease in dogs and cats include neoplasia, fungal rhinitis, foreign body inhalation, dental-related disease, and idiopathic or inflammatory rhinitis, which is a diagnosis of exclusion.
- Clinical signs are similar for all etiologies and include sneezing, nasal discharge, epiphora, and possibly facial pain or asymmetry.
- Diagnostic testing can include serology for certain diseases, imaging (preferably computed tomography), rhinoscopy, and sample collection for histopathology, culture, and sometimes polymerase chain reaction (PCR).

Sample Collection

Indications include chronic nasal discharge, sneezing, epiphora, facial pain or deformity, exophthalmia, palatal defect, and reduced or absent nasal airflow. Imaging should be performed before the collection of a nasal sample, and an assessment of primary and secondary hemostasis should also be considered.

Methodology

- Samples from the external nasal nares
  - A microscope slide pressed firmly on a nasal mass or mucoid discharge can produce an impression smear of cytologic value in the diagnosis of

---

https://doi.org/10.1016/j.yasa.2022.05.008
2666-450X/22/ Published by Elsevier Inc.

cryptococcosis, but is of little value in dogs with aspergillosis [1].

○ Culture of the exterior nasal discharge is of no value and could lead to the inappropriate use of antimicrobials.

Procedure for internal sampling

• General anesthesia is required to place any item into the nose for sampling.

• Additional local anesthesia can be provided by an infraorbital block using 0.25 to 1.00 mL of bupivacaine.

• Topical anesthesia with intranasal instillation of lidocaine via an atomizer can help to decrease reactivity during the procurement of samples.

Equipment and technique

• *Cytology brush*: Sterile microbial or DNA collection brush (Cytosoft) (Fig. 1).

○ In a dog, the stem of the brush should be measured on the outside of the skull to the level of the medial canthus, which approximates the end of the nasal cavity and the beginning of the brain. In a cat, the brush portion approximates this length. After insertion of the brush, it is gently twirled inside the nasal cavity and then placed in a red top tube or transport media for submission.

• *Flush*: A 5F to 10F red rubber catheter, with 2 to 5 mL of sterile, warmed nonbacteriostatic saline.

○ A red rubber catheter is inserted into the ventral meatus of the nasal cavity to the level of the rostral soft palate.

○ Two fingers are placed in the mouth, pressing the soft palate into the nasopharynx to trap fluid in the nasal cavity.

○ Approximately 2 to 3 mL of sterile saline are injected followed by 2 mL of air to clear the catheter.

○ After gentle manipulation of the palate, fluid is aspirated by house or wall suction.

○ Both cytology and culture can be performed on nasal flush fluid, although caution is warranted in interpretation owing to the wide variety of normal flora that can be encountered. Cytology evidence of septic, suppurative inflammation might be of greater value in documenting a bacterial component to disease.

• *Biopsy*: A 2-, 3-, or 4-mm cup biopsy forceps, histopathology cassettes, and Eppendorf tubes if frozen sections or DNA extraction are desired

○ Visualization of the site of the lesion during the biopsy procedure is beneficial for ensuring a diagnostic sample.

○ A mass lesion or fungal plaque (Fig. 2) should be grasped tightly with the forceps. A firm tug on the instrument will obtain the biopsy.

○ An impression smear can be made to obtain early diagnostic information, although correlation of cytology with histopathology is low in some diseases.

○ Bleeding is common.

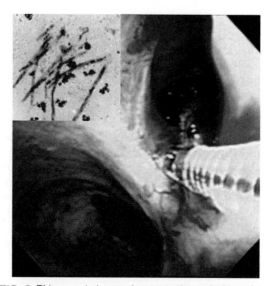

FIG. 2 Rhinoscopic image demonstrating collection of a fungal plaque with flexible through-the-scope biopsy forceps. Inset: Microscopic image of fungal hyphae. Wright Giemsa stain, 40X.

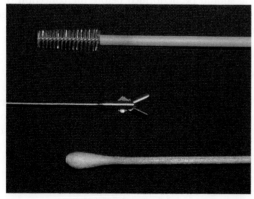

FIG. 1 Sterile Cytosoft (TM) brush and 3 mm Karl Storz cup biopsy forceps compared with a standard cotton-tipped applicator.

Sample handling

- Cytology A brush cytology sample, cytospin from a flush sample, or impression smear of a biopsy sample can be examined cytologically, although caution is warranted in interpretation given the superficial nature of the sample.
- Microbiology
  - A brush sample can sometimes yield important microbiologic information in a cat with rhinitis, such as the identification of resistant bacteria in a cat that has been treated with multiple antibiotics [2].
  - Culture of external nasal discharge is rarely of value, although the collection of a sample from the frontal sinus or the nasopharynx can sometimes be helpful in dogs or cats. These regions are more protected from external contamination and thus might yield information that is of value in documenting a bacterial or fungal infection. Access to these areas is more challenging, requiring both anesthesia and endoscopic or surgical intervention.
  - The nasopharynx can be accessed in a dog or cat by using a flexible endoscope (Fig. 3) and passing a microbiology brush through the biopsy channel.
  - Access to the frontal sinus of a dog can sometimes be achieved through a rostral approach using a

flexible endoscope, as long as marked turbinate destruction is present.
  - Trephination into the frontal sinus can be used to obtain a sample for culture.
- Histopathology
  - Cryptococcus organisms are readily observed in standard biopsy samples.
  - Histopathology is diagnostic of aspergillosis in cases in which a plaque lesion has been sampled by direct visualization [3], although blind sampling of the nasal mucosa may not contain fungal elements, leading to a false negative biopsy sample.
- PCR
  - Molecular diagnostics can be applied to paraffin embedded material if desired, although a role for infectious organisms in inflammatory rhinitis (feline herpesvirus [FHV-1] and *Bartonella* in cats; *Bartonella*, *Chlamydophila*, *Mycoplasma*, and specific fungi in dogs) has not been supported by clinical studies [2,4–7].

Aftercare

- Slow recovery from anesthesia is advised to avoid perpetuating hemorrhage after biopsy, and judicious use of acepromazine (0.01–0.02 mg/kg subcutaneously, intramuscularly, or intravenously [IV] every 4–6 hours) can be useful for sedation and to lower blood pressure.
- Pain control after the procedure can be achieved with narcotic agents and nonsteroidal anti-inflammatory drugs as indicated.
- The use of ice packs on the nose might limit bleeding. Intranasal decongestant sprays are used by some clinicians, but they are often diluted by ongoing hemorrhage and expelled by sneezing.

SPECIFIC DISEASE CONSIDERATIONS

Viral Infections

- Viral infection of the upper respiratory tract most often occurs as part of a complex of infections by multiple organisms. Acute signs of sneezing and oculonasal discharge are typical.
- In the cat, FHV-1 is most commonly implicated as the etiologic agent for acute rhinitis, although feline calicivirus, *Mycoplasma*, *Bordetella*, and commensal bacteria can also be involved. The importance of viral detection in a cat is difficult to assess because of the ubiquitous nature of many of the upper respiratory viruses.
  - Young kittens are affected most commonly and disease is characterized by systemic signs of

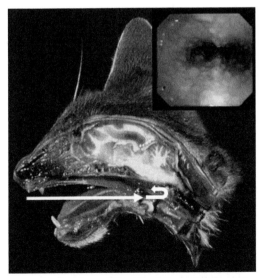

FIG. 3 Cross-section of a cat skull illustrating the path taken by a flexible endoscope (*white arrows*) for examination of the nasopharynx. Inset: Endoscopic view of the openings of the choanae in a cat that has proliferative pharyngitis.

illness, including fever, anorexia, and dehydration. Older cats can suffer acute exacerbation of disease owing to stress or concurrent illness.

○ It has been proposed that early FHV-1 infection in kittens could contribute to the development of idiopathic rhinosinusitis in the cat by causing turbinate destruction [8] and predisposing the epithelial surface to recurrent bacterial infection, although clinical evidence is lacking to date.

• In the dog, organisms associated with canine infectious respiratory disease (canine distemper virus, canine adenovirus, canine parainfluenza virus (CPIV), canine herpesvirus, canine influenza virus, *Mycoplasma*, *Bordetella*) can result in acute upper respiratory tract signs, although with the exception of canine herpesvirus, most cause cough more commonly than oculonasal discharge.

• Molecular tests can be performed on conjunctival, nasal, or oropharyngeal swabs, with the purpose of amplifying nucleic acids of potential pathogens; however, it is important to note that the presence of viral DNA or RNA is not an indication that disease is associated with that organism.

• Use of quantitative PCR might be of benefit in future investigations of disease causation, although additional studies are needed.

Fungal Infections

• The most common infecting organisms include *Cryptococcus neoformans* in the cat and *Aspergillus fumigatus* in the dog, although either fungus can invade the alternate species.

• Serology
  ○ The only diagnostic blood test available for nasal disease is the cryptococcal latex agglutination titer. This test is both sensitive and specific for the diagnosis of cryptococcosis in dogs and cats. The quantitative latex agglutination titer can also be used to monitor response to therapy.
  ○ A recent study confirmed the usefulness of 2 different point-of-care tests (CrAg LFA, Immy [Norman, OK] and the Crypto PS, Biosynex [Strasbourg, France]) for rapid, patient-side diagnosis of disease with 92% and 93% sensitivity and specificity for the Immy test and 80% and 95% sensitivity and specificity for the Crypto PS assay [9].
  ○ Agar gel immunodiffusion (AGID) for canine nasal Aspergillus uses an *Aspergillus* antigen prepared from combined cultures of *A fumigatus*, *A niger*, and *A flavus*, the most common fungal species involved, to detect serum antibody.

○ A positive AGID was 68% sensitive and 98% specific for the diagnosis in 1 study, with positive and negative predictive values of 94% and 84%, respectively [2]. Therefore, positive serology can be taken as evidence that *Aspergillus* is the likely cause of nasal discharge; however, a negative test does not rule it out.

○ It is unclear how long dogs remain positive on the AGID throughout the course of disease; therefore, it cannot be used to monitor response to treatment.

○ Serum aspergillus galactomannan antigen has relatively poor diagnostic value for nasal aspergillosis in dogs and cats [10,11].

○ A better screening test for aspergillosis in the cat is the IgG enzyme-linked immunosorbent assay (ELISA), which can detect more than 90% of cases when an appropriate cutoff value is used [12]. This test has 7% to 8% false-positive results, but could be used to prioritize the need for a diagnostic workup, including fungal culture or molecular analysis of nasal samples in cats with upper respiratory tract signs.

• Cytology
  ○ In dogs with sinonasal aspergillosis, fungal hyphae were observed in smears of nasal exudates or in blind swabs of the nasal cavity in only 13% to 20% of cases, although cytology of a swab or biopsy sample collected endoscopically demonstrated fungal elements in more than 90% of cases [1].
  ○ A nasal swab sample or impression of nasal discharge can occasionally provide a cytologic diagnosis of cryptococcosis because the characteristic polysaccharide coat of the organism excludes stain and is readily visible in most cytologic preparations. The organism itself is generally 2 to 5 microns in diameter, but the halo of the outer coat approaches 20 to 30 microns in diameter.
  ○ Lymph node aspiration from a site near the lesion or an impression smear of a biopsy sample can sometimes yield a diagnosis in cryptococcosis, but reactive inflammation is typically found in *Aspergillus* infection.

• Culture
  ○ Fungal culture is not typically used to make a diagnosis of cryptococcosis because subclinical infection or asymptomatic carriage of cryptococcus has been documented [13]. Fungal culture might be warranted for speciation or for susceptibility testing.

○ Fungal culture for aspergillosis can be of value when a visualized plaque is sampled [3], although false negatives are possible (sensitivity of 77%, but specificity of 100%). A blindly collected mucus or epithelial sample is of little diagnostic value [1].

Bacterial Infections

- Bacterial infections in the nasal cavity typically are secondary to either dental-related disease, foreign body inhalation, or potentially destruction from previous viral damage (idiopathic or chronic rhinosinusitis).
- In 1 small prospective study, potential pathogens were isolated more commonly from cats with chronic rhinosinusitis than from control cats [2]. Bacterial isolates included *Pasteurella, Bordetella, Mycoplasma, Staphylococcus, Streptococcus, Pseudomonas, Actinomyces, Corynebacterium*, and anaerobes, with isolation of multiple species from most of the cats.
- In one of the author's experience (L.R.J.), cats that have had multiple courses of antibiotics, can have resistant species of *E coli* and *Pseudomonas* isolated.

INTRODUCTION TO AIRWAY AND PARENCHYMAL INFECTIONS

Infections typically lead to cough, with or without fever, and difficulty breathing. Tracheal sensitivity and variable changes in lung sounds are expected. Animals with parenchymal infection tend to be more systemically ill and have alterations in the respiratory pattern when compared with those with uncomplicated airway infections.

Sample Collection

Indications include acute or chronic cough and diffuse or focal radiographic infiltrates. A tracheal wash collects a global, central sample from the carinal region, and bronchoscopy can access focal and distal lesions. Bronchoscopy is typically advised if there is nonresolving disease or the suspicion of superinfection or a foreign body and can be used to collect a guided bronchoalveolar lavage (BAL) sample from a specific lung region. Fine needle aspiration (blind or ultrasound guided) can be useful for investigating focal lesions near the chest wall.

Methodology

- Tracheal wash
  ○ Tracheal wash involves insertion of a sterile catheter into the airway of a dog or cat, injection of sterile saline, and subsequent aspiration of the fluid that has contacted the airway lining. Fluid is submitted for culture and cytology.
  ○ The catheter can be inserted via a transoral approach using a sterile endotracheal tube, or via a transtracheal approach between tracheal rings.
- Bronchoscopy with BAL
  ○ Provides both visual assessment of the airways and allows collection of a sample from specific lung segments.
  ○ Might be less susceptible to upper airway contamination of the sample.
- Nonbronchoscopic, blind BAL
  ○ Provides equivalent cytologic assessment of the lower airways to bronchoscopic BAL [14,15].
  ○ Fine needle lung aspiration.
    ○ Collects a small sample that might only allow cytology, although, in some instances, material for culture can also be obtained.

Contraindications for all sample collection methods

- Bleeding disorders.
- Anesthetic contraindications.
- Severe tracheal sensitivity.

Potential complications

- Any anesthetic complication.
- Subcutaneous emphysema from tracheal trauma.
- Pneumomediastinum or pneumothorax.
- Hemorrhage.
- Chondroma formation from a transtracheal wash.

Before the procedure

- Imaging (orthogonal radiographs or a computed tomography scan) is performed before the evaluation of the lower airways.
- A complete blood count, serum biochemistry profile, and urinalysis are typically performed as part of the respiratory workup and to assess general health for anesthesia.
- Thrombocytopenia represents a contraindication to airway sampling.
- Pulse oximetry can be used to screen for hypoxemia although arterial blood gas analysis is more accurate.
- An anesthetic plan should be devised that allows a comprehensive laryngeal examination for animals undergoing transoral tracheal wash or bronchoscopy. Doxapram should be available to stimulate respiration.

- Terbutaline (0.01 mg/kg subcutaneously) should be available for use in cats before tracheal wash and BAL to counteract the tendency for bronchoconstriction.

Equipment
- Laryngoscope or rigid telescope for laryngoscopy.
- Transoral tracheal wash: Local anesthesia (lidocaine), sterile endotracheal tube, sterile catheter or tubing, syringes, sterile saline, and suction. A suction trap device with house suction can be useful to maximize return.
- Transtracheal wash: Sedation protocol that allows intubation, jugular catheter or over-the-needle catheter, sterile tubing, syringes, sterile saline, and suction.
- Flexible endoscope with a biopsy channel and at least 2-way flexion for bronchoscopy
- Cats and small dogs (<8 kg): 2.8 to 3.8 mm outer diameter endosope (jet ventilation).
- Larger dogs (>8 kg): Less than 5 mm outer diameter endoscope (intubation and gas anesthesia).

Technique
- Animals are preoxygenated for 5 minutes before sedation or anesthesia and placed in sternal recumbency.
- Transoral tracheal wash.
  - Is appropriate for use in any sized animal.
    - Laryngeal examination is performed to confirm abduction of the corniculate processes of the arytenoids on inspiration.
    - If abduction is not apparent despite adequate thoracic expansion, administer doxapram (1 mg/kg IV) as a bolus and watch immediately for abduction.
      - The anesthetist will need to increase the depth of anesthesia before doxapram administration, because doxapram is stimulatory.
      - If abduction is still absent or if paradoxic laryngeal motion is noted (adduction on inspiration) after 2 to 3 doses of doxapram, laryngeal paralysis can be diagnosed.
  - The sterile endotracheal tube is passed into the trachea, taking care to avoid the oral mucosa or larynx with the end of the tube to limit contamination with oropharyngeal commensal bacteria.
  - An assistant holds the endotracheal tube in place, and a 5F to 8F sterile polypropylene catheter or

red rubber catheter is passed to the level of the carina (as estimated at the fourth rib).
  - An aliquot of nonbacteriostatic saline (5–10 mL) is instilled into the trachea followed by 1 to 2 mL of air to clear the catheter, and suction is used to retrieve the fluid and cells from the lower airways.
  - Removal of fluid can be enhanced by having the assistant coupage the chest or by stimulating a cough during suction.
  - Instillation and aspiration of fluid can be repeated 2 to 3 times until an adequate sample has been retrieved (1–2 mL is usually sufficient for culture and cytology).
- Transtracheal wash
  - Is appropriate for use in dogs larger than 8 to 10 kg.
    - The ventral portion of the neck is clipped and lightly scrubbed with antiseptic solution followed by alcohol wipes. Lidocaine (0.25–0.50 mL) is injected subcutaneously at site of entry to the skin, and a more complete surgical preparation is performed.
    - The short catheter is inserted into the skin with the bevel of the needle facing downward; the catheter is advanced off the needle, and the needle is withdrawn.
    - The sterile tubing or catheter is passed down the trachea through the short catheter.
    - An aliquot of nonbacteriostatic saline (5–10 mL) is injected into the catheter followed by 1 to 2 mL of air and then suction is applied.
    - Stimulation of a cough or coupage can facilitate retrieval of a cellular sample.
    - Instillation and aspiration of fluid can be repeated 2 to 3 times until an adequate sample has been retrieved.
- Bronchoscopy with BAL
  - Bronchoscopy is typically performed in sternal recumbency and general anesthesia is required.
  - Balanced anesthesia should include premedication followed by induction agents that allow assessment of laryngeal function. Consider midazolam combined with propofol or alfaxalone IV to effect.
  - Gas anesthesia and an endotracheal tube adaptor for the bronchoscope can be used in dogs large enough to accept a 7.5F endotracheal tube.
  - Small dogs and cats require intravenous infusion of an anesthetic agent such as propofol and supplemental administration of oxygen via jet ventilation or placement of a tracheal catheter.

- o Examine the trachea, lobar, and segmental airways in a systematic manner.
- o After a complete visual examination of the airways, the scope is withdrawn from the airways, the outside of the endoscope is wiped with sterile saline-soaked gauze pads, and the biopsy channel is flushed with sterile saline.
- o On the second entry to the airway, the scope should be kept in the center of the airways to minimize upper airway and mucosal contamination when approaching the site(s) chosen for lavage.
- o Success in retrieving BAL fluid will depend on the ability to wedge the bronchoscope in a bronchus and isolate a segment of alveolar volume (Fig. 4). The goal is to flood this small wedge of lung, float the resident inflammatory cells, and gently aspirate back the fluid using a combination of tip deflection and slight withdrawal of the scope.
- o Instill approximately 1 mL/kg of sterile nonbacteriostatic saline per site, but do not exceed 20 mL/site. Hand suction or wall suction can be used to retrieve fluid. Expect 35% to 80% return. An adequate sample is usually cloudy or foamy, indicating the presence of surfactant.
- Nonbronchoscopic BAL
  - o Nonbronchoscopic BAL can be performed with an animal in sternal or lateral recumbency. It can be done through an endotracheal tube or directly via a tube placed through the larynx, depending on the size of the animal.
  - o A sterile, long, soft catheter is passed caudally until it wedges in the distal lung as in Fig. 4. A red rubber catheter is suitable for cats and small dogs, or a modified foal gastroscopy tube (16F) can be used in dogs between 9 and 26 kg [15].
  - o The catheter should be premeasured against the thorax to the caudal border of the rib and not passed further than that length to avoid puncturing the lung. The tube should be passed slowly and wedged gently in the distal airway.
  - o Lavage can be performed with 5 to 20 mL of fluid. Enough air needs to be passed slowly through the catheter to clear all fluid from the length of the tube, and then aspiration is applied to retrieve fluid.
- Fine needle lung aspiration
  - o Is often performed with ultrasound guidance. Similar sedation can be used as for a tracheal wash.
    - o The animal is initially placed in lateral recumbency to collapse the affected, dependent lung

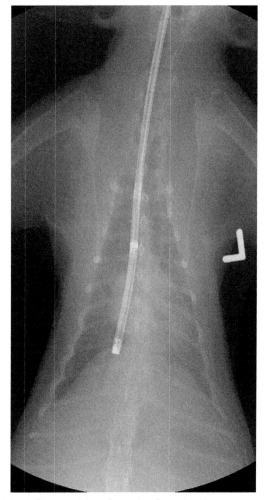

FIG. 4 Dorsoventral radiographs demonstrating the location of a bronchoscope in the wedged position for BAL. Use of a long catheter or tubing for nonbronchoscopic BAL would have a similar appearance.

then the affected lung is oriented upwards for aspiration using a 27G needle.
  - o Typically, the volume of fluid retrieved is very small therefore a decision must be made whether to submit culture or cytology or to obtain several aspirates.
  - o If a fungal infection is suspected, cytology is generally sufficient to identify the organism or to determine the need for additional assays. If a bacterial infection is considered likely, a culture of the material acquired from an aspirate can provide a diagnosis.

○ After aspiration, the animal is placed in the opposite recumbency for 20 to 30 minutes for recovery to facilitate sealing of the aspiration site. Ultrasound examination is used to check for bleeding or air accumulation.

Sample handling
- Airway samples are submitted for cytology and bacterial culture.
- Aerobic bacterial and *Mycoplasma* cultures are used to rule out infection in animals suspected of bronchial disease, and anaerobic bacterial culture should also be performed in animals with pneumonia, because viscid secretions can create an environment conducive to growth of anaerobes.
- Some laboratories require specialized medium for *Mycoplasma* or anaerobic cultures.
- Fungal culture and susceptibility should be considered on a case-by-case basis. Culture in coccidioidomycosis suspects is not recommended owing to the zoonotic nature of the laboratory isolate.

Interpretation
- Cytology
  - Tracheal wash samples in normal animals have ciliated respiratory epithelial cells and rare inflammatory cells or macrophages.
  - Normal BAL cytology is characterized by approximately 400 cells per microliter comprised primarily of macrophages (70%–75%) with 5% to 10% neutrophils, lymphocytes, and eosinophils, and few mast cells.
    - ○ Higher percentages of eosinophils (≤17%) are considered normal in the cat.
    - ○ Degenerate neutrophils and intracellular bacteria are typically found in infectious processes (Fig. 5).
    - ○ Airway parasites, fungal organisms, or protozoa can be evident on cytology and confirm the diagnosis.
- Culture
  - Bacterial culture of airway fluid in healthy dogs and cats can reveal light growth of various types of bacteria including *Pasteurella, Streptococcus, Staphylococcus, Acinetobacter, Moraxella, Enterobacter, Pseudomonas, E coli,* and *Klebsiella.*
  - Fungal cultures are rarely performed because alternate means are used for the diagnosis.
- Respiratory PCR panels
  - Respiratory PCR panels are available to detect organismal nucleic acids in dogs (influenza,

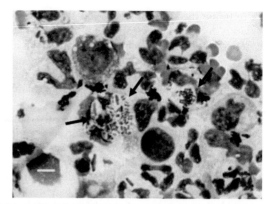

FIG. 5 Bronchoalveolar lavage sample revealing septic, suppurative airway neutrophilia (*black arrows*). The yellow bar represents 5 microns. Wright Giemsa stain, 100X.

Bordetella, canine adenovirus 2, canine distemper, parainfluenza, respiratory coronavirus, *Mycoplasma, Streptococcus equi* subsp *zooepidemicus*) and cats (*Bordetella,* herpesvirus, calicivirus, and *Mycoplasma*); however, these outcomes do not prove causation of disease and they also do not provide susceptibility information.
  - The primary benefit of a PCR panel would be to identify DNA of canine distemper virus, which can carry a guarded prognosis.

Conditions that alter results or complicate procedures
- Corticosteroids decrease the influx of inflammatory cells into the airways and can worsen infection.
- Consider the withdrawal of antimicrobials 3 to 7 days before the procedure depending on clinical circumstances to avoid antibiotic suppression of bacterial growth, although studies have demonstrated positive growth in the face of antibiotic use [16,17].
- Upper airway contamination indicated by the presence of squamous cells or *Conchiformibius* (previously *Simonsiella*) bacteria on cytology increases the likelihood of growth of bacteria but should not influence interpretation of cytology.

SPECIFIC DISEASE CONSIDERATIONS
Viral Pneumonia
- Etiologic agents.
  - Etiologic agents in the dog include canine distemper virus, canine adenovirus-2 virus CPIV, canine respiratory coronavirus virus, canine influenza

virus, canine pneumovirus, and canine herpes virus-1.

  o Viral infections in the cat, such as FHV-1 and calicivirus, are most commonly associated with upper respiratory disease but can cause primary pneumonia.

- Primary viral pneumonia is uncommon in adult animals (with the exception of canine influenza virus) as compared with young animals, but can predispose any animal to secondary bacterial pneumonia.

- A recent small study identified a potential role for underlying CPIV in 30% of dogs with bacterial pneumonia based on PCR evaluation of BAL samples [18].

- In a second study, nasopharyngeal swabs were positive for CPIV in more dogs with acute respiratory disease (38%) than in dogs without (8%), indicating the importance of underlying viral infection in resultant clinical presentation [19].

  o These findings also highlight the importance of infection control in dogs with serious respiratory illnesses, because viruses can be readily spread among populations of animals held in confined circumstances, such as a hospital intensive care units or patient wards.

  o It is interesting to speculate on whether coinfection with viruses could be universal or confined to certain geographic areas because viral prevalence in different regions of the country and world are quite variable. For example, in a study performed in US shelters, CPIV was found in only 3% of dogs, and these dogs did not have clinical respiratory disease [20].

Bacterial Pneumonia

- Animals with bacterial pneumonia usually have a history of a moist, productive cough, tachypnea, and respiratory distress; however, some animals present with more vague signs such as malaise, lethargy, anorexia, and weight loss.

  o These general rules are followed much more closely in dogs than in cats, in which bacterial pneumonia can cause clinical presentation similar to chronic bronchitis [21].

- Thoracic auscultation is typically abnormal with loud or harsh lung sounds; crackles are variably detected. Fever may or may not be present.

- Animals with bacterial pneumonia generally have peripheral blood leukocytosis, with or without a left shift. Elevated C-reactive protein has been reported [22].

- Pneumonia typically results in interstitial to alveolar radiographic pulmonary infiltrates.

- In dogs and cats with bacterial pneumonia, aerobic bacteria are most commonly isolated (Table 1); however, anaerobes can be detected in 17% to 20% of cases [16,21].

  o Most lung infections are polymicrobial [16,21,25], although 1 study reported a preponderance of infection by a single microbe [26].

  o Some clinicians believe that *Bordetella* or *Mycoplasma* can result in primary lung infection and particularly that *Mycoplasma* should be considered a pathogen [16,21,27]. However, in a retrospective immunohistochemical study of cats with pneumonia, *Mycoplasma* spp. were only found in association with other organisms, suggesting a secondary role in infection [28].

- Interpretation of susceptibility data for organisms isolated in lower respiratory tract infection is hampered by the lack of breakpoint measurements for most species [29].

  o Minimum inhibitory concentrations are often established by commercial laboratories using agar dilution methods recommended by the Clinical and Laboratory Standards Institute, and are used to interpolate susceptibility and resistance patterns.

- Susceptibility data reported in the literature can be used for initial empirical antibiotic therapy or for patients that cannot have airway sampling completed [16,30]; however, animals that have chronic, nonresolving pneumonia require specific assessment, and a consultation with a microbiologist, infectious disease, or respiratory specialist can be required.

  o Resistance to empirically administered antibiotics has been demonstrated in 57% to 100% of isolates from dogs with pneumonia [24,25], although the collection of airway samples has demonstrated retention of susceptibility to commonly administered antimicrobials for most organisms [16,26].

  o In an animal with nonresolving pneumonia, the possibility of a foreign body or pulmonary abscess should be considered.

- Recurrent disease could indicate structural respiratory tract disease, perhaps owing to bronchiectasis, or reinfection owing to aspiration.

FUNGAL PNEUMONIA

- Fungal pneumonias are typically caused by dimorphic fungi that have disseminated hematogenously to multiple organs.

TABLE 1
Organisms Identified in Dogs and Cats with Bacterial Pneumonia

	No. of Samples of Dog Isolates: % [Reference]	No. of Samples of Cat Isolates: % [Reference]
Enteric group	21/105: 20% [16] 16/40: 40% [24]	2/26: 8% [21]
E coli	17/105: 17% [16] 11/40: 28% [24]	5/40: 12% [23] 1/26: 4% [21] 30/485: 6% [26]
Klebsiella pneumonia	2/105: 2% [16] 4/40: 10% [24] 20/157: 13% [25] 164/1504: 11% [26]	
Proteus	2/105: 2% [16] 1/40: 2% [24]	
Pasteurella	22/105: 21% [16] 0/40: 0% [24] 38/157: 24% [25] 208/1504: 14% [26]	9/40: 22% [23] 8/26: 31% [21] 92/485: 19% [26]
Bordetella	23/105: 22% [16] 20/40: 50% [24] 5/157: 3% [25] 157/1504: 10% [26]	12/40: 30% [23] 1/26: 3% [21] 3/485: 1% [26]
Mycoplasma	29/99: 29% [16]	6/20: 15% [23] 11/26: 42% [21] 13/485: 3% [26]
Pseudomonas	6/105 (6%) [16] 2/40 (5%) [24] 9/157 (6%) [25] 136/1504 (9%) [26]	2/26: 8% [21] 29/485: 6% [26]
Stenotrophomonas	2/105: 2% [16]	
Actinomyces	5/105: 5% [16]	
Staphylococcus	6/105: 6% [16] 5/40: 12% [24] 15/157: 10% [25] 54/1504: 4% [26]	1/26: 4% [21] 7/485: 1% [26]
Streptococcus	10/105: 10% [16] 4/40: 10% [24] 21/157: 13% [25] 46/1504: 3% [26]	6/40: 15% [23] 9/26: 35% [21] 18/485: 4% [26]
Corynebacterium	2/105: 2% [16]	2/26: 4% [21]
Anaerobes	18/104: 17% [16] 12/1504: 1% [26]	7/24: 29% [21] 10/485: 4% [26]

- Chronic inflammation can result in neutrophilic leukocytosis, monocytosis, hyperglobulinemia, hypoalbuminemia, and nonregenerative anemia.

- Thoracic radiographic findings (Fig. 6) include hilar lymphadenopathy, interstitial to nodular infiltrates, mass lesions, and lobar infiltrates [31,32].

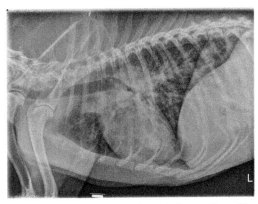

FIG. 6 Left lateral thoracic radiograph from a dog with fungal pneumonia (coccidioidomycosis) reveals hilar lymphadenopathy and a prominent bronchial pattern.

Specific Fungal Characteristics
Blastomycosis
- The etiologic agent *Blastomyces dermatitidis* has an ecological niche in the Ohio and Mississippi river valleys of the United States, Wisconsin, and Minnesota.
- Disease sites include the lungs, bones, reproductive organs, central nervous system, lymph nodes, and the skin in dogs.
- Serology cannot be relied on for diagnosis of blastomycosis, but disease can be confirmed by identification of 20 to 30 μm broad based budding yeasts in airway fluid or lymph node aspirations, or by urine antigen testing (Mira Vista Labs, Indianapolis, IN) [33].

Coccidioidomycosis
- The etiologic agent *Coccidioides immitis* has an ecological niche in the San Joaquin river valley, Arizona, New Mexico, and Texas in the United States and in Central and South America.
- Disease sites include the lung, pericardium, bones, and central nervous system. Cats more often present with dermatologic rather than pulmonary disease.
- Serology for IgM and IgG using gel immunodiffusion in dogs can aid in the diagnosis, although dogs living in endemic regions will naturally develop antibody production over time [34]. Heat-treated AGID assays are considered most reliable in dogs with appropriate clinical signs. If initial titers are negative but a high suspicion for coccidioidomycosis remains, convalescent titers should be repeated in 2 to 3 weeks. An antibody enzyme immunoassay

that detects canine IgG can aid in the diagnosis in a time-efficient manner, particularly when combined with an antigen immunoassay [35].
- Diagnosis can be confirmed by identification of a 7- to 80-μm doubled-walled spherule, although organisms are typically sparse in cytology.

Histoplasmosis
- The etiologic agent *Histoplasma capsulatum* has an ecological niche in the Ohio and Mississippi river valleys of the United States, with pockets of infection noted in California, as well as in Africa, Latin America, and China
- Other than the lung, disease sites include the liver, spleen, gastrointestinal tract, lymph nodes, bone marrow, and the skin in cats.
- Serologic diagnosis is confused by false positive and false negative results, but diagnosis can be confirmed by identification of 4 to 6 μm intracellular yeasts located within macrophages in airway fluid or in other sites. Urine antigen testing (Mira Vista Labs) is highly useful for the diagnosis, with a sensitivity of 80% and specificity of 100% [36].

Pneumocystis canis
- Pneumocystis canis is distributed world-wide and seems to be associated with immune dysfunction.
- Breed predilection is recognized in Cavalier King Charles Spaniels and miniature Dachshunds. Dogs are typically young, approximately 1 year of age [37,38].
- Common clinical signs include cough, weight loss, tachypnea, and cyanosis. Fever is uncommon.
- Thoracic computed tomography scans reveal a ground-glass appearance that can appear similar to interstitial pulmonary fibrosis [39].
- This fungal infection can be diagnosed through cytologic identification of 5- to 10-μm cysts in airway fluid or tissue samples. Special stains can be required because cysts are easily missed on cytology.
- Quantitative PCR on airway fluid has been used to establish a diagnosis [40].

Parasitic Pneumonia
- Several nematode parasites target the pulmonary parenchyma and airways; potential pathogens vary based on geographic location.
- Peripheral eosinophilia can be present on a complete blood count and radiographic patterns are highly variable.

- *Aelurostrongylus* and *Trogolostrongylus* cause airway infection in cats, whereas *Filaroides* is the most common cause in the dog.
- Diagnosis can sometimes be made by cytologic identification of parasites on airway lavage or in fecal samples using the Baermann sedimentation method [41], although testing is insensitive owing to intermittent shedding and parasite migration. Serology and PCR testing for feline lungworm have been performed in research studies, but are not commercially available in most regions.
- *Dirofilaria immitis* causes pulmonary vascular infection in both dogs and cats. In the dog, heartworm antigen testing is the recommended screening test, whereas in the cat antibody tests are often used to assess exposure. Disease in the dog is relatively straightforward to document; however, cats can have negative antibody and antigen tests yet be infected with heartworm. Also, it has been suggested that developing, migrating larval stages can cause pulmonary disease in cats that leads to cough, resulting in a challenging diagnosis.
- *Angiostrongylus vasorum* is an emerging vascular infection that could ultimately have worldwide implications. Larval migration induces a granulomatous pneumonitis and thrombotic disease, as well as hemorrhagic diathesis. Fecal Baermann can provide the diagnosis, although multiple fecal samples are typically required. PCR or ELISA antibody testing on airway lavage can aid in diagnosis of *Angiostrongylus* if the parasite is not identified on cytology and a high index of suspicion remains [42].

Protozoal Infections

- *Toxoplasma gondii* infection can result in acute or chronic pneumonic signs in cats, but is rarely associated with pneumonia in the dog.
- Clearance of toxoplasmosis is usually not possible and reactivation can occur, especially in the face of immunosuppression.
- Thoracic radiographs typically display an interstitial pattern. Diagnosis can be achieved by serologic testing for IgG and IgM or by airway sampling revealing typical tachyzoites approximately 2×6 μm.

INTRODUCTION TO PLEURAL INFECTION AND EMPYEMA

- Bacterial pyothorax typically results from migration of an inhaled or ingested foreign body into the pleural space, penetrating bite wounds or other injuries, and occasionally via extension of pneumonia (pleuropneumonia).
- Pneumothorax can be found concurrently owing to lung lobe or pleural rupture.
- Nonseptic suppurative to pyogranulomatous inflammation in cats often reflects feline infectious peritonitis (FIP).

Thoracocentesis
Indications

- Clinical signs include respiratory difficulty or tachypnea, although chronic nonspecific signs such as lethargy, inappetence, and weight loss can predominate in some cases. Cough is reported less commonly and is likely due to airway compression.
- Physical examination often reveals rapid, shallow respirations and decreased heart and lung sounds ventrally. Fever may or may not be present.

Before the procedure

- Thoracic ultrasound examination can be used to confirm the presence of fluid, although in animals with marked respiratory distress, immediate thoracocentesis should be performed when physical examination findings suggest pleural fluid.
- If the animal is stable enough for thoracic radiographs, pleural fissure markings and loss of the cardiac silhouette are often noted. Dorsoventral positioning should be used to avoid patient distress, although ventrodorsal positioning improves visualization of scant amounts of fluid.
- Sedation is often required depending on patient stability.
- Oxygen supplementation during the procedure can help alleviate respiratory distress; however, removal of the fluid is more important for improving ventilation and oxygenation.

Equipment

- Butterfly catheter (21G–23G) or 14G (large dog) to 20G (cat or small dog) over-the-needle IV catheter attached to an extension set, 3-way stopcock, and syringe.
- Clippers, lidocaine with sodium bicarbonate added.
- Sterile scrub, fenestrated drape, and surgical gloves.
- Collection tubes (red and purple top tubes), culturette, and collection bowl.

Technique

- Thoracocentesis is best performed with at least 2 but preferably 3 personnel.

- Place an IV catheter if possible and administer appropriate sedation and pain control.
- Position the animal in sternal recumbency and clip the ventral thorax near the seventh to ninth intercostal space. The side of thorax and specific site is chosen based on auscultation or use of point-of-care ultrasound examination to find the largest pocket of fluid.
- Perform sterile preparation of the site with alternating wipes of chlorhexidine scrub and alcohol.
- Local subcutaneous anesthetic block at the site of catheter or needle placement (lidocaine with sodium bicarbonate in 9:1 ratio) can be considered.
- With sterile gloves, select a site for the catheter that avoids the caudal margin of the rib where intercostal vessels and nerves travel. Make a stab incision using a #11 scalpel blade and insert the needle through the skin, subcutaneous tissue, and intercostal muscles until it penetrates the pleural space.
- If using an over-the-needle catheter, advance the catheter off the needle, withdraw the needle stylet, and rapidly attach the extension set to evacuate the chest.
- An assistant withdraws as much fluid as needed for diagnostic testing (usually 3–5 mL). If marked pleural effusion is present, therapeutic thoracocentesis should also be performed to withdraw as much fluid as possible; an over-the-needle catheter is preferable to a butterfly catheter for large volumes.
- Depending on the chronicity and amount of fibrin present, using gravity to remove a large volume of effusion can be more effective than continued aspiration with a syringe because the latter can pull fibrin strands and visceral pleura against the catheter tip, interrupting flow. A second extension set is attached to the 3-way stopcock and the end of the second extension set is placed into a collection bowl below the site of thoracocentesis to allow gravity-assisted flow.

Sample handling

- Samples should be placed into EDTA and sterile collection tubes for fluid analysis and cytology, and into a culturette for bacterial aerobic and anaerobic culture.
- Fungal culture can be considered if there is high suspicion for fungal pyothorax on imaging (eg, perihilar lymphadenomegaly) or cytology.
- Samples should be saved for possible PCR testing, if indicated based on cytology.
- Pyothorax or empyema is characterized by increased protein concentration (>3.5 g/dL) and increased total nucleated cell count (>5000/μL) on fluid analysis.

Aftercare

- Monitor respiratory rate and effort, as well as thoracic auscultation and ultrasound examination, to detect the development of iatrogenic pneumothorax or recurrence of pleural effusion.
- Administer oxygen as needed.
- Limit activity until fully recovered from sedation or anesthesia.
- If pleural effusion reaccumulates rapidly, placement of indwelling unilateral or bilateral chest tubes should be considered.

SPECIFIC DISEASE CONSIDERATIONS
Bacterial Pyothorax
- Cytologic analysis is critically important to confirm infection. In one study, bacteria were visualized via cytology in 68% of samples from dogs and 91% of samples from cats [43].
- Samples should be submitted for both aerobic and anaerobic cultures with anaerobic media. Organisms isolated from dogs and cats in 1 study (Table 2) revealed polymicrobial infections in a majority of cats and dogs [43]; however, a study from the UK found monomicrobial infection in 85% of dogs [45].

Viral Infection: Feline Infectious Peritonitis
- The enteric feline coronavirus, an enveloped RNA virus, typically causes mild gastrointestinal signs but occasionally mutates in vivo to the more virulent FIP virus and spreads systemically leading to vasculitis, serositis, and pyogranulomatous inflammation and the syndrome of FIP [46].
- Cats less than 2 years tend to be affected, although some studies show a bimodal distribution with cats aged more than 10 years also at risk. Males are predisposed [46,47].
- Approximately 80% of cats with FIP have the effusive form of the disease; of these, 21% have pleural effusion [47].
- Effusions from cats with FIP are grossly straw yellow in color (icteric) and viscous (ie, proteinaceous).
- Fluid analysis is uniquely characterized by having a high protein concentration (>3.5 g/dL) with a comparatively low total nucleated cell count (<5000/μL).
- Diagnosis can be confirmed with positive real-time qPCR for feline coronavirus in pleural fluid, or

TABLE 2
Organisms Identified in Dogs and Cats with Pyothorax

	Dog: No. of Samples of Dog Isolates: % [Reference]	Cat: No. of Samples of Dog Isolates: % [Reference]
Aerobes		
Enteric bacteria – *E coli*, *Klebsiella, Enterobacter*	6/47: 22% [43] 9/99: 9% [45]	1/45: 4% [43]
Nonenteric bacteria – *Pasteurella, Acinetobacter, Pseudomonas*	10/47: 37% [43] 9/99: 9% [45]	19/45: 70% [43] 11/38: 29% [44]
Actinomyces	5/47: 19% [43] 5/99: 5% [45]	4/45: 15% [43] 3/38: 8% [44]
Anaerobes		
Peptostreptococcus	18/47: 27% [43] 7/99: 7% [45]	17/45: 20% [43]
Bacteroides	17/47: 25% [43] 7/99: 7% [45]	20/45: 24% [43] 6/38: 16% [44]
Fusobacterium	14/47: 21% [43]	14/45: 17% [43] 1/38: 3% [44]
Porphyromonas	6/47: 9% [43]	10/45: 12% [43]

positive immunocytochemistry or immunofluorescence for feline coronavirus within macrophages in pleural fluid.

Fungal Pyothorax and Empyema
Coccidioidomycosis

- *Coccidioides immitis* and *Coccidioides posadasii* are dimorphic soil fungi endemic to the Southwestern United States, Mexico, and Central and South America.
- Pericarditis or pericardial effusion with subsequent pleural effusion has been reported [48], and there are rare reports of eosinophilic pleural effusion [49].
- Cytology has low sensitivity for identifying the tissue form of the fungus, the spherule, despite its relatively large size (8–70 μm) and culture is also insensitive, as well as a public health hazard.
- Positive quantitative (heat-treated) AGID serology is considered diagnostic for disease in conjunction with appropriate clinical signs [32].

Opportunistic molds

- Opportunistic molds including *Aspergillus* spp., *Penicillium* spp., and *Rasamsonia* spp. can lead to systemic

disease including pleural effusion in immunocompromised breeds such as the German Shepherd dog.
- Pyogranulomatous exudate and neutrophilic-eosinophilic exudate without fungal elements was reported in dogs with systemic *Rasamsonia* spp. infections, with diagnosis confirmed by DNA sequencing as well as urine culture [50].
- Pyogranulomatous pleural effusion, sometimes with fungal hyphae, has also been reported in dogs with systemic aspergillosis [51].
- Serum and urine galactomannan antigen ELISA assay for *Aspergillus* is the noninvasive test of choice for diagnosing disseminated mold infections in dogs, particularly immunocompromised dogs. This assay is highly sensitive but not specific for aspergillosis; cross-reactivity was noted in dogs with *Rasamsonia* spp., *Paecilomyces* spp., *Geotrichum* spp., *Cryptococcus neoformans*, and *Penicillium* spp. infections [50,52].
- Pleural fluid analysis and fungal culture of effusions are recommended for definitive diagnosis of species and for susceptibility patterns, as many of these opportunistic molds will cross-react with the *Aspergillus* galactomannan antigen ELISA assay.

CLINICS CARE POINTS

- Nasal samples submitted for bacterial or fungal cultures or for PCR can establish a diagnosis in certain nasal conditions however caution is warranted in patient selection and in interpretation of results.

- Radiographic and clinical presentations of many infectious pneumonias can overlap, but history, signalment, and nonrespiratory clinical signs can help prioritize the list of differential diagnoses and the diagnostic work up.

- Bronchoscopy can be diagnostic for many infectious pneumonias, but minimally invasive diagnostics, such as Baermann fecal evaluation, fungal antigen testing, and some PCR analyses, could be indicated initially based on clinical suspicion.

- Pleural fluid samples should be submitted for aerobic and anaerobic culture when neutrophilic cytology is found. If fluid is pyogranulomatous, consideration should be given to the diagnosis of FIP in the cat and for fungal empyema in dogs or cats.

DISCLOSURE

The authors have no commercial or financial conflicts of interest. All authors are employed by the University of California, Davis. Partial funding was provided by the Bailey Wrigley Foundation.

REFERENCES

[1] De Lorenzi D, Bonfanti U, Masserdotti C, et al. Diagnosis of canine nasal aspergillosis by cytological examination: a comparison of four different collection techniques. J Small Anim Pract 2006;47:316–9.

[2] Johnson LR, Foley JE, De Cock HEV, et al. Assessment of infectious organisms associated with chronic rhinosinusitis in cats. J Am Vet Med Assoc 2005;227:579–85.

[3] Pomrantz JS, Johnson LR, Nelson RW, et al. Use of serologic evaluation via agar gel immunodiffusion and fungal culture of tissue for diagnosis of nasal aspergillosis in dogs. J Am Vet Med Assoc 2007;230:1319–23.

[4] Berryessa NA, Johnson LR, Kasten RW, et al. Microbial culture of blood samples and serologic testing for bartonellosis in cats with chronic rhinosinusitis. J Am Vet Med Assoc 2008;233:1084–9.

[5] Hawkins EC, Johnson LR, Guptill L, et al. Failure to identify an association between serologic or molecular evidence of Bartonella infection and idiopathic rhinitis in dogs. J Am Vet Med Assoc 2008;233:597–9.

[6] Windsor RC, Johnson LR, Sykes JE, et al. Molecular detection of microbes in nasal tissue of dogs with idiopathic lymphoplasmacytic rhinitis. J Vet Intern Med 2006;20: 250–6.

[7] Mercier E, Peters IR, Billen F, et al. Potential role of Alternaria and Cladosporium species in canine lymphoplasmacytic rhinitis. J Small Anim Pract 2013;54(4):179–83.

[8] Hoover EA, Griesemer RA. Bone lesions produced by feline herpesvirus. Lab Invest 1971;25(5):457–64.

[9] Reagan KL, McHardy I, Thompson GR 3rd, et al. Evaluation of the clinical performance of 2 point-of-care cryptococcal antigen tests in dogs and cats. J Vet Intern Med 2019;33:2082–9.

[10] Billen F, Peeters D, Peters IR, et al. Comparison of the value of measurement of serum galactomannan and Aspergillus-specific antibodies in the diagnosis of canine sino-nasal aspergillosis. Vet Microbiol 2009;133:358–65.

[11] Whitney J, Beatty JA, Martin P, et al. Evaluation of serum galactomannan detection for diagnosis of feline upper respiratory tract aspergillosis. Vet Microbiol 2013;162: 180–5.

[12] Barrs VR, Ujvari B, Dhand NK, et al. Detection of Aspergillus-specific antibodies by agar gel double immunodiffusion and IgG ELISA in feline upper respiratory tract aspergillosis. Vet J 2015;203:285–9.

[13] Malik R, Wigney DI, Muir DB, et al. Asymptomatic carriage of Cryptococcus neoformans in the nasal cavity of dogs and cats. J Med Vet Mycol 1997;35:27–31.

[14] Hawkins EC, Kennedy-Stoskopf S, Levy J, et al. Cytologic characterization of bronchoalveolar lavage fluid collected through an endotracheal tube in cats. Am J Vet Res 1994;55:795–802.

[15] Hawkins EC, Berry CR. Use of a modified stomach tube for bronchoalveolar lavage in dogs. J Am Vet Med Assoc 1999;215:1635–9.

[16] Johnson LR, Queen EV, Vernau W, et al. Microbiologic and cytologic assessment of bronchoalveolar lavage fluid in dogs with lower respiratory tract infection. J Vet Intern Med 2013;27:259–67.

[17] Graham AM, Tefft KM, Stowe DM, et al. Factors associated with clinical interpretation of tracheal wash fluid from dogs with respiratory disease: 281 cases (2012-2017). J Vet Intern Med 2021;35:1073–9.

[18] Viitanen SJ, Lappalainen A, Rajamäki MM. Co-Infections with respiratory viruses in dogs with bacterial pneumonia. J Vet Int Med 2015;29:544–51.

[19] Schulz BS, Kurz S, Weber K, et al. Detection of respiratory viruses and Bordetella bronchiseptica in dogs with acute respiratory tract infections. Vet J 2014;201:365–9.

[20] Lavan R, Knesl O. Prevalence of canine infectious respiratory pathogens in asymptomatic dogs presented at US animal shelters. J Small Anim Pract 2015;56:572–6.

[21] Dear JD, Vernau W, Johnson EG, et al. Clinicopathologic and radiographic features in 33 cats with aspiration and 26 cats with bronchopneumonia (2007-2017). J Vet Intern Med 2021;35:480–9.

[22] Viitanen SJ, Laurila HP, Lilja-Maula LI, et al. Serum C-reactive protein as a diagnostic biomarker in dogs with bacterial respiratory diseases. J Vet Intern Med 2014;28:84–91.

[23] Bart M, Guscetti F, Zurbriggen A, et al. Feline infectious pneumonia. a short literature review and a retrospective

immunohistological study on the involvement of *Chlamydia* spp. and distemper virus. Vet J 2000;159:220–30.

[24] Proulx A, Hume DZ, Drobatz KJ, et al. In vitro bacterial isolate susceptibility to empirically selected antimicrobials in 111 dogs with bacterial pneumonia. J Vet Emerg Crit Care (San Antonio) 2014;24:194–200.

[25] Qekwana DN, Naidoo V, Oguttu JW, et al. Occurrence and predictors of bacterial respiratory tract infections and antimicrobial resistance among isolates from dogs presented with lower respiratory tract infections at a referral veterinary hospital in South Africa. Front Vet Sci 2020;7:304.

[26] Mavrides DE, Morgan AL, Na JG, et al. Antimicrobial resistance profiles of bacteria associated with lower respiratory tract infections in cats and dogs in England. Vet Rec 2021;e779.

[27] Foster SF, Martin P, Allan GS, et al. Lower respiratory tract infections in cats: 21 cases (1995-2000). J Feline Med Surg 2004;6:167–80.

[28] Schmal-Filius E, Nedorost N, Weissenbacher-Lang C, et al. A retrospective study on the presence of selected infectious agents in lung samples of cats with pneumonia. Acta Vet Hung 2020;68:275–84.

[29] Moyaert H, de Jong A, Simjee S, et al. Survey of antimicrobial susceptibility of bacterial pathogens isolated from dogs and cats with respiratory tract infections in Europe: ComPath results. J Appl Microbiol 2019;127: 29–46.

[30] Lappin MR, Blondeau J, Boothe D, et al. Antimicrobial use guidelines for treatment of respiratory tract disease in dogs and cats: antimicrobial guidelines Working Group of the International Society for Companion Animal Infectious Diseases. J Vet Intern Med 2017;31: 279–94.

[31] Crews LJ, Feeney DA, Jessen CR, et al. Radiographic findings in dogs with pulmonary blastomycosis: 125 cases (1989-2006). J Am Vet Med Assoc 2008;232:215–21.

[32] Johnson LR, Herrgesell EJ, Davidson AP, et al. Clinical, clinicopathologic, and radiographic findings in dogs with coccidioidomycosis: 24 cases (1995-2000). J Am Vet Med Assoc 2003;222:461–6.

[33] Spector D, Legendre AM, Wheat J, et al. Antigen and antibody testing for the diagnosis of blastomycosis in dogs. J Vet Int Med 2008;22:839–43.

[34] Shubitz LF, Butkiewicz CD, Dial SM, et al. Incidence of *Coccidioides* infection among dogs residing in a region in which the organism is endemic. J Am Vet Med Assoc 2005;226:1846–50.

[35] Holbrook ED, Greene RT, Rubin SI, et al. Novel canine anti-*Coccidioides* immunoglobulin G enzyme immunoassay aids in diagnosis of coccidioidomycosis in dogs. Med Mycol 2019;57:800–6.

[36] Cunningham L, Cook A, Hanzlicek A, et al. Sensitivity and specificity of *Histoplasma* antigen detection by enzyme immunoassay. J Am Anim Hosp Assoc 2015; 51:306–10.

[37] Lobetti R. Common variable immunodeficiency in miniature dachshunds affected with *Pneumocystis carinii* pneumonia. J Vet Diagn Invest 2000;12:39–45.

[38] Watson PJ, Wotton P, Eastwood J, et al. Immunoglobulin deficiency in Cavalier King Charles Spaniels with *Pneumocystis* pneumonia. J Vet Int Med 2006;20:523–7.

[39] Schiborra F, Scudder CJ, Littler RM, et al. CT findings in *Pneumocystis carinii* pneumonia in five dogs. J Small Anim Pract 2018;59:508–13.

[40] Danesi P, Ravagnan S, Johnson LR, et al. Molecular diagnosis of *Pneumocystis* pneumonia in dogs. Med Mycol 2017;55:828–42.

[41] Lacorcia L, Gasser RB, Anderson GA, et al. Comparison of bronchoalveolar lavage fluid examination and other diagnostic techniques with the Baermann technique for detection of naturally occurring *Aelurostrongylus abstrusus* infection in cats. J Am Vet Med Assoc 2009;235:43–9.

[42] Canonne AM, Billen F, Losson B, et al. Angiostrongylosis in dogs with negative fecal and in-clinic rapid serological tests: 7 Cases (2013-2017). J Vet Intern Med 2018;32: 951–5.

[43] Walker AL, Jang SS, Hirsh DC. Bacteria associated with pyothorax in dogs and cats: 98 cases (1989-1998). J Am Vet Med Assoc 2000;216:359–63.

[44] Krämer F, Rainer J, Bali MS. Short- and long-term outcome in cats diagnosed with pyothorax: 47 cases (2009-2018). J Small Anim Pract 2021;62:669–76.

[45] Eiras-Diaz A, FrykforsvonHekkel A, Hanot E, et al. CT findings, management and short-term outcome of dogs with pyothorax: 101 cases (2010 to 2019). J Small Anim Pract 2021;62(11):959–66.

[46] Barker EN, Tasker S. Advances in molecular diagnostics and treatment of Feline Infectious Peritonitis. Adv Small Anim Care 2020;1:161–88.

[47] Riemer F, Kuehner KA, Ritz S, et al. Clinical and laboratory features of cats with feline infectious peritonitis - a retrospective study of 231 confirmed cases (2000-2010). J Feline Med Surg 2016;18:348–56.

[48] Heinritz CK, Gilson SD, Soderstrom MJ, et al. Subtotal pericardectomy and epicardial excision for treatment of coccidioidomycosis-induced effusive-constrictive pericarditis in dogs: 17 cases (1999-2003). J Am Vet Med Assoc 2005;227:435–40.

[49] Piech TL, Jaffey JA, Hostnik ET, et al. Bicavitary eosinophilic effusion in a dog with coccidioidomycosis. J Vet Int Med 2020;34:1582–6.

[50] Dear JD, Reagan KL, Hulsebosch SE, et al. Disseminated *Rasamsonia argillacea* species complex infections in 8 dogs. J Vet Intern Med 2021;35:2232–40.

[51] Schultz RM, Johnson EG, Wisner ER, et al. Clinicopathologic and diagnostic imaging characteristics of systemic aspergillosis in 30 dogs. J Vet Intern Med 2008;22:851–9.

[52] Garcia RS, Wheat LJ, Cook AK, et al. Sensitivity and specificity of a blood and urine galactomannan antigen assay for diagnosis of systemic aspergillosis in dogs. J Vet Intern Med 2012;26:911–9.

Advances in Small Animal Care 3 (2022) 177–220

ADVANCES IN SMALL ANIMAL CARE

Canine Leptospirosis – Global Distribution, Diagnosis, and Treatment

Christine Griebsch, Dr med vet, DipECVIM-CA, GradCertEdStud (HigherEd), FHEA, PhD Candidate*,
Michael P. Ward, BVSc(Hons), MSc, MPVM, PhD, DVSc, FANZCVS,
Jacqueline M. Norris, BVSc, MVS, PhD, FASM, RCVS (Microbiology), GradCertEdStud (HigherEd)
Sydney School of Veterinary Science, University of Sydney, New South Wales 2006, Australia

---

KEYWORDS

• Leptospirosis • *Leptospira* • Canine • Microscopic agglutination test • Zoonosis

KEY POINTS

- Serovars responsible for canine leptospirosis vary between geographic regions.
- Diagnosis of acute canine leptospirosis can be difficult due to false-negative PCR in dogs pretreated with antibiotics or insufficient time for seroconversion in microscopic agglutination test (MAT).
- The MAT lacks sensitivity and specificity to determine the causative Serovar. Therefore, new molecular methods are being developed to diagnose infecting Serovars.
- Vaccines contain Serovars known to cause disease in their respective geographic region. While they offer a high level of Serogroup specific protection, fully vaccinated dogs can develop leptospirosis.

INTRODUCTION

Leptospirosis is a potentially fatal zoonotic bacterial disease affecting dogs worldwide. Clinical disease is characterized by acute kidney injury in most, hepatic involvement in many and hemorrhagic and pulmonary involvement in some cases. Transmission occurs by direct contact with infected urine or via urine-contaminated environments. Rodents are the reservoir host that most frequently transmit leptospires, but the primary reservoir host can vary between geographic regions, likely contributing to differences in seroprevalence [1,2].

While identification of the infecting Serovar has historically been based on the magnitude of antibody titers via the microscopic agglutination test (MAT) – with the Serovar with the highest titer nominated as the infecting Serovar [3] – this diagnostic approach remains unverified in dogs [4,5]. In dogs with similarly high titers to multiple Serovars, the causative Serovar is usually not reported. Other studies take possible cross-reactivity between Serovars within the same Serogroup into account hence report the causative Serogroup rather than Serovar [6–9]. Furthermore, comparison of seroprevalence study results is complicated by differences in study design and inclusion of different Serovars in MAT. Therefore, new molecular methods are being developed to determine infecting Serovars and their global distribution more accurately, to improve disease control via vaccination. Vaccination is part of the preventive strategy; however, its impact in preventing disease is inconsistent and influenced by the infecting Serovar(s) and valency of the vaccine. Prevention strategies more broadly need to include a suite of measures tailored to different geographic regions taking epidemiological data (including distribution and control [eg, pest control] of reservoir hosts, nature of the terrain, community

---

*Corresponding author, *E-mail address:* christine.griebsch@sydney.edu.au

https://doi.org/10.1016/j.yasa.2022.06.001

awareness and infection prevention measures) into account. Outcomes of infection differ between geographic regions and available epidemiological data and might be due to variation in virulence of infecting Serovars, availability of vaccines, index of suspicion, availability of diagnostic testing, speed of diagnosis, rapid treatment with antibiotics and in the most severe cases, availability of advanced treatment options such as hemodialysis.

BACTERIAL PROPERTIES, TAXONOMY, AND TRANSMISSION

Leptospira spp. are thin (0.1 µm diameter), flexible, highly motile, spiral-shaped gram-negative spirochete bacteria with a hook-shaped end (*leptos* = thin, *spira* = coiled) [10]. The genus *Leptospira* is considered to have 2 clades (pathogenic [P] and saprophytic [S]), with each clade further divided into 2 subclades (P1, P2, S1 and S2). P1 contains >60 pathogenic species affecting humans and animals [11]. The two main species causing clinical disease in dogs are *Leptospira interrogans* and *L. kirschneri*, with other species such as *L. borgpetersenii*, [12,13] *L. noguchii* [14] and *L. santarosai* [15] occasionally reported in focal geographic locations. There are more than 20 different Serogroups and 250 different Serovars. Antigenically related Serovars are grouped within the same Serogroup. Serovars can be distinguished by differences in the carbohydrate component of their lipopolysaccharide (LPS) antigens [16]. Within each Serovar there are different strains, which are specific isolates of a defined leptospiral Serovar, and these strains are used in the MAT. The classification of leptospires has become even more complex with the availability of genotyping as Serovars of the same Serogroup may belong to different genomic species [2]. (Table 1).

Each Serovar is adapted to different wild or domestic animal reservoir hosts. Reservoir hosts experience limited subclinical or asymptomatic disease, usually maintaining leptospires in their renal tubules for prolonged periods of time, excreting them in their urine and hence act as a source of infection for other animals and humans (hence reservoir hosts are sometimes termed "silent shedders"). Incidental hosts can develop a range of clinical manifestations from mild febrile illness to severe multisystemic disease following infection. Dogs are reported to be reservoir hosts for Serovar Canicola [17]. However, clinical leptospirosis due to infection with Serovar Canicola has been described in dogs (Table 3), prompting reconsideration of the concept of a reservoir versus incidental host of *Leptospira*. Reservoir hosts vary between different regions. Rodents are regarded as one of the major reservoir hosts worldwide (including Serovars Icterohemorrhagiae, Copenhageni, Ballum, Grippotyphosa) [18]. Other important reservoir hosts include horses (Serovar Bratislava) [19,20], cattle (Serovar Hardjo) [21,22], sheep (Serovar Hardjo) [22], pigs (Serovar Pomona, Bratislava) [23], racoons [24–26], hedgehogs (Serovar Australis) [27] and opossums [26].

PATHOGENESIS

Once excreted in urine, leptospires immediately require moisture to survive and remain infectious. Under these conditions they can stay infectious for weeks to months [28]. They do not replicate outside of the host and are inactivated when exposed to heat, freezing, ultraviolet irradiation and a variety of disinfectants.

TABLE 1
Examples of How Pathogenic *LEPTOSPIRA* (Subclade P1) Are Classified By Species, Serogroup, Serovar and Strain

Genus	Clade	Species	Serogroup	Serovar	Strain
Leptospira	Pathogenic (P1)	*Leptospira interrogans*	Serjoe	Hardjo Serjoe Saxkoebing Wolfii	Hardjoprajitano M 84 Mus 24 3709
		Leptospira borgpetersenii		Hardjo	Hardjobovis Lely 607

Serovar Hardjo is in the serogroup Serjoe together with Serovars Serjoe, Saxkoebing, and Wolfii. Serovar Hardjo has different strains which are used in the MAT. Depending on MAT results and genotyping, the serovar can either belong to species *L. interrogans* or *L. borgpetersenii*.
   Strains used for MAT in a study by Jorge S, Schuch RA, de Oliveira NR, et al. Human and animal leptospirosis in Southern Brazil: A five-year retrospective study. *Travel Medicine and Infectious Disease.* 2017;18:46-52.

Dogs become infected by direct contact with urine or indirectly via contaminated environments such as soil and water through intact mucus membranes, abrasions, or ingestion of infected tissue [1]. Venereal and placental transfer [1,29,30] have also been described. Following transmucosal passage, bacteraemia occurs for up to 10 days followed by vasculitis, organ ischemia and invasion of the kidneys and liver, resulting in the shedding of leptospires into urine [1,2,31]. Systemic inflammation, immune-mediated, direct leptospiral effects, and endothelial activation and dysfunction are thought to affect multiple body systems, and can result in leptospiral pulmonary hemorrhage syndrome (LPHS) in some dogs [32–35].

GLOBAL DISTRIBUTION

Leptospirosis has a worldwide distribution. Evidence of exposure via serological studies and prevalence of disease vary widely between different regions, likely due to differences in climate and environmental conditions and the presence of reservoir hosts. To estimate seroprevalence and determine the causative Serovar in clinical disease, the MAT is widely used. The Serovar with the highest titer is usually considered to be the causative Serovar [3]. Recent studies have challenged this assumption (see Serological Diagnostics: Microscopic Agglutination Test section). Comparison of the seroprevalence and Serovars causing disease between regions is difficult due to differences in diagnostics and study design including the number and type of Serovars used in MAT, paradoxical reactions especially during the acute phase of infection [36], discordancy of results between different laboratories [4], inclusion/exclusion of vaccinated dogs, differences in the demographics of the sampled population (e.g, age profile, inclusion of stray or shelter dogs), reporting of Serogroups versus Serovars and choice of cut-off titers (see MAT).

Table 2 summarizes the global data on the seroprevalence in healthy dogs, and Table 3 the global data on most common Serovars causing disease. The most commonly identified Serogroup causing disease in Europe is Australis [37–48]. In North America Serogroups Autumnalis [49–54], Pomona [55–59] and Grippotyphosa [6,7,58,60–62] are the most commonly reported to cause disease. Serogroup Icterohemorrhagiae is the most commonly identified Serovar causing disease in Southern Europe [63], the British Isles [20,64,65], the Caribbean [9,66], South America [67–69] and Oceania (Australia, NSW) [70]. In East Asia (China, Japan) Serogroups Australis [71–73], Canicola [73] and Hebdomanis [71,73] have been reported, whereas in South Asia

Serovars Grippotyphosa [74,75], Australis [74–76], Autumnalis [74,76] (India), Bataviae [13] and Javanica [13] (Malaysia) have been found.

PREVALENCE OF SILENT SHEDDERS

"Silent shedders" are identified based on positive urine polymerase chain reaction (PCR) in the absence of clinical signs of disease. The prevalence of silent shedders varies widely in different countries and is summarized in Table 4.

Concerningly, a study investigating 126 healthy dogs from Brazil (PCR and MAT negative at enrolment) found that 49% became PCR positive at some timepoint over a 1 year period, suggesting that healthy dogs can intermittently shed leptospires [77]. The extent of longitudinal shedding has not been determined globally.

EPIDEMIOLOGY

A seasonal pattern has been described with most cases of leptospirosis reported in late summer [42,50,78,79] and autumn [42,50,78–80], and an increase in cases in areas with higher average annual temperature [42,81] and rainfall [42,53,78,79,82,83]. In contrast, some studies found that the seasonal pattern for canine leptospirosis differed by geographic region (North America [53,84,85] and Scotland [81], with higher case numbers during cool temperatures [81,83]) and distinct spatial and space-time clusters for individual Serovars [85].

Sex, breed and use of dogs play a role in the likelihood of disease. Male [61,83,86,87] adult [61,86,87] dogs seem to be at an increased risk in most studies. Herding dogs, hounds, working dogs and mixed breed dogs had a significant greater risk than companion dogs in the US [86], while Cocker Spaniels, Collies, and Lurchers seem to be at increased risk to develop leptospirosis in the UK [20].

Whereas dogs in urban areas had an increased risk to develop leptospirosis in Canada [50], Kansas and Nebraska [88], dogs in periurban areas [62], dogs who had been walked in rural areas [56] or dogs in close proximity to university/college and parks/forests [89] had a greater risk of leptospirosis in other parts of North America.

Contact with water [53] as determined by high hydrographic density [56,90], high percent of wetlands [56], frequently flooded areas [90], swimming in or drinking from outdoor water [56] and a lack of

TABLE 2
Prevalence of Antibody Titers As Measured By Microscopic Agglutination Test (MAT) in Healthy Dogs Tested Worldwide Since 2000 (Or Most Recent Report If There Are No Studies After 2000)

Region	Sample No.	Types of Dogs Sampled	Vaccination Status	MAT Cut-Off	Serovars Tested	Prevalence[a]	Most Common Serovars	Study Reference
Europe								
Eastern Europe								
Poland	130	Healthy	Unvaccinated	1/100	18	22%	Serovars Sejroe, Canicola	Krawczyk [191], 2005
Western Europe								
Germany (South)	200	Healthy	Not reported	1/100	Not reported	17%	Not reported	Llewellyn et al [192], 2014
Switzerland	377	Healthy	Vaccinated/unvaccinated	1/100	12	25%	Serovars Australis, Bratislava, Copenhageni, Canicola	Delaude et al [19], 2017
Netherlands	86	Healthy	Unknown	1/20	16	72%	Serovars Copenhageni, Patoc, Icterohemorrhagiae	Houwens et al [193], 2011
	100	Healthy	Unknown			32%	Serovar Copenhageni	
	26	Healthy, hunting	Unvaccinated			87%	Serovars Patoc, Copenhageni, Bratislava	
Southern Europe								
Greece	855	Healthy (88.2%) + sick (11.8%)	81.5% Vaccinated (CAN + ICT)	1/10	5	13%	Serogroup Pomona (Serovar Altodouro, Mozdok, Pomona), Serogroup Australis (Serovar Bratislava)	Arent et al [194], 2013
	254	Healthy randomly selected	Not reported	1/100	18	11%	Serogroup Icterohemorrhagiae (Serovars Copenhageni, Icterohemorrhagiae), Serovar Canicola	Burriel et al [195], 2003
Italy	1296	Owned and kennel dogs	88% Vaccinated (CAN + ICT)	1/100	9	13%	Serogroup Icterohemorrhagiae, Serovar Bratislava, Canicola, Grippotyphosa	Piredda et al [196], 2021
	1144	Healthy	Not reported	1/100	8	9%	Serogroups Icterohemorrhagiae, Australis	Bertelloni et al [197], 2019
	3028	Healthy	Unknown	1/100	8	30%	Serovars Bratislava, Copenhageni, Icterohemorrhagiae, Canicola	Tagliabue et al [198], 2016
	244	Healthy (34)	73% Vaccinated	1/100; 1/800 for CAN + ICT	8	3%	Serovar Canicola	Scanziani et al [199], 2002
		Stray (33)	Unknown			30%	Serovars Icterohemorrhagiae, Bratislava, Grippotyphosa, Canicola	
		Kennel (63)-good hygiene	95% Vaccinated			14%	Serovar Bratislava	
		Kennel (57)	100% Vaccinated			39%	Serovars Grippotyphosa, Bratislava, Icterohemorrhagiae	
		Kennel (58)	86% Vaccinated			49%	Serovars Bratislava, Canicola, Grippotyphosa, Icterohemorrhagiae	
Spain	1310	Samples submitted for testing	Unknown	1/100	8	26%	Serovars Icterohemorrhagiae, Bratislava, Grippotyphosa, Australis	Lopez et al [200], 2019
	28	Healthy rural	Unvaccinated	1/100	14	36%	Serovars Icterohemorrhagiae, Canicola, Australis	Millan et al [201], 2009
	864	Random sampling (clinic, kennels)	Not reported	Not reported	12	20%	Not reported	Fernandez et al [202], 2005
British Isles								
Ireland	474	Client owned dogs	Unknown	1/10	10	7%	Serogroups Ballum, Australis, Pomona, Sejroe	Schuller et al [203], 2015

Location	N	Population	Vaccination status	No. serovars	MAT titer cutoff	Seroprevalence	Serovar(s)/Serogroup(s)	Reference
Scotland	511	Urban dogs	Unvaccinated	9	1/10	24% 28%	Serovars Canicola, Icterohemorrhagiae, Bratislava, Ballum	Van den Broek et al [204], 1991
North America								
North America - general								
Washington State	158	Healthy	17 Unknown 141 Unvaccinated	7	1/100	17% (29% Unknown, 16% Unvaccinated) 3%	Serovars Autumnalis, Icterohemorrhagiae, Canicola	Davis et al [54], 2008
Appalachia	219	Shelter	Unknown	7	1/800	18%	Serovars Icterohemorrhagiae, Autumnalis, Bratislava	Spangler et al [205], 2020
Illinois	1260	Samples submitted to laboratory; 87 titer>1/800	Unknown	6	1/100	19%	Serovars Canicola, Icterohemorrhagiae, Bratislava, Grippotyphosa	Boutilier et al [92], 2003
Michigan	1241	Healthy at least 4 months old	Vaccinated and Unvaccinated (ICT + CAN)	6	1/200; Vaccinated: 1/1600 ICT; 1/3200 CAN	25%	Serovars Grippotyphosa, Bratislava, Canicola, Icterohemorrhagiae	Stokes et al [206], 2007
Mexico	61	Farm dogs	Not reported	10	1/100	36%	Serovars Canicola, Icterohemorrhagiae	Cardenas-Marrufo et al [207], 2011
	323	Household (181)	Not reported	9	1/100	17%	Serovars Canicola, Hardjo, Icterohemorrhagiae, Pomona	Dominguez et al [208], 2013
		Stray (142)				27%	Serovars Canicola, Icterohemorrhagiae, Pomona, Bataviae	
	106	Living with seropositive humans	Not reported	12	1/100	17%	Serovars Wolffi, Bratislava, Australis, Canicola	Hernandez-Ramirez et al [209], 2020
	400	Stray	Unknown	10	1/100	35%	Serogroups Canicola, Icterohemorrhagiae, Panama, Pyrogenes	Jimenez-Coello et al [8], 2008
	224	Stray	Unknown	10	1/100	5%	Serovars Pyrogenes, Tarassovi	Jimenez-Coello et al [210], 2010
	350	Stray	Unknown	10	1/100	34%	Serovars Canicola, Icterohemorrhagiae	Ortega-Pacheco et al [211], 2008
	103	Stray	Unknown	Not reported	Not reported	52%	Serovar Canicola	Abdoel et al [212], 2011
Caribbean								
Barbados	78	Healthy unwanted	Unknown	22	1/100	62%	Serogroup Autumnalis (Serovars Bim, Fortbragg), Serogroup Icterohemorrhagiae (Serovar Copenhageni), Serogroup Australis (Serovars Bajan, Barbadensis, Bratislava), Serogroup Pomona (Serovar Pomona)	Weekes et al [66], 1997
Saint Kitts	101	Domestic dogs	Vaccinated (23) Unvaccinated (78)	21	1/100	56% Vaccinated 69% Unvaccinated	Serovars Autumnalis, Icterohemorrhagiae, Canicola, Djasiman	Pratt et al [213], 2017
Trinidad	207	Stray	Unknown	23	1/20	15%	Serogroup Icterohemorrhagiae (Serovars Copenhageni, Icterohemorrhagiae, Mankarso)	Suepaul et al [9], 2014
	419	Healthy	Vaccinated and Unvaccinated	17	1/100	15% (6% house dogs, 4% stray, 20% farm, 26% hunting)	Serogroup Icterohemorrhagiae (Serovars Mankarso, Icterohemorrhagiae, Copenhageni)	Adesiyun et al [214], 2006
	25	Stray	Unknown	Not reported	Not reported	4%	Serovar Copenhageni	Abdoel et al [212], 2011
South America								
Brazil	145	Zoonosis Control Center	Unknown	19	1/100	64%	Serogroups Djasiman, Canicola, Cynopteri, Icterohemorrhagiae	Da Rocha Albuquerque et al [215], 2020
	414	Healthy owned	Unvaccinated <12 months	23	1/50	12%	Serogroups Icterohemorrhagiae, Autumnalis, Pomona, Grippotyphosa	Bernardino et al [216], 2021

(*continued on next page*)

TABLE 2
(continued)

Region	Sample No.	Types of Dogs Sampled	Vaccination Status	Serovars Tested	MAT Cut-Off	Prevalence[a]	Most Common Serovars	Study Reference
	729	Healthy owned	Dogs vaccinated <6 months excluded	10	1/100	21%	Serogroups Canicola, Autumnalis (Serovar Butembo), Serogroup Australis (Serovar Bratislava), Serogroup Grippotyphosa	Do Nascimiento Benitez et a.[217], 2020
	161	Healthy	Unvaccinated	13	1/100	6%	Serovars Grippotyphosa, Copenhageni, Pomona	Ornellas et al [218], 2020
	331 373 347	Healthy	During 2nd collection (year2) vaccinated with polyvalent vaccine (Serovars CAN, ICT, GRIP, COP, POM)	24	1/100	11% (year 1) 7% (year 2) 14% (year 3)	Serogroup Cynopteri (Serovar Cynopteri), Serogroup Autumnalis (Serovar Butembo), Serogroup Sejroe (Serovar Hardjoprajitno)	Seva et al [219], 2020
	48 16	Healthy CKD	Unvaccinated	8	1/100	25% 75%	Serogroups Icterohemorrhagiae, Canicola	Sant'Anna et al [94], 2019
	192	Healthy	Not reported	23	1/100	10%	Serovars Australis, Bratislava, Cynopteri, Canicola	De Abreu et al [220], 2019
	384	Dogs attending vet clinic	Not vaccinated < 6 months	20	1/100	12%	Serogroups Icterohemorrhagiae, Grippotyphosa, Canicola, Djasiman	De Lima Brasil et al [221], 2018
	181	Stray	Unknown	22	1/100	17%	Serovars Canicola, Butembo, Grippotyphosa, Pomona	Hafemann et al [222], 2018
	106	Healthy	Not reported	12	1/100	6%	Serovars Canicola, Autumnalis, Grippotyphosa	Latosinski et al [223], 2018
	131	Healthy	Unvaccinated	8	1/100	32%	Serogroup Icterohemorrhagiae (Serovars Icterohemorrhagiae, Copenhageni), Canicola	Sant'Anna et al [224], 2017
	425	Stray	Unknown	22	1/100	17%	Serovars Canicola, Autumnalis, Icterohemorrhagiae. Butembo	De Freitas Siquiero et al [225], 2017
	274	Kennel, shelter, zoonosis control center, domestic	Unknown	25	1/100	17%	Serovars Canicola, Patoc, Icterohemorrhagiae, Copenhageni	Paz et al [226], 2015
	36	Rural	Not reported	22	1/100	25%	Serovars Butembo, Autumnalis	De Oliveira et al [227], 2016
	175	Stray	Unknown	22	1/100	20%	Serovars Canicola, Bratislava, Tarrassovi, Hardjo	Dreer et al [228], 2013
	335	Stray	Unknown	29	1/100	12%	Serovars Pyrogenes, Canicola, Copenhageni	Fonzar and Langoni [229], 2012
	282	Healthy	Vaccinated (n = 20, 3/20 positive titers)	24	1/100	7%	Serovars Copenhageni, Autumnalis, Grippotyphosa, Bratislava	Lavinsky et al [230], 2012
Chile	192	Healthy	Not disclosed	6 in all, additional 12 Serovars in 26 dogs	1/100 in unvacc 1/400 in vacc within 1-3 months; 1/200 vacc >3 months	13%	Serovars Ballum, Canicola, Icterohemorrhagiae, Pyrogenes	Azocar-Aedo et al [231], 2018
	265	Healthy overall Farm (82) Rural village (94) Urban slums (71)	No history of vaccination	20	1/100	25% 11% 22% 45%	Serovars Canicola, Autumnalis, Bratislava	Lelu et al [232], 2015
Argentina	143	Stray	Not reported	Not reported	Not reported	51%	Serovars Canicola, Pyrogenes, Autumnalis	Myers [233], 1980 (abstract)

Region	N	Population	Vaccination status		MAT titer	Seroprevalence	Serovars/Serogroups	Reference
Colombia	92	Working dogs	Vaccinated	24	1/400	57%	Serogroups Canicola, Panama	Murcia et al [234], 2020
	192	Domestic dogs	Unvaccinated	16	1/100	35%	Serovars Autumnalis, Canicola, Pomona, Bratislava	Cardenas et al [235], 2018
	54	Domestic dogs living on a farm	Unvaccinated	13	1/100	35%	Serovars Grippotyphosa, Pomona, Australis, Tarrassovi	Calderon et al [236], 2014
	83	Healthy + sick from area with reported human cases	Unvaccinated	21	1/100	23% (19/83) 15/19 = clinical leptospirosis	Serogroups Icterohemorrhagiae, Tarrassovi, Louisiana	Romero-Vivas et al [69], 2013
French Guiana	95	Not reported	Unvaccinated	27	1/160	12%	Serogroups Icterohemorrhagiae, Australis, Canicola	Roqueplo et al [237], 2019 (abstract)
Oceania								
Australia	956	Healthy QLD = 123 NSW = 431 VIC = 111 SA = 100 WA = 101 NT = 90	No known history of vaccination	22	1/50 Unvaccinated 1/100 uncertain vaccination history	3% 2% 3% 0% 1% 1%	Serovars Ballum, Arborea, Australis Serovars Copenhageni, Canicola, Arborea Serovars Pomona, Arborea Serovar Ballum Serovars Ballum, Arborea	Zwijnenberg et al [238], 2008
	98	Healthy pig hunting dogs	Unvaccinated (87) Vaccinated (11) (AUS or COP)	23	1/50	26% (Unvaccinated) 73% (Vaccinated)	Serovars Australis, Topaz	Orr et al [135], 2022
New Zealand	466	Healthy	Unknown	5	1/100	14%	Serovars Copenhageni, Hardjo	O'Keefe et al [239], 2002
Pacific Islands								
Fiji	100	Healthy, used complement fixation test (CFT)	Unknown	12		57%	Serogroups Icterohemorrhagiae, Ballum, Australis	Collings et al [240], 1984
New Caledonia	78	Healthy urban and rural	Unknown	12	1/100	31%	Serogroup Icterohemorrhagiae	Gay et al [131], 2014
Asia								
South Asia								
India	423	Healthy	Unvaccinated	16	1/100	29%	Serovars Icterohemorrhagiae, Grippotyphosa, Pyrogenes, Javanica	Behera et al [143], 2021
	250	Healthy and suspected leptospirosis	Vaccinated 185(CAN + ICT) Unvaccinated 65	12	1/100	6% (apparently healthy)	Serovars Grippotyphosa, Autumnalis, Australis, Pomona	Sathiyamoorthy et al [74], 2017
	205	Healthy vaccinated (35); Healthy unvaccinated (30); suspected leptospirosis (unknown vaccination status) (140)	Vaccine used CAN + ICT	9	1/100	71% (healthy unvaccinated negative, healthy vaccinated positive to CAN + ICT)	Serovars Autumnalis, Australis, Pomona, Canicola	Ambily et al [76], 2013
	124	Vaccinated (42), Unvaccinated-semiowned (48), Stray (10)		5	1/40	Vaccinated: 57% Unvaccinated 29% Stray: 35%	Serovars Icterohemorrhagiae, Canicola, Pomona, Grippotyphosa	Senthil et al [241], 2013
Thailand	273	Stray (119), client-owned (154) [rural (139), urban (134)]	Unvaccinated	19	1/20	12%	Serogroup Icterohemorrhagiae (Serovars Copenhageni, Icterohemorrhagiae)	Altheimer et al [149], 2020
	230	Stray	Unknown	21	1/100	84%	Serovars Bataviae, Patoc, Tarassovi, Sejroe	Jittapalong et al [242], 2009
	210	Presented to vet clinic	Not reported	24	1/20	11%	Serovars Bataviae, Canicola, Bratislava, Icterohemorrhagiae	Meeyam et al [243], 2006
	153	Rural	Unvaccinated	24	1/50	58%	Serovars Tarassovi, Ranarum, Saigon, Bratislava	Niwetpathomwat and Assarasakorn [244], 2007
	55	Healthy	Unvaccinated	24	1/100	11%	Serovar Canicola	Punpiputt and Suwannarong [245], 2016

(continued on next page)

TABLE 2
(continued)

Region	Sample No.	Types of Dogs Sampled	Vaccination Status	Serovars Tested	MAT Cut-Off	Prevalence[a]	Most Common Serovars	Study Reference
Malaysia	100	Stray	Unknown	20	1/100	32%	Serovars Javanica, Bataviae, Icterohemorrhagiae, Autumnalis	Goh et al [246], 2021
	127	Shelter, healthy	Unvaccinated	20	1/100	21%	Serogroup Ballum, Icterohemorrhagiae, Bataviae, Lai	Rani et al [247], 2020
	266	Working(73) +shelter dogs (193)	152 Vaccinated (49 working dogs, 103 shelter dogs), 113 = ICT + CAN; 39 = ICT + CAN + POM + GRIP	20	1/100	22% (6% working, 16% shelter)	Serovars Icterohemorrhagiae, Ballum, Bataviae, Australis	Goh et al [159], 2019
	80	Shelter	Vaccinated (ICT + CAN + POM + GRIP)	10	1/80	4%	Serovar Bataviae	Hua et al [248], 2016
	96	Working dogs	Vaccinated (ICT + CAN + POM + GRIP)	11	1/80	3%	Serovars Javanica, Australis, Bataviae	Lau et al [249], 2017
	57	Healthy (38) Kidney disease (19)	35 healthy Vaccinated 15 kidney disease Vaccinated	10	1/80	3% 16%	Serovar Icterohemorrhagiae Serovar Canicola	Lau et al [250], 2016
	142	Stray	Not reported	Not reported	1/100	33%	MAT, Serovar Pomona	Phumoona et al [251], 2009
East Asia								
Japan	801	Healthy and treated for disease unrelated to leptospirosis	243 Unvaccinated	5	1/80	27% (17% unvaccinated)	Serovars Icterohemorrhagiae, Autumnalis, Canicola, Hebdomanis	Iwamoto et al [252], 2009
Middle East								
Turkey	116	Healthy stray	Not reported	5	1/100	44%	Serovars Bratislava, Canicola, Grippotyphosa	Aslantas et al [253], 2005
Iran	149	Rural (100) Urban (49)	Unvaccinated	6	1/100	5%	Serovars Hardjo, Ballum, Icterohemorrhagiae, Grippotyphosa	Avizeh et al [254], 2009
Africa	475	Sudan (62) Gabon (255), Ivory Coast (158; Vaccinated = 93)	Vaccinated (CAN + ICT) + Unvaccinated	16	1/320	Overall: 41% Ivory Coast Vaccinated = 59%; Ivory Coast, Unvaccinated = 48%	Serogroups Grippotyphosa, Sejroe Sudan: Icterohemorrhagiae, Canicola	Roqueplo et al [255], 2015
Central Africa								
Gabon	255	Urban (99) Rural (156)	Not reported	16	1/320	9% 35%	Serovars Icterohemorrhagiae, Autumnalis, Grippotyphosa Serovars Icterohemorrhagiae, Australis, Autumnalis, Panama	Roqueplo et al [255], 2015
Southern Africa								
South Africa	530	Stray + Owned	Not reported	15	Not reported	5%	Serovars Canicola, Pyrogenes	Roach et al [256], 2010 (abstract)
East Africa								
Uganda	105	Collected during rabies vaccination program	Unvaccinated	14	1/200	27%	Serovars Canicola, Pyrogenes, Tarrassovi, Grippotyphosa	Millan et al [257], 2013
Sudan	62	Healthy	Not reported	16	1/320	74%	Serovars Icterohemorrhagiae, Sejroe, Canicola, Grippotyphosa	Roqueplo et al [255], 2015
Egypt	168	Stray	Unknown	24	1/200	58%	Serovars Canicola, Icterohemorrhagiae	Samir et al [258], 2015

a Decimal places rounded off; AUS, Australis; CAN, Canicola; COP, Copenhageni; GRIP, Grippotyphosa; ICT, Icterohemorrhagiae; POM, Pomona.

TABLE 3
Prevalence of Serum Antibody Titers as Measured by Microscopic Agglutination Test (MAT) in Dogs with Confirmed or Suspected Leptospirosis Tested Worldwide Since 2000 (Or Most Recent Report If There Are No Studies After 2000) and Studies Identifying Species and Serovars Via Molecular Methods

Region	Sample No.	Types of Cases Sampled	Vaccination Status	No. of Serovars Tested	Diagnostic Criteria	Seroprevalence	Most Common Serovars	Study reference
Europe								
Eastern Europe								
Croatia	60	Clinical leptospirosis	Vaccinated (13), Unvaccinated (41)	13	≥1/800 against nonvaccine Serogroups OR 4-fold rise in titer (45); positive PCR blood and/or urine (15); positive culture	85% (positive MAT or seroconversion)	Serogroups Pomona, Icterohemorrhagiae, Grippotyphosa, Australis	Habus et al [100], 2020
	364	Suspected leptospirosis	Unknown	12	≥1/800	23%	Serogroups Pomona, Icterohemorrhagiae, Grippotyphosa	Habus et al [259], 2017
	151	Suspected leptospirosis, samples submitted to laboratory	Unknown	12	≥1/1000 OR seroconversion considered leptospirosis (n = 26) 1/100 to <1/1000 considered seropositive but not necessarily diseased (n = 54)	17% 38%	Serovars Pomona, Grippotyphosa, Icterohemorrhagiae, Australis	Stritof Majetic at el [260], 2012
Western Europe								
Germany (North-East)	50	Clinical leptospirosis	34 Vaccinated (CAN + ICT)	16	≥1/800 against nonvaccine Serovars; 2-fold rise in titer within 2–3 weeks (37); positive PCR blood and/or urine (15); histopathology (6)	74% (positive MAT or seroconversion)	Serovars Bratislava, Grippotyphosa, Pomona	Kohn et al [37], 2010
	329	Suspected leptospirosis	>80% (CAN + ICT)	17	≥1/100 against nonvaccine Serovars	25% positive to nonvaccine Serovars	Serogroups Australis (Serovar Bratislava), Grippotyphosa, Pomona	Mayer-Scholl et al [38], 2013
	99	Clinical leptospirosis	80 Vaccinated (CAN + ICT)	17	≥1/800 (72); 4-fold rise in titer (71); PCR (73); Levaditi staining (11)	73% (positive MAT or seroconversion)	Serogroups Australis, Grippotyphosa, Pomona, Icterohemorrhagiae	Knopfler et al [39], 2017
	442	Suspected leptospirosis (confirmed in 39)	Unknown	10	≥1/800 (39)	9%	Serovars Bratislava, Copenhageni, Grippotyphosa, Icterohemorrhagiae	Gerlach and Stephan [40], 2007

(continued on next page)

TABLE 3
(continued)

Region	Sample No.	Types of Cases Sampled	Vaccination Status	No. Of Serovars Tested	Diagnostic Criteria	Seroprevalence	Most Common Serovars	Study reference
Germany (South)	42	Clinical leptospirosis	25 Vaccinated <12 months (CAN + ICT), 6 not regularly vaccinated, 6 never vaccinated, 5 unknown	8	≥1/1600 to nonvaccine Serogroups (15); 4-fold increase in titer (10); ELISA: IgM > IgG (15); PCR positive in urine (2)	60% (positive MAT or seroconversion)	Serogroups Grippotyphosa, Saxkoebing, Icterohemorrhagiae, Canicola	Geisen et al [3], 2007
	337	Suspected leptospirosis (42 confirmed, see Geisen 2007 [3])	Not reported	8	≥1/100	48%	Serovars Copenhageni, Canicola, Grippotyphosa, Bratislava	Geisen et al [261], 2008 (abstract)
	1401	Suspected leptospirosis	Unknown (usually vaccinated)	8	Not reported	49%	Serovars Grippotyphosa, Bratislava, Saxkoebing	Brem et al [262], 1990 (abstract)
Switzerland	18	Clinical leptospirosis	Not reported	12	≥1/800 (13); 4-fold increase in titer (11); positive IgM (12)	72% (positive MAT at presentation)	Serovars Australis, Bratislava, Pomona, Autumnalis	Keller et al [41], 2016
	298	Clinical leptospirosis	239/251 (95.2%) Vaccinated	11	≥1/800 (127); 4-fold increase in titer(132); IgM ELISA (6); PCR (11); histopathology (22)	87% (positive MAT or seroconversion)	Serogroups Australis (Serovars Australis, Bratislava), Serovars Grippotyphosa, Pomona	Major et al [42], 2014
	28	Clinical leptospirosis	Not reported	Not reported	≥1/400 nonvaccine Serovars, ≥1/1600 vaccine Serovars	Not reported	Serovars Australis, Bratislava, Autumnalis	Francey [43], 2006 (abstract)
	30	Clinical leptospirosis	99% Vaccinated	11	4-fold increase in titer (30)	100%	Serovars Australis, Bratislava, Autumnalis, Grippotyphosa	Fraune et al [44], 2013
France	727	Suspected leptospirosis	580 Vaccinated (ICT + CAN) 147 Unvaccinated	16	≥1/40 Unvaccinated; ≥1/320 Vaccinated	*report no overall prevalence but prevalence for individual Serovars*	Serovars Icterohemorrhagiae, Australis, Sejroe, Grippotyphosa (unvacc) Serovars Icterohemorrhagiae, Canicola, Australis, Sejroe (vacc)	Andre-Fontaine and Triger [180], 2018
	27	Clinical leptospirosis	17 Vaccinated (CAN + ICT), 6 Unvaccinated, 4 Unknown	19	≥1/800 nonvaccine Serovars (12), ≥1/1600 vaccine Serovars; 4-fold increase in titer (2); positive PCR in blood and/or urine PCR (5)		Serogroups Australis, Icterohemorrhagiae, Autumnalis	Magnin et al [45], 2020
	35	Clinical leptospirosis	97% Vaccinated (ICT + CAN)	13	≥1/800 nonvaccine Serovars (25), ≥1/1600 vaccine Serovars; 4-fold increase in titer (5), positive urine and/or blood PCR (5), combination of MAT and PCR results (8)	52%	Serogroups Australis, Autumnalis, Panama	Barthelemy et al [46], 2017

Country	n	Population	Vaccination		Criteria	%	Serovars	Reference
	232	Clinical leptospirosis (samples submitted to "Laboratoire de Leptospires," clinical and clinicopathological signs and with titer >1:640)	Unknown		≥1/640 against nonvaccine Serovars	100%	Serogroups Australis, Grippotyphosa, Sejroe	Ayral et al [47], 2014
	517	Suspected leptospirosis (302) and increased risk (215)	Not reported	4	≥1/10	26% for Serovar Bratislava	Serogroups Australis (Serovar Bratislava), Grippotyphosa	Renaud et al [48], 2013
Belgium	7	Clinical leptospirosis	2 Vaccinated (ICT + CAN)	20	MAT (3/3), immunohistochemistry (1), Antibody test (BioRad) (7)	100%	Serovar Pomona	Claus et al [166], 2008
Southern Europe								
Greece	855	Healthy (88%) + sick (12%)	82% Vaccinated (CAN + ICT)	5	≥1/10	13%	Serogroup Pomona (Serovar Altodouro, Mozdok, Pomona), Serogroup Australis (Serovar Bratislava)	Arent et al [194], 2013
Italy	47	Clinical leptospirosis	Not reported		≥1/800 in unvaccinated dogs; 4-fold increase in titer within 1–2 weeks (27); positive PCR blood and/or urine (20)	57%	Serovars Icterohemorrhagiae, Canicola, Pomona	Lippi et al [63], 2021
Spain	1310	Samples submitted for testing	Unknown	8	≥1/100	26%	Serovars Icterohemorrhagiae, Bratislava, Grippotyphosa, Australis	Lopez et al [200], 2019
British Isles								
England	38	Clinical leptospirosis	21 Vaccinated (15 CAN + ICT, 6 unknown vaccine used), 2 puppies received first dose of vaccination, 8 Unvaccinated, 7 unknown vaccination status		≥1/800 in nonvaccinated <4 months, ≥1/1600 in recently vaccinated or serology by immunofluorescence (27); 4-fold increase in titer (7), positive PCR blood, urine or tissue (2), positive FISH (2)	Not reported	Serovars Copenhageni	Raj et al [64], 2021
	1715	Samples submitted for testing (IDEXX)	Unknown		≥1/800	6%	Serogroups Icterohemorrhagiae, Sejroe, Australis	Taylor et al [20], 2021
Ireland	1	Clinical leptospirosis	Vaccinated <6 months	3	Seroconversion	100% (1 case)	Serogroup Icterohemorrhagiae	Juvet et al [65], 2011
North America								
Canada								
Ontario	31	Clinical leptospirosis	Vaccination history not obtained but anecdotal evidence suggests not vaccinated	6	≥1/320	100%	Serovars Autmnalis, Bratislava, Grippotyphosa, Pomona	Prescott et al [49], 2002
	474	Submitted samples	Unknown	7	≥1/100	39%		

(continued on next page)

TABLE 3
(continued)

Region	Sample No.	Types of Cases Sampled	Vaccination Status	No. Of Serovars Tested	Diagnostic Criteria	Seroprevalence	Most Common Serovars	Study reference
	1	Clinical leptospirosis	Vaccinated (CAN + ICT)	7	1/1280, culture and immunofluorescence	1 case only	Serovars Canicola, Icterohemorrhagiae, Bratislava, Autumnalis	Prescott et al [263], 1991
	2	Clinical leptospirosis	Not reported	Not reported	Titers, however, do not mention which method used	2 cases only	Serovar Pomona	Prescott et al [263], 1991
Guelph							Serovars Grippotyphosa, Pomona	Hrinivich and Prescott [264], 1997
Quebec	3	Clinical leptospirosis	Vaccinated	6	Titers were ≥1/3200	3 cases only	Serovar Pomona	Kalin et al [265], 1999
	1406	Suspected leptospirosis (serologic submission reports)	Unknown	6	≥1/800	57%	Serovars Autumnalis, Bratislava, Grippotyphosa, Icterohemorrhagiae	Alton et al [50], 2009
	19	Suspected leptospirosis	Unvaccinated	5	1/400–1/12800	79%	Serovars Grippotyphosa, Pomona	Ribotta et al [266], 2000
North America - general	33119	Submitted to commercial laboratory	Unknown	7	≥1/1600	8%	Serovars Autumnalis, Grippotyphosa, Pomona, Bratislava	Gautam et al [51], 2010
	23005	Submitted to commercial laboratory	Unknown	7	≥1/400, ≥1/800, ≥1/1600	Calculate prevalence for individual Serovars; eg Autumnalis (9.1%, 6.5%, 4.7%, respectively)	Serovars Autumnalis, Grippotyphosa, Bratislava, Pomona	Moore et al [52], 2006
Oregon	72	Clinical leptospirosis	95% Unvaccinated	Not reported	MAT ≥1/800 with no history of vacc (30), seroconversion (13), positive PCR blood and/or urine (29)	60% (positive MAT or seroconversion)	Serovars Autumnalis, Pomona, Bratislava, Grippotyphosa	Grayzel and De Bess [53], 2016
Washington State	816 tested in 2006	Clinical cases	Not reported	7	≥1/800	11%, 8%, 8%	Serovars Autumnalis, Bratislava, Pomona	Davis et al [54], 2008
California	36	Clinical leptospirosis	Not reported	6	≥1/800 (26), seroconversion (10)	100%	Serovars Pomona, Bratislava	Adin and Cowgill [55], 2000
	43	Clinical leptospirosis	Not vaccinated < 3 months	Not reported	≥1/800 and not vacc in last 3 months	100%	Serovars Pomona, Canicola, Bratislava	Ghneim et al [56], 2007
	67	Clinical leptospirosis	24 Vaccinated or unknown vaccination history	6	≥1/800 (21); 4-fold increase in titer (44); renal immunohistochemistry (2) positive PCR (2)	97% (positive MAT or seroconversion)	Serovars Pomona, Bratislava	Hennebelle et al [57], 2013
	55	Clinical leptospirosis	Not reported	Not reported	Not reported	Not reported	Serovar Pomona	Sykes et al [58], 2007 (abstract)
Arizona	54	Clinical leptospirosis	41 Unvaccinated; 7 unknown vaccination history; 6 Vaccinated	Not reported, different laboratories used	MAT ≥1/400 in nonvaccinated, ≥1/800 vacc >6 months ago, higher titers if vaccinated <6 months ago (confirmed with MAT n = 13); positive PCR (36), positive MAT + PCR (5)	33%	Serovars Canicola, Djasiman	Iverson et al [91], 2021

New York	36	Clinical leptospirosis	25 Vaccinated (CAN + ICT); 7 Unvaccinated; 4 unknown vaccination history	Not reported	MAT ≥1/3200 (28), clinical signs + MAT ≥1:1600 to nonvaccinal Serovars with titers<1:800 for CAN + ICT (5); 4-fold rise in titer; positive urine FAT (1); postmortem diagnosis (FAT) (2)	92% (positive MAT or seroconversion)	Serovars Grippotyphosa, Pomona	Birnbaum et al [60], 1998
	55	Clinical leptospirosis	Not reported, likely not vaccinated	7	≥1/800 to nonvaccinal Serogroups; >2-fold increase in convalescent titer to nonvacc Serogroups ≥1/3200 against vacc Serogroups; positive urine or tissue FAT (1); positive culture	98%	Serovars Grippotyphosa, Pomona, Autumnalis, Bratislava	Goldstein et al [6], 2006
Pennsylvania	51	Clinical leptospirosis	18% Vaccinated	5-7	≥1/1600 in vaccinated or ≥1/800 in nonvaccinated (28); 4-fold rise in titer (23)	100%	Serovars Grippotyphosa, Icterohemorrhagiae, Pomona	Tangeman and Littman [7], 2013
New Jersey and Michigan	17	Clinical leptospirosis	Not reported	Not reported	Not reported	Not reported	Serovars Pomona, Grippotyphosa, Autumnalis	Harkin and Gartrell [267], 1996 (abstract)
Illinois	87	Samples submitted to laboratory with titer>1/800	Unvaccinated	6	≥1/800 +clinical signs	17% clinical leptospirosis	Serovars Grippotyphosa, Bratislava	Boutillier et al [92], 2003
Indiana	90	Clinical leptospirosis	Not reported	6	≥1/800	20/30 MAT tested (67%)	Serovar Grippotyphosa	Ward et al [61], 2004a
	36	Clinical leptospirosis	Not reported	6	Clinicopathological findings, response to treatment, MAT ≥1/800 (8); ≥1/400 (4); ≥1/200 (1); ≥1/100 (2); <1/100 (1): 4-fold rise in titer (11); 2- to 3-fold rise in titer (2); FAT urine (1), liver + kidney (1), urine + liver + kidney (1), silver staining liver + kidney (1)		Serovar Grippotyphosa	Ward et al [62], 2004b
Massachusetts	17	Clinical leptospirosis	12 Vaccinated (CAN + ICT)	5	MAT ≥1/3200; 4-fold rise in titer	100% (positive MAT or rise in titer)	Serovars Pomona, Grippotyphosa	Renko et al [59], 1992
Minnesota	35	Clinical leptospirosis	Not reported	Not reported	4-fold rise in titer	Not reported	Serovars Grippotyphosa, Pomona	Sykes et al [58], 2007 (abstract)
Caribbean								
Barbados	61	Suspected leptospirosis	Not reported	22	MAT ≥1/800; 4-fold titer rise; IgM >320 ELISA	75% (positive MAT)	Serogroup Icterohemorrhagiae (Serovar Copenhageni), Serogroup Australis (Serovars Bajan, Barbadensis, Bratislava)	Weeks et al [66], 1997
Saint Kitts	1	Clinical leptospirosis, stray	Unknown	20	PCR + culture positive, MAT negative, whole genome sequencing	1 case only	Serovar Copenhageni	Larson et al [268], 2017
Trinidad	50	Suspected leptospirosis	Not reported	23	Clinical signs suggestive of leptospirosis, MAT ≥1/20	72%	Serogroup Icterohemorrhagiae (Serovars Copenhageni, Icterohemorrhagiae, Mankarso)	Suepaul et al [9], 2014

(continued on next page)

TABLE 3
(continued)

Region	Sample No.	Types of Cases Sampled	Vaccination Status	No. Of Serovars Tested	Diagnostic Criteria	Seroprevalence	Most Common Serovars	Study reference
South America								
Brazil	57	Suspected leptospirosis	1/3 of confirmed vaccination (CAN + ICT or CAN + ICT + POM + GRIP)	24	PCR urine (32), culture (12), MAT ≥1/800 (15), genotyping (MLVA) – 38 confirmed	26%	Serogroups Icterohemorrhagiae, Australis, Canicola, Pomona; Serogroup Icterohemorrhagiae confirmed with MLVA in 12/38 with confirmed leptospirosis	Paz et al [67], 2021a
	31	Suspected leptospirosis	2 Vaccinated (one no detectable titers)	24	≥1/800, positive PCR blood and/or urine, culture (confirmed in 17 dogs)	36%	Serogroups Autumnalis (Serovar Butembo), Icterohemorrhagiae (Serovars Copenhageni, Icterohemorrhagiae), Canicola MLSA: Canicola (1), Icterohemorrhagiae (3)	Santos et al [269], 2021
	1	Stray, confirmed leptospirosis					L. noguchii (sequencing from kidney)	Silva et al [14], 2009
	92	Suspected leptospirosis	Unvaccinated < 6 months	8	Clinicopathological abnormalities, MAT ≥1/400	100%	Serogroups Icterohemorrhagiae, Australis	Penna et al [68], 2017
	1176	Suspected leptospirosis	Not reported	55	≥1/100	28% 13% 10% 9%	Serogroup Canicola (Serovar Canicola), Serogroup Icterohemorrhagiae (Serovar Copenhageni), Serogroup Ballum (Serovar Ballum), Serogroup Autumnalis (Serovar Butembo)	Jorge et al [82], 2017
	1195	Submitted to laboratory	Unknown	12	≥1/100	10%	Serovars Canicola, Copenhageni, Icterohemorrhagiae, Autumnalis	Kikuti et al [80], 2012
Argentina	8	Clinical leptospirosis	Not reported				MLVA: Serovars Canicola, Icterohemorrhagiae, Pomona	Loftis et al [105], 2014
	1	Aborted dog fetus	Unvaccinated	38	Culture of mixed liver + kidney tissue, Serovar identification with Cross-Agglutination Absorption test (CAAT), species determination by sequencing.		Serogroup Djasiman, Serovar Buenos Aires	Rossetti et al [29], 2005
Colombia	83	Healthy + sick from area with reported human cases	Unvaccinated	21	≥1/100 (19), positive urine culture, positive urine PCR (2)	23% (19/83) 15/19 = clinical leptospirosis	Serogroups Icterohemorrhagiae, Tarassovi, Louisiana	Romero-Vivas et al [69], 2013
	2	Cases from Romero Vivas 2013a, do not report if clinical signs were present, one MAT positive			Urine PCR positive, isolation and genotyping (PFGE)		new Serovar closely related to Leptospira Noguchii	Romero-Vivas et al[270] 2013

Location	No. of dogs	Clinical presentation	Vaccination status	Diagnostic criteria	No. of serovars tested	Seropositivity	Serovars / serogroups identified	Reference
Oceania								
Australia	40	Clinical leptospirosis	Not reported	≥1/200	14	100%	Serovars Australis, Zanoni, Hardjo Copenhageni	Miller et al [79], 2007
Australia	17	Clinical leptospirosis	1 Vaccinated (COP)	Clinical signs, ≥1/800 (8) or 4-fold increase in titer (3); positive PCR on blood (1), urine (4), kidney (1) blood and urine (9)	23	67%	Serovar Copenhageni (7), Hardjo (1)	Griebsch et al [70], 2022
New Zealand	655	Submissions to laboratory	Unknown	≥1/96	4	15%	Serovars Copenhageni, Hardjo, Pomona, Ballum	Harland et al [271], 2013
Asia								
South Asia								
India	250	Healthy and suspected leptospirosis	Unvaccinated	≥1/100	12	28% (overall) 38% (sick) 6% (healthy)	Serovars Grippotyphosa, Autumnalis, Australis, Pomona	Sathiyamoorthy et al [74], 2017
India	40	Suspected leptospirosis	Not reported	≥1/80	10	17.5%	Serovar Pyrogenes	Patil et al [272], 2014
India	205	Healthy vaccinated (35); Healthy unvaccinated (30); suspected leptospirosis (vaccination status unknown) (140)	Vaccine used CAN + ICT	≥1/100	9	Overall 71% (healthy unvaccinated negative)	Serovars Autumnalis, Australis, Pomona, Canicola	Ambily et al [76], 2013
India	300	Suspected leptospirosis	No history of vaccination	≥1/50	5	33%	Serovars Canicola, Icterohemorrhagiae, Grippotyphosa, Australis	Kumar et al [75], 2013
Thailand	6	Confirmed leptospirosis	2 Unvaccinated 4 unknown vaccination history	PCR, direct genotyping, sequencing (16S rRNA, LipL32), MLST	6		L. interrogans (6); Identified by MLST: Serogroup Bataviae (2)	Paungpin et al [273], 2020
Malaysia	124	Kidney ± liver disease	Vaccinated 52 Nonvaccinated 72	≥1/100 (53); PCR blood (42), PCR urine (36/113), kidney (2/23), liver (2/23), abdominal effusion (4), partial 16S rRNA sequencing, culture: blood (3), urine (7), abdominal effusion (1)	20	43%	Serovars in unvaccinated dogs: Bataviae, Javanica; vaccinated dogs: Icterohemorrhagiae); 16S rRNA sequencing: L. interrogans (62), bongpetersenii (17), kirschneri (6), kmetyi (1) (likely contaminant); Characterization of isolates from culture (11 from 8 dogs): Serovars Bataviae, Javanica, Australis	Rahman et al [13], 2021
Malaysia	19	kidney disease	Vaccinated and Unvaccinated	≥1/80, PCR plasma (1)	10	16% (3/19), 2/3 vaccinated (CAN + ICT)	Serovar Canicola	Lau et al [250], 2016
East Asia								
Japan	283	Suspected leptospirosis	29% Vaccinated	≥1/800 (29); 4-fold rise in titer; (30); PCR (44), blood culture (45) = 83 cases confirmed (31 hunting dogs, 50 companion dogs). MLST and/or PFGE	Not reported	36% (30/83)	Serogroups Hebdomanis, Australis, Autumnalis (genetic heterogeneity in all, in Serogroup Hebdomanis unique mortality rate for each genotype)	Koizumi et al [71], 2013
Japan	11	Suspected leptospirosis	8/11 Vaccinated	≥1/800 (2/6); Clinical signs (5). PCR blood (1) and/or urine (1). IgM+ (4)	5	33%	Serovar Australis	Saeki and Tanaka [72], 2021
China	24	Suspected leptospirosis	Not reported	16SrRNA sequencing from kidney or whole blood (species identification), MAT (serogroup identification)	15	Only reported positive cases	L. interrogans Serogroups Australis (n = 11), Canicola (n = 10), Hebdomanis (n = 3),	Zhang et al [73], 2019

Abbreviations: CAN, Canicola; COP, Copenhageni; ELISA, enzyme linked immunosorbent assay; FISH, fluorescent in situ hybridization; ICT, Icterohemorrhagiae; MAT, microscopic agglutination test; MLST, multilocus sequence typing; MLVA, multilocus variable number of tandem repeat analysis; PCR, polymerase chain reaction; PFGE, pulse field gel electrophoresis.

TABLE 4
Prevalence of Dogs that Are Silent Shedders of Leptospires Worldwide

Region	Sample No	Type of Dogs Sampled	Test Used	Prevalence	Study Reference
Europe					
Germany	200	Owned	real-time PCR (LipL32) MLST	1.5% (3/200) L. interrogans (2) L. borgpetersenii (1)	Llewellyn et al [274], 2014
	26	Owned	urine culture (EMJH)	19.2% (5/26)	Ruehl-Fehlert et al [275], 2000
Switzerland	408	Owned	quantitative real-time PCR (LipL32)	0.2% (1/408)	Delaude et al [19], 2017
Italy	64	Kennel	PCR (16S rRNA)	7.8%	Vicari et al [276], 2007
Ireland	525	Kennel and teaching hospital	quantitative real-time PCR (LipL32)	7.1% (37/525)	Rojas et al [126], 2010
North America					
Appalachia	198	Shelter	TaqMan-based quantitative PCR (LipL32) rpoB gene sequencing	13.1% (26/198) L. interrogans (21)	Spangler et al [205], 2020
Kansas	500	Owned	PCR (23S rDNA) urine culture	8.1% (41/500) 0%	Harkin et al [93], 2003
South America					
Brazil	123	Stray and shelter	qPCR (LipL32) 16S rRNA and secY phylogenetic analysis Culture (EMJH) MLST	10.5% (13/123) L. interrogans (10) L. santarosai (3) 2/3 PCR positive L. interrogans Serogroup Canicola L. santarosai Serogroup Sejroe (not virulent)	Miotto et al [128], 2018
	106	Owned	PCR (16S rRNA)	0.9% (1/106)	Latosinsky et al [223], 2018
	131	Owned	PCR (LipL32)	19.8% (26/131)	SanT'Anna et al [224], 2017
	16 / 48	CKD / healthy	PCR (LipL32)	75% (12/16) 20.8% (10/48)	SanT'Anna et al [94], 2019

Country	N	Population	Method	Result	Reference
	126	Healthy – PCR negative – longitudinal study over 1 year (5 timepoints)	PCR (LipL32) Sequencing (secY gene) (22)	48.8% (62/126) PCR positive at some time point *L. interrogans* Serovar Icterohemorrhagiae (20) *L. noguchii* (2)	SanT'Anna et al [77], 2021
	1	Stray	Culture (EMJH) Sequencing (secY gene) MLST	*L. kirschneri* Serogroup Pomona Serovar Mozdok	Da Cunha et al [277], 2016
Colombia	92	Vaccinated police dogs	Culture (EMJH)	58.7% (54/92)	Murcia et al [234], 2020
Oceania					
Pacific Islands: New Caledonia	82 kidneys 13 urine samples	Shelter Healthy dogs from various tribes	PCR (LipL32) Genotyping (lfb 1 gene)	4.4% (3 kidney, 1 urine) Icterohemorrhagiae (2) Pomona (2)	Gay et al [131], 2014
Asia					
India	236	Healthy	qPCR (LipL32)	0%	Rohilla et al [278], 2020
	40 kidneys	Submitted for postmortem	PCR (seqY)	22.5% (9/40) – only 4 dogs renal changes	Dash et al [279], 2018
Thailand	237	119 Stray 154 Client owned	qPCR (LipL32) culture (EMJH)	4.4% (12/273) 0.4% (1/273)	Altheimer et al [149], 2020
	58	Healthy	rrs nested PCR culture (EMJH) MLST	10.36% (6/58) 4/58 *L. interrogans* (2) *L. weilii* (2)	Kurilung et al [280], 2017
Malaysia	100	Stray	Culture (EMJH) blood, urine, kidney, liver PCR (16S rRNA, LipL32) MAT on isolates	3% (3/100); urine (2), kidney (2), liver (2) Bataviae (5), Autumnalis/Pomona (1)	Goh et al [246], 2021
	150	Stray	PCR (16S rRNA + secY) DNA sequencing	7.3% (11/150) Serovar Canicola (9) Serovar Icterohemorrhagiae (2)	Benacer et al [281] 2017

(continued on next page)

TABLE 4
(continued)

Region	Sample No	Type of Dogs Sampled	Test Used	Prevalence	Study Reference
Middle East					
Iran	90	Healthy + sick, not suspected leptospirosis	PCR-RFLP	31% (28/90)	Khorami et al [130], 2010
Africa					
Algier	104	Stray	Real-time PCR (rrs, hsp) Partial PCR sequencing (rpoB gene)	4.8% (5/104) *L. interrogans*	Zaidi et al [282], 2018

Abbreviations: EMJH, Ellinghausen–McCullough–Johnson–Harris; MAT, microscopic agglutination test; MLST, Multilocus Sequence Typing; RFPL, restriction fragment length polymorphism; PCR, polymerase chain reaction.

TABLE 5
Clinical Signs Reported in Dogs with Clinical Leptospirosis Worldwide

Common	Lethargy [3,6,7,13,37,39,40,49,53,55,59,60,67,79,100,104,115,166] Inappetence [3,6,7,13,37,39,40,49,53,55,59,60,79,100,104,115,166] Vomiting [3,6,13,37,39,40,49,53,55,59,60,79,100,104,115,166] Diarrhea [3,6,7,13,37,39,40,53,55,59,60,79,104,115] Abdominal pain [3,6,37,39,49,53,55,59,60,79,100,104,115,166] Jaundice [3,6,13,37,39,40,49,53,60,67,79,100,104,115,166] Pyrexia [3,6,13,37,39,40,49,53,55,59,60,67,79,100,104,166] Labored breathing/dyspnea, tachypnea (+/− coughing, hemoptysis) [7,37,39,49,57,59,60,100,104,115,167] Oliguria/anuria [7,13,39,55,60,104,115,166] PU/PD [6,7,13,37,39,40,49,53,59,60,104] Hypothermia [3,37,39,55,59,79,100,104,115,166] Dehydration [3,6,37,49,60,79,100], prolonged CRT [37,39], pale mucus membranes [6,39,53,79]
Less common	Hemorrhagic diathesis [79,104,115,166], petechiae [49,104], melena [6,60,67,104,166], hematochezia [60] Pigmenturia/hematuria [3,37,39,59,60,104] Renomegaly [6,49,59] Peripheral lymphadenopathy [39,49,60] Weight loss [3,6,7,39,49,53,59,60,79] Stiff gait [37,39,49,55,59], reluctance to move [37,39,59], myalgia [53], musculoskeletal pain [60], lumbar pain [49] Nasal, ocular or oculonasal discharge [59,60,104]
Uncommon	Panuveitis [108,109,283], scleral injection [55] Hypertension [59] Peripheral edema [6,166] Recumbency [104], weakness [3,55,60], posterior paresis [69], ataxia [7] Disorientation [60] Adipsia [39,60] Ascites [49] Cardiac murmur [6,115,166] Tachycardia [104,166], bradycardia [59,166], arrhythmia [104] Abortion [100] Calcinosis cutis [284,285]

plumbing facilities [89] has been associated with clinical leptospirosis.

Other identified risk factors associated with leptospirosis were low socioeconomic status of the owner [89], close contact with other dogs (e.g, day-care boarding facilities, kennels) [91], and contact with reservoir hosts such as wildlife [53].

CLINICAL MANIFESTATIONS

Clinical signs are often nonspecific and have been summarized in Table 5. Cases can be classified based on the predominant clinical manifestations (renal, hepatic,

pulmonary, hemorrhagic syndromes) (Table 6), and one or all four of these manifestations can be present [42].

The kidneys play an important role in the life cycle and transmission of leptospires, with shedding occurring in symptomatic and asymptomatic infections. Therefore, reports of leptospirosis without renal involvement are rare [42,49,60,92]. Leptospiral shedding was found in dogs with chronic kidney disease (CKD), indicating a possible association between CKD and asymptomatic leptospiral infection in dogs in endemic regions [93,94]. Nonazotemic polyuria/polydipsia (PU/PD) has been described in dogs testing

TABLE 6
Clinical Manifestations of Canine Leptospirosis

Clinical Manifestation	Definition
Renal	Acute kidney injury (AKI): documented AKI (historical, clinical, laboratory, imaging evidence), oliguria (<1 mL/kg/h) or anuria (no urine production), and progressive increase in creatinine concentration of >26.4 µmol/L within 48 hours according to IRIS guidelines. Severity of AKI is based on the IRIS grading system [286].
Hepatic	Elevated liver enzymes and hyperbilirubinemia; one study suggested classification based on serum bilirubin concentration as mild (bilirubin 10–20 µmol/L), moderate (bilirubin 20–30 µmol/L), or severe (bilirubin >30 µmol/L) [42]
Pulmonary	Leptospiral pulmonary hemorrhage syndrome (LPHS): labored breathing, dyspnoea, and hemoptysis or radiographic evidence of moderate to severe peribronchial, interstitial, or alveolar infiltrates
Hemorrhagic syndrome	Evidence of hemorrhage (other than LPHS) or the presence of DIC (≥3 of the following criteria: thrombocytopaenia, prolonged PT or aPTT, reduced AT-activity or fibrinogen concentration, high FDPs or D-dimer concentration [287]

Abbreviations: aPTT, activated partial thromboplastin time; AT, antithrombin; FDPs, fibrin degradation products; DIC, disseminated intravascular coagulation; IRIS, International Renal Interest Society; PT, prothrombin time

positive for leptospirosis via PCR and rapidly responding to doxycycline treatment, which is thought to be due to tubular dysfunction or secondary nephrogenic diabetes insipidus [93].

Hepatic involvement alone is rare [7,64,92]. While some studies found leptospires in the liver of dogs with chronic hepatopathies [95–97], other studies failed to identify an aetiological role for *Leptospira* in dogs with acute or chronic hepatitis [98] or granulomatous hepatitis [99]. Pancreatitis is a known complication in canine leptospirosis, and can cause cholestasis further contributing to a cholestatic hepatopathy [31,49]. Further studies are needed to determine the role of leptospirosis in chronic hepatopathies.

Hemorrhagic syndrome was diagnosed in up to 45% of reported cases of clinical leptospirosis [3,42,45,46,70]. A hypocoagulable thromboelastometry (TEM) profile, but not the presence of DIC, was significantly associated with hemorrhagic diathesis and higher mortality rate in one study [46].

A specific form of hemorrhage localized to the lungs with an unknown etiology (LPHS) has been described in up to 70% of dogs with leptospirosis [37,39,42,45,63,70,100]. The relationship between impaired liver function and pulmonary involvement (LPHS) has not been determined but hyperbilirubinemia was associated with increased risk of LPHS in one study [63]. Severe lung involvement is associated with

high mortality [39,45,63,101]. Other causes of respiratory signs include pulmonary edema due to fluid overload, pain or acidosis.

Other clinical manifestations of leptospirosis include disease within the gastrointestinal tract, muscle, heart and eyes. Gastrointestinal dysfunction with acute diarrhea or vomiting is likely a consequence of systemic rather than primary gastrointestinal disease. Ultrasonographic findings consistent with gastritis or enteritis can be present [45]. Small intestinal intussusception has also been described as a complication of leptospirosis [102,103]. Muscle involvement based on elevations in creatinine kinase (CK) has been described in 50 to 70% of dogs with leptospirosis [49,104]. However, mild increases in CK can be seen with minor muscle trauma such as restraint, recumbency or blood collection. Therefore, a definition of muscle involvement should be based on clinical signs such as myalgia in combination with a markedly elevated CK. Cardiac involvement-defined as increased cardiac troponin 1 (cTNI) [41,104] and presence of ventricular premature complexes (VPCs) [41] has been described in up to 69% of canine leptospirosis cases [104]. The number of VPCs was reflective of disease severity and predictive of outcome [41]. On postmortem examination, myocarditis [105], myocardial necrosis [106], epicarditis and endocarditis [107] have been described. While commonly seen as a primary clinical sign in species such as horses, uveitis is infrequently seen in dogs with leptospirosis [108–110].

Immune-mediated disease, presumed to be secondary to leptospirosis, has been infrequently described [111–114]. In two dogs with polyarthritis, leptospires were identified in synovial fluid of one [111], and polyarthritis in the other was presumed to be immune-mediated or reactive [112]. Two dogs with immune-mediated hemolytic anemia (IMHA) had severely elevated liver enzymes and hyperbilirubinemia but not azotemia on presentation; one dog subsequently developed azotemia. Diagnosis was confirmed via fluorescent in situ hybridization (FISH) in the first case [113], by positive urine PCR in the second [114] and was supported by positive MATs in both dogs [113,114].

DIAGNOSIS

Clinicopathologic Changes

The most common hematology finding in leptospirosis cases is thrombocytopenia [3,6,37,39,40,46,49,55,59,60, 64,70,100,104,115]. The proposed pathophysiological mechanisms for thrombocytopenia include vasculitis due to circulating leptospires causing endothelial injury with subsequent platelet adhesion and activation of the coagulation cascade [55], DIC [3,37], immune-mediated destruction [116] or splenic sequestration [37]. Mild to moderate anemia is thought to be the result of systemic inflammatory disease or blood loss via the respiratory or gastrointestinal tract; hemolysis due to effects of leptospiral toxins on the erythrocyte membrane is thought to be rare in dogs [117]. A leukocytosis with neutrophilia is present in most dogs with leptospirosis [6,37,39,49,55,59,70,104] and is reflective of systemic inflammation.

Most dogs will be azotemic and hyperphosphatemic at presentation [3,6,7,37,39,40,42,49,55,60,64,67, 70,79,100,104]. Glucosuria with normoglycemia is a sign of tubular damage and should raise the index of suspicion for leptospirosis in azotemic dogs [6,7,37,39,55,59,60,64,104]. Proteinuria can be due to high molecular weight proteins consistent with glomerular damage and low molecular weight proteins consistent with tubular damage [104,118].

Elevated urinary Kidney Injury Molecule-1 (uKIM-1), a transmembrane glycoprotein expressed in renal damage, was able to detect naturally occurring acute and subacute leptospirosis accompanied by tubular injury in early nonazotemic infections [119].

Hyperkalemia is a common complication of anuric/oliguric kidney failure and can cause severe bradyarrhythmias and cardiac arrest. Hypokalemia [6,39,100] can be refractory [120] in some cases due to severe kaliuresis [121] which is thought to result from decreased reabsorption of sodium and potassium in the proximal tubules, upregulation of the Na^+-K^+-$2Cl^-$ cotransporter in the thick ascending loop of Henle and increase in Na^+/K^+ exchange pump in the distal segment which reabsorbs more sodium in exchange for increased urinary loss of potassium. Elevated liver enzyme activities can be detected in 30 to 80% of dogs [40,59,67]. Most dogs will have a cholestatic liver profile with an increase in ALP greater than that of ALT and AST [3,6,7,37,39,49,60,64,70,79,100,104]. Hyperbilirubinemia is present in 15 to 94% of dogs [3,6,7,37,39,40,49,55,60,64,70,79,100,104] and was associated with a poor outcome in one study [42].

Increased CK has been described in 44 to 71% of dogs with leptospirosis and could be due to myositis [49,70,79,104]. An increased cTNI (a marker for cardiac damage) was found in 69% of dogs [104].

Increased lipase and amylase activity can be found in up to 50% of dogs [49,64,70,104], is nonspecific and could be due to pancreatitis, decreased renal excretion or gastrointestinal disease. An increase in the acute phase proteins C-reactive protein (CRP) [100,104] and haptoglobin [104] indicates a severe systemic inflammatory response.

Abnormalities found on coagulation profile include prolonged aPTT [6,7,37,39,64,70,104,115], PT [6,7,37,39,70,104], decreased antithrombin (AT) concentration [104], increased D-dimers [104], increased fibrin degradation products (FDPs) [7] and increased fibrinogen concentration [104].

Diagnostic Imaging

In dogs with LPHS, typical findings on thoracic radiographs include an interstitial (mild), reticulonodular interstitial (moderate) and patchy alveolar (severe) lung pattern [37]. These changes are often diffuse, accentuated caudodorsally and can be symmetric or asymmetric [122]. Even in the absence of respiratory signs, radiographs are recommended to detect early lesions. However, radiological changes often have a poor correlation with clinical manifestations [45,63,101]. In dogs with respiratory signs, chest radiographs should be performed to differentiate LPHS from other causes, including fluid overload (eg, pleural effusion, pulmonary vein enlargement) [45].

Findings on abdominal radiographs can include lack of serosal detail [37,39,59], hepatomegaly [37,39,59,60], splenomegaly [37,39,59,60] and

TABLE 7
Ultrasonographic Findings in Dogs with Leptospirosis

	Findings
Kidney	Retroperitoneal/peri-renal effusion [39,64,65,288]
	Renomegaly [7,39,59,60,64,288]
	Pyelectasia [7,39,59,60,64,166,288]
	Hyperechoic renal cortex [7,39,55,59,60,64,104,166,288]
	Medullary rim sign [64,288]
	Decreased renal corticomedullary junction distinction [7]
	Irregular renal surface [7]
Liver	Hepatomegaly [7,39,55,64]
	Heterogeneous parenchyma [7,39,64]
	Hypoechoic parenchyma [7,64]
	Hyperechoic parenchyma [64]
	Thickened gallbladder wall [39]
	Gallbladder sludge [7,39]
Spleen	Splenomegaly [7,39,55]
	Heterogeneous parenchyma [39]
Pancreas	Hypoechoic parenchyma [7,39,64]
	Hyperechoic parenchyma [7,64]
	Heterogeneous parenchyma [64]
	Pancreatic enlargement [64]
Gastrointestinal tract	Changes in wall layering [7,39]
	Wall thickening [7]
	Changes consistent with gastritis or enteritis [45]
Other	Mesenteric lymphadenopathy [7,39,64]
	Mild to moderate ascites [7,39,55,64,104]

renomegaly [59,60]. Typical ultrasonographic findings are summarized in Table 7.

Criteria Used to Establish a Diagnosis

Criteria used to establish a diagnosis of canine leptospirosis vary between different countries depending on test availability, prevalence of disease and vaccination status. Generally, at least one of the criteria summarized in Table 8 is used in conjunction with typical clinicopathological findings (azotemia, elevated liver enzymes, hyperbilirubinemia).

The combined use of PCR and MAT is recommended to increase the positive predictive value to diagnose leptospirosis in clinically affected dogs [123] (Box 1).

Molecular Diagnostics

The most commonly used molecular method to diagnose leptospirosis is polymerase chain reaction (PCR). While conventional PCRs target the 16sRNA or 23SrDNA, most new PCR assays target the LipL32 gene [124–126] and some the LigA and LigB genes [127] which are present only in pathogenic *Leptospira* species.

Diagnosis can be confirmed with PCR testing of blood, urine or tissue. While the PCR is usually positive in blood during the first 10 days after infection, followed subsequently by positive PCR results in the urine, it is recommended to submit both blood and urine concurrently to increase the sensitivity of testing, as the day of infection is generally unknown.

TABLE 8	
Criteria Used to Establish a Diagnosis of Canine Leptospirosis Used in Different Studies	
Test	**Sample Required/Criteria for Diagnosis**
MAT (single titer)	Serum: ≥1/800 against any Serovar in nonvaccinated dogs [6,7,37,39,41,42,45,53,56,57,63,64,67,137] ≥1/800 [42,45,46] or ≥1/1600 [3,7,60] against nonvaccine Serovars in vaccinated dogs with negative or low vaccination titers [37] ≥1/3200 [59,60] regardless of vaccination status ≥1/1600 [45,46,64] or ≥1/3200 in vaccinated dogs against vaccine Serovars [6,37,39]
MAT (seroconversion)	A greater than 2-fold [6,37] or 4-fold [3,7,39,41,42,45,46,59,60,63,64,137] rise of titers within 1–2 [63], 1–3 [42] or 2–3 [3,39,41] weeks regardless of vaccination status
PCR	Blood [37,39,45,46,53,63,64,137], DNA detection Urine [3,37,39,45,46,53,63,64,67,137], DNA detection Tissue [64], DNA detection
Culture	Urine or blood using Ellinghousen McCullough Johnson Harris (EMJH) culture medium [6,67,71]; positive culture
Levaditi-staining/silver staining	Tissue [37,39,64], organism detection
Fluorescent in situ hybridisation (FISH)	Tissue [64], DNA detection
Fluorescent antibody test (FAT)	Tissue [6,60], positive fluorescence
Immunohistochemistry	Tissue [57], antigen detection
Immunofluorescence assay (IFA)	Serum: High immunoglobulin M (IgM) (>1/320) in combination with low immunoglobulin G (IgG) titer in dogs for which the last vaccination against leptospirosis had occurred at least 3 months ago [3] OR single antibody titer of ≥1/800 not vaccinated in the last 4 months [64]
Urine fluorescent antibody test (FAT)	Urine, positive result [6,60]
Point-of-care canine IgM ELISA (Test-it®)	Serum, positive result [41] in dogs not vaccinated within 5 months of presentation [42]

Although several studies have shown positive urine PCR results in healthy dogs (silent shedders) [93,126,128–131], a positive result in a dog with consistent clinical signs and clinicopathologic changes confirms leptospirosis [1].

False-negative PCR results can be encountered due to low bacterial loads, especially after the administration of antimicrobials [1,44]. PCR from whole blood is more affected by previous antibiotic treatment than PCR from urine [91]. False-positive PCR results could occur due to the contamination of the sample. While the 16sRNA PCR is highly specific using aseptically collected urine samples, it could yield false-positive results in free-catch urine samples due to unrelated bacteria [132,133]. As vaccines are inactivated or recombinant and not live attenuated, vaccination does not interfere with PCR results [134]. Sensitivity and specificity of PCR is summarized in Table 9.

Loop-mediated isothermal amplification method (LAMP) is a molecular method which offers accurate and sensitive results in a range of resource restrained environments, however, it is currently not commercially available to the authors knowledge (Box 2).

New molecular methods used predominantly to characterise populations and inform vaccine strategies are available. They are expensive, resource intensive and require a high level of expertise so currently are more suitable for research projects (Box 3).

BOX 1
Suggested Confirmatory Testing Regime to Diagnose Canine Leptospirosis

Supportive evidence from serum biochemistry and hematology plus:

- Dual blood and urine PCR
- Serum MAT at the time of presentation
- A convalescent titer obtained 1 to 2 weeks later (4-fold increase in titer confirms the diagnosis)

SEROLOGICAL DIAGNOSTICS
Microscopic Agglutination Test

The MAT is the most widely used test to diagnose lepto-spirosis worldwide and requires specific equipment, highly trained staff and the maintenance of live cultures of several reference strains of *Leptospira* for use as antigens which undergo reaction with patient serum samples to detect agglutinating antibodies. Antibodies are directed against immunogenic carbohydrate antigens of leptospiral lipopolysaccharide (LPS). Serovars within the same Serogroup can cause cross-reaction with each other in the MAT. The highest serum dilution

---

TABLE 9
Sensitivity and Specificity of PCR for the Diagnosis of Canine Leptospirosis as Reported in Different Studies

Test	Sensitivity	Specificity	Diagnosis Established[a]	Reference
PCR (23S rDNA)	100%	88%	MAT Seroconversion	Harkin et al [110], 2003
qPCR (LipL32)	91.6%	100%	PCR (16sRNA)	Miotto et al [125], 2018
qPCR (LipL32)	68% (urine) 83% (blood)	97% (urine) 84% (blood)	Culture	Blanchard et al [289], 2021
qPCR (LipL32)	13.5%	92%	MAT Rapid point of care tests	Troia at al [137], 2018
FRET-PCR (LigA, LigB)	100x more sensitive compared to qPCR (LipL32) 10x more sensitive compared to 16sRNA TaqMan		qPCR (LipL32) 16sRNA TaqMan	Xu et al [127], 2014
Multiplex qPCR (3 regions of 16sRNA)	99.8%	100%	qPCR (TaqMan)	Perez et al [290], 2020
qPCR TaqMan (multi-gene targeted: LipL32, secY, ompL1) to differentiate *L. interrogans*, kirschnerii, borgpetersenii, noguchii	100%	100%	Culture	Ferreira at al [291], 2014

Abbreviations: FRET, fluorescent resonance energy transfer; PCR, polymerase chain reaction.

[a] Standard against which the PCR result was verified.

BOX 2
Loop-Mediated Isothermal Amplification Method (LAMP)

LAMP was developed in 2000 as a method to amplify DNA with high specificity, efficiency, and rapidity under isothermal conditions without the need for special laboratories or expensive equipment, allowing its use in resource-restricted environments and making it more user friendly than PCR [293]. A systematic review article comparing LAMP and PCR in clinical samples of humans with leptospirosis concluded that LAMP is more sensitive and has better diagnostic accuracy compared to PCR [294]. Similar to PCR, LAMP targeting the 16S rRNA yielded more false-positive results in field samples compared to LAMP targeting lipL32. It was concluded that LAMP 16S rRNA could be used as a screening test in endemic areas; however, confirmation using LAMP lipL32 is needed in positive samples [295]. In another study, PCR and LAMP showed the same sensitivity for the diagnosis of leptospirosis in canine sera [296]. PCRun is a commercially available molecular assay based on the isothermal amplification of part of the *Hap*I gene and is intended for the qualitative detection of pathogenic *Leptospira* species (Biogal-Galed Labs, Kibbutz Galed, Israel). One study showed a close correlation between PCRun and qPCR assays [297]. In conclusion, LAMP can be a useful easy-to-use screening test in dogs with suspected leptospirosis in endemic areas with limited resources.

---

causing the agglutination of 50% of leptospires is reported.

Comparison of MAT results between different studies is difficult. Generally, Serovars tested include those commonly encountered in the environment of different geographic regions. Therefore, the type as well as the number of Serovars tested can vary widely between different studies with as few as six [55,92] and as many as 23 Serovars tested [70,135] in the past two decades. Furthermore, MAT results can be discordant across different laboratories in dogs recently vaccinated against leptospirosis and in dogs with clinical leptospirosis [4]. Similarly, the cut-off for reported minimum titers can differ with most studies reporting MAT titers of 1/100 as the lowest titer while other studies report titers as low as 1/10 [136] or 1/40 [49].

Diagnostic criteria similarly vary between different studies with different cut-off titers used for acute (eg, 1/800 vs 1/1600) and convalescent (2-fold to 4-fold increase) MAT titers as well as different timings between obtaining acute and convalescent MAT samples (see Table 8).

The sensitivity of MAT in the diagnosis of leptospirosis is likely influenced by the time of infection and the host reaction to the Serovar involved. While experiments using intraperitoneal and conjunctival inoculation of virulent cultures of Canicola Serovar resulted in elevations of MAT titers after 5 days, peaking at 14 days, the extent to which these findings correspond generally to other Serovars and natural infection in the dog is unknown. Convalescent MAT can have a sensitivity as high as 100%, [44] whereas the sensitivity

---

BOX 3
New Molecular Methods Used to Characterize Causative *Leptospira* Serovars

In the past two decades, different molecular methods have been explored to better identify causative Serovars in different geographic regions and inform vaccine strategies. In *Multilocus Sequence Typing (MLST)* [12,71,125,273,277,298,299] several housekeeping genes are amplified and sequenced. *Multispacer Sequence typing (MST)* [300] is based on the sequencing of several intergenic regions. *Variable Number Tandem Repeat (VNTR)* [300,301] or *Multilocus Variable Number of Tandem Repeat Analysis (MLVA)* [12,302,303] evaluates numerous repeated insertion sequences in the genome occurring in variable copy numbers. Other methods used include *mass spectrometry (MALDI-TOF)* [304] and *Restriction Fragment Length Polymorphism (RFLP)* based on *Pulse Field Gel Electrophoresis (PFGE)*. Through the assignment of sequence types (STs), the above methods permit objective comparisons between strains of *Leptospira* and provide a specific pattern for each serovar. Interpretation of results relies on the availability of data from previously sequenced *Leptospira* strains [305,306].

While these molecular methods are promising tools for more precise characterization of infecting serogroups and Serovars their use is currently reserved for research settings due to high costs and high level of expertise needed to perform these and are unsuitable for diagnosis of individual dogs in the clinical setting. Further studies are needed to increase the genomic database and the sensitivity of available test methods.

of acute MAT titers can be as low as 18.2% [123]. The low sensitivity of acute MAT titers can be explained by insufficient time for seroconversion after infection. False-negative titers may occur if the infecting Serovar is not included in the MAT panel. The specificity of acute MAT can be as high as 100% [44,137], while convalescent titers had a specificity of 92% in one study [44]. False-positive titers may occur due to interference with postvaccinal titers hence vaccination (including time of last vaccination) always needs to be taken into account when interpreting MAT results.

Most studies assume that the infecting Serovar is the Serovar with the highest MAT [3]. If similar high titers to multiple Serovars are present, the causative Serovar is usually not reported but the overall result is considered positive. Other studies report the causative Serogroup rather than Serovar based on the assumption of possible cross-reactivity between Serovars within the same Serogroup [6–9]. Based on the results of a recent study, even this assumption may be problematic. Dogs were experimentally inoculated (orally, conjunctivally and intranasally) with Serovars Canicola, Grippotyphosa, Icterohemorrhagiae, and Pomona and MAT against these Serovars and Serovars Autumnalis, Bratislava and Hardjo were measured on day of exposure and 4, 7, 10, and 14 days after exposure. The Serovar with the highest MAT titer was often different from that of the infecting Serovar and strong cross-agglutination was observed among all Serovars except Hardjo [5]. One study evaluated the usefulness of MAT to determine the infecting Serovar by serological responses of 7 different Serogroups to 4 specific culture-proven *Leptospira* Serovar isolates. The overall sensitivity of MAT to predict the infecting Serovar was 46% at a cut-off of 1/100 and 44% at a cut-off of 1/800. The overall specificity for all Serogroups was 65% for acute titers and 75% when only convalescent samples with titers $\geq 1/800$ were considered [36]. Results for the same dog can be discordant between different laboratories, further complicating the prediction of the infecting Serovar by MAT [4]. In conclusion, MAT is useful to diagnose leptospirosis and the sensitivity increases when convalescent samples are used. MAT is variable in its ability to identify the infecting Serovar, which is less important for the individual patient but more important for the epidemiology of disease within a population.

Another simple and inexpensive serological test which has potential value as a screening test under field conditions – however, is currently not commercially available to the authors' knowledge – is the latex agglutination test (LAT) (Box 4).

Enzyme-Linked Immunosorbent Assay

Multiple different indirect enzyme-linked immunosorbent assays (ELISA) have been developed for the use of antibody detection (IgG, IgM or both) against *Leptospira* spp. in dogs. IgM antibodies increase during the first week of infection, IgG antibodies 1 to 3 weeks after infection. ELISAs either detect antibodies against the whole bacterial cell [68,138] or against specific antigens from the bacterial surface which are expressed by pathogenic leptospires [75,139–148]. These might be useful to differentiate between vaccinated and infected dogs [144].

Multiple studies have compared MAT and ELISA and overall found a good [68,138,142,143,146] to fair [141,145,147–149] agreement between tests depending on the ELISA used. The advantages of ELISA compared to MAT include that live *Leptospira* cultures and therefore high biosecurity measures are not needed and that ELISA detecting IgM antibodies might be useful in the early detection of infection when MAT is still negative due to insufficient time for seroconversion.

BOX 4
Latex Agglutination Test (LAT) for Diagnosis of Leptospirosis by Antibody Detection

LAT is a simple and inexpensive rapid recombinant protein-based diagnostic test that can be applied as a screening test for the detection of antileptospiral antibodies in sera in field conditions. Proteins used as antigens include recombinant outer membrane protein (OMP) A-like protein (rLoa22) of *Leptospira interrogans* serovar Hardjo [307], immunoglobulin-like protein B (LigB) [143], rLipL41+rLipL32 [148] and LipL32 [308]. Compared to MAT results, sensitivities of 94 to 98% [148,307,308] and specificity of 96 [308] to 98% [148] have been reported. Using LigB – which is only expressed during natural infection – as an antigen the capability of LAT to differentiate infected from vaccinated animals (DIVA) was explored. Out of 60 vaccinated dogs, MAT was positive in 46 and LAT in 8/46. While positive titers in those 8 dogs were thought to be due to vaccination failure and natural infection rather than vaccination titers this could not convincingly be proven hence further studies are needed to evaluate the DIVA capability of this test [143]. Overall, while LAT could be used as an inexpensive screening test providing rapid results under field conditions, this test is currently not commercially available to the authors' knowledge.

Box 5

Evaluation of the Performance of Commercially Available Point-of-Care Tests for Diagnosis of Leptospirosis

Box 5a. Summary of results: Dogs were experimentally infected with Serovars Canicola, Grippotyphosa, Icterohemorrhagiae, or Pomona [5].

Comparison of WITNESS Lepto, SNAP Lepto and MAT:

Day Postinfection	WITNESS Lepto	Sensitivity[a]	MAT	Sensitivity[a]	SNAP Lepto	Sensitivity[a]
	Positive		Positive		Positive	
0	0/32		0/32		0/32	
4	0/32		0/32		0/32	
7	28/32	50–100%	21/32	25–100%	1/32	12.5%
10	31/31	100%	29/31	87.5–100%	3/31	12.5–14.3%
14	24/24	100%	23/24	83.3–100%	0/24	

[a]Depending on serovar.

Box 5b. Summary of results from a study evaluating acute sera of dogs with confirmed (n = 42), negative (n = 36), and unconfirmed (n = 11) leptospirosis based on the results of MAT on admission, convalescent MAT, and PCR results. While none of the negative leptospirosis cases were positive with Witness Lepto, 27% were positive with SNAP Lepto [137].

	WITNESS Lepto	MAT	SNAP Lepto
Sensitivity	71.4%	76.2%	78.5%
Specificity	100%	100%	72.2%

Box 5c. Summary of results from a study comparing the performance of SNAP Lepto and MAT in a broad population of canine samples submitted to a commercial laboratory. Only 1/52 serum samples positive for *Borrelia burgdorferi* antibodies and negative on MAT tested positive on SNAP Lepto hence cross-reactivity with other spirochete bacteria seems to be low [183].

Comparison of *SNAP Lepto* and *MAT*:

MAT Titer	MAT Positive	SNAP Lepto Positive	Positive Percent Agreement
>1/100	259	205	79.2%
1/100–1/400	57	37	64.9%
>1/800	202	168	83.2%
>1/3200	115	106	92.2%

Box 5d. Summary of results from a study comparing results of MAT and SNAP Lepto postvaccination. It was concluded that SNAP Lepto demonstrated similar performance to MAT and both give false-positive results due to vaccination [183].

Week Postvaccination	MAT Positive	SNAP Lepto Positive
3	27/28	15/28
4	28/28	22/28
52	3/21	5/21
56	15/19	16/19

Box 5e. Summary of results from a study comparing results of SNAP Lepto and MAT on initial presentation in dogs with confirmed leptospirosis (n = 22), suspected leptospirosis (n = 9), and dogs with other illnesses (n = 131). There was an overall agreement with the clinical diagnosis of 80% for SNAP Lepto and 78% for MAT [309].

(continued on next page)

	MAT (≥1/100)	SNAP Lepto
	MAT (≥1/100)	SNAP Lepto
Confirmed leptospirosis	18/22	15/22
Suspected leptospirosis	6/9	4/9
Dogs with other disease	29/131	20/131

Box 5f: Summary of results from a study comparing WITNESS Lepto and MAT which showed a sensitivity and specificity of 98% and 93.5% for WITNESS, respectively [310].

Comparison of *WITNESS Lepto* and *MAT*:

MAT	WITNESS Lepto
Positive ≥1/800	49/50
Borderline <1/800	10/35
Negative: negative or vaccinal ≤1/400	0/50

Box 5g: Summary of results from a study comparing WITNESS Lepto and MAT in dogs with confirmed leptospirosis, dogs with other disease, and healthy dogs. In vaccinated dogs WITNESS Lepto was positive 4 weeks postvaccination in 64% and 12 weeks postvaccination in 24%; 26 weeks postvaccination all tested samples were negative [311].

	MAT	Witness Lepto	Diagnostic Performance Witness	Overall Agreement
Acute-phase sera				
Confirmed leptospirosis (n = 37), acute-phase sera	9/37	28/37	Sensitivity 75.7%	89.7%
Dogs with other disease (n = 15)		0/15	Specificity 98.3%	
Healthy dogs with incomplete history of vaccination (n = 45)		1/45		
Convalescent-phase sera				
Confirmed leptospirosis (n = 9)	9/9	9/9		100%

Box 5h: Summary of results from a study that evaluated the usefulness of Test-it and WITNESS Lepto in the early diagnosis of leptospirosis using samples taken at admission in 108 dogs with confirmed leptospirosis and 53 control dogs. If weak positive results were considered positive Test-it had a sensitivity of 82% and specificity of 91%, WITNESS Lepto had a sensitivity of 76% and specificity of 100%. Some technical difficulties were encountered with Test-it [312].

Comparison of *Test-it* and *WITNESS Lepto*:

	Test-it (n = 118)	WITNESS Lepto (n = 69)
Confirmed leptospirosis (n = 108)		
Negative	14	10
Weakly positive	10	10
Strongly positive	48	21

(continued on next page)

	Test-it (n = 118)	WITNESS Lepto (n = 69)
Control (n = 53)		
Negative	38	28
Weakly positive	4	0
Strongly positive	0	0

Box 5i: Summary of results of a study that evaluated Test-it using another IgG/IgM test as a reference test in 23 dogs with confirmed leptospirosis and 107 random samples and found a sensitivity of 100% and specificity of 95.3%. To rule out cross-reactivity 59 samples from dogs with infectious diseases and 40 healthy dogs were tested and the test was negative in 98% of dogs [212].

Comparison of *Test-it* and another IgG/IgM test:

Test-it

Confirmed acute		
leptospirosis (n = 23)	23/23	Sensitivity 100%
Healthy control (n = 107)	5*/107	
*vaccinated <5 months		Specificity 95.3%

* indicates that 5 of the dogs have been vaccinated <5 months

One disadvantage is the lack of information about the possible causative Serovar.

Commercially Available In-House Tests

Multiple commercially available rapid point-of care tests have become available in recent years and have been evaluated in multiple studies (Box 5). These tests determine the presence of IgG and/or IgM antibodies against any *Leptospira* species and therefore do not provide any information about the possible causative Serovar. They are useful in the clinical setting as they provide real time results which aids in the early diagnosis and implementation of biosecurity measures. A positive result in a dog with typical clinicopathological findings is highly suggestive of leptospirosis; however, a negative result does not exclude leptospirosis. False-positive results can occur during the first 3 months postvaccination. False-negative results can occur in acute leptospirosis due to insufficient time for seroconversion, especially if the test is designed to detect IgG antibodies. Confirmation of the diagnosis relies on further testing including PCR tests and acute and convalescent MAT titers.

The following commercial canine tests are currently available:

- *SNAP Lepto (IDEXX)*: LipL32-based ELISA, detects IgG and IgM antibodies with higher affinity for IgG antibodies.
- *WITNESS Lepto (Zoetis)*: immunochromatographic test, detects IgM antibodies.
- *Test-IT (Prodivet)*: *Leptospira* specific antigen-based immunochromatographic test, detects IgM antibodies.
- *Immunocomb (Biogal-Galed Labs)*: detects IgG antibodies against Serovars Canicola, Icterohemorrhagiae, Grippotyphosa and Pomona. As Immunocomb has not been independently evaluated for the use in dogs this test is not discussed further.

Culture

Culture in Ellinghausen–McCullough–Johnson–Harris (EMJH) medium is still regarded as the gold standard for the identification of the causative Serovar. Culture is technically difficult and necessary safety and biosecurity measures limit its use to research or reference laboratory settings only. Finally, culture takes several months, which is impractical in the clinical setting [1].

Histopathology

Spirochete organisms can be identified in tissue using silver stains [150] such as Levaditi [37,39,60] or Warthin–Starry stains [7]. To confirm the presence of leptospires, FISH [64], immunofluorescence [60,106] or immunohistochemistry [106] can be used. Common histopathological findings in the kidney include mixed interstitial inflammation [49,60,67,103,104,106,107], acute tubular necrosis [7,49,67,103,105,151] and the presence of casts [49,67,104]. Common findings in the liver include hepatocellular necrosis [7,49,103,105–107] and mixed inflammation [49,60,64,103,107]. In dogs with LPHS, acute alveolar hemorrhage and alveolar wall necrosis with hyaline membrane formation can be found [151]. Cardiac changes include myocarditis, endocarditis, epicarditis, myocardial degeneration, necrosis and hemorrhage [105,107]. Other systemic changes include diffuse hemorrhage, vasculitis and thromboemboli [7].

Treatment

The mainstay of treatment involves antibiotics to reduce or eliminate the bacteria and supportive care to treat significant organ damage, such as acute kidney injury or hepatopathy. In dogs with suspected leptospirosis, antibiotic treatment should never be delayed pending results. In the acute phase of infection when the administration of oral medication is not possible, penicillin derivatives should be used IV (penicillin G [20,000-40,000 U/kg q6-8h], ampicillin [20-30 mg/kg q 6-8h], amoxicillin [20-30 mg/kg q 6-8h]. In dogs with decreased renal function the dose should be adapted, e.g. double the administration interval in dogs with a creatinine concentration >440 μmol/L [2]. To clear the infection from the renal tubules and thus avoid a carrier state, a 14-day course of doxycycline (5 mg/kg q 12h or 10 mg/kg q 24h PO or IV) needs to be given, which can be commenced as soon as oral medications can be administered.

Treatment of acute kidney injury involves the administration of intravenous fluid therapy while closely monitoring "ins" (fluids) and "outs" (urine). A urinary catheter should be placed to monitor urine output and avoid contamination of the environment with infectious urine. Urine output should be monitored every 2 to 4 hours, body weight, blood pressure, electrolytes and acid–base status should be checked at least twice daily, renal function every 24 hours and CBC every 48 hours during hospitalization. Fluid therapy should be adjusted accordingly to avoid fluid overload and correct electrolyte abnormalities [31].

In oliguric patients, the administration of diuretics such as frusemide and mannitol should be considered. Indications for hemodialysis [37,39,45,55,104,115] include fluid overload, anuria or oliguria during the first 6 hours after admission in a dog with adequate volume status, being refractory to diuretics, absence of decreased plasma urea and creatinine concentrations after 24 hours of adequate intravenous fluid therapy and hyperkalemia refractory to conventional medical treatment [55,115]. Availability of hemodialysis can vary widely between jurisdictions. Hypertensive patients (repeated measurements with systolic BP > 160 mm

Hg) should be treated with antihypertensive medication (e.g, amlodipine) [152].

Other symptomatic treatment includes antiemetics (maropitant, ondansetron, metoclopramide), gastroprotectants (H2-receptor blockers: ranitidine, famotidine, cimetidine; proton pump inhibitors: omeprazole) and analgesics (eg, buprenorphine, methadone).

Suggested preventive measures to avoid LPHS include the minimization of manipulation and stress, overhydration/hypervolemia and control of systemic hypertension [2]. Treatment includes supportive care, oxygen therapy and in severe cases mechanical ventilation. Treatment with glucocorticoids, desmopressin, bronchodilators (theophylline) and frusemide has been attempted in earlier studies, but improved outcome was not demonstrated [37,153], and further studies are needed before recommending these treatments [2].

Early aggressive treatment and supportive care are important to counteract the development of DIC. Transfusion with fresh frozen plasma (FFP) is recommended in dogs with DIC and signs of bleeding [2].

Treatment of Dogs in Close Contact with Cases

Dogs living in the same household as dogs with confirmed leptospirosis should be prophylactically treated with doxycycline 5 mg/kg q 12hr or 10 mg/kg q 24hr for 14 days [31].

Zoonotic Risk

Leptospirosis is a zoonosis of global importance and is an occupational hazard for people who work outdoors or with animals. In two studies evaluating veterinarians, veterinary technicians and dog owners who had been in contact with patients with canine leptospirosis, all tested negative for leptospirosis [154,155] despite bare skin contact with blood or urine from infected dogs being common and inconsistent infection control being practiced [155]. Another study estimated a seroprevalence of 2.5% in veterinarians attending a conference in the US. [156]. Importantly, while it is generally considered that urinary shedding ceases approximately 48 to 72 hours after initiating appropriate antibiotic treatment, there are occasional reports of ongoing shedding beyond this [65,91,157]. While dog-to-human transmission seems to be rare, cases of transmission have been described. A parasitology researcher dissecting dogs tested positive for leptospirosis in Malaysia [158]. Similarly, dog handlers in Malaysia had a higher risk of being seropositive, which increased with dog contact time [159]. During human outbreaks, an association has been found between contact with seropositive dogs and human leptospirosis [160] and in Chile, an association was found between the presence of dogs and *Leptospira* positive puddles [161]. Due to the zoonotic potential of leptospirosis, appropriate biosecurity measures need to be put in place (Box 6).

Prognosis

Fatality rates of 18%-84% have been described [3,37,39,42,55,60,70,79,104,162] and depend on many different factors including host immune response, inoculation dose and virulence of the infecting strain [2].

The main causes for euthanasia include respiratory distress due to LPHS [37], acute renal failure [37,39,60], progression of disease [39] or financial reasons [39,42,60]. An increased case fatality rate has been found in dogs with pulmonary [42,45,63], hepatic [42,79] and hemorrhagic [42,45,55] organ involvement. More severe renal failure has been associated with a poor outcome [79] and hemodialysis improves the outcome [55]. Case fatality increases if $\geq$ 3 clinical manifestations are present [45]. Acute necrotizing pancreatitis has been associated with leptospirosis [55] and increases mortality.

Clinicopathological changes associated with increased case fatality include significantly higher cTNI (marker of cardiac involvement), C-reactive protein (CRP) [163] or haptoglobin (acute phase proteins), urine albumin/creatinine (UAC) ratio, urine protein/creatinine (UPC) ratio, and significantly lower albumin and total protein concentration [104], a stress leukogram and metabolic acidosis [79].

Prevention

Risk mitigation methods are the most important measures to prevent leptospirosis infection. Contact with sources of infection should be limited. This includes limiting contact with, swimming in, and drinking out of stagnant water and avoiding contact with possible reservoir hosts such as rodents and farm animals, which can be achieved by fencing and rodent control [31]. Similarly, contact with leptospire-infected dogs should be avoided. In endemic areas – especially during leptospirosis outbreaks – close dog-to-dog contact, for example, doggy daycare and boarding in kennels should be reconsidered [91].

Vaccination is another important part of prevention. It appears that currently available vaccines induce Serogroup-specific immunity and only partial immunity to heterologous Serogroups [2,164]. Licensed inactivated vaccines against canine leptospirosis have been on the market since the 1960s and include bivalent vaccines against Serovars Canicola and Icterohemorrhagiae in most countries [165,166]. Available vaccines differ between countries depending on which Serovars are thought to cause clinical disease in the respective geographic area and the willingness of companies to offer vaccines in a country based on the prevalence of disease (Table 10).

Leptospira vaccines are noncore in most countries according to WSAVA guidelines and should be used in geographical areas where a risk of exposure has been established or for dogs whose lifestyle places them at risk [167]. However, leptospirosis is considered a core vaccine in some countries including Germany and the UK.

BOX 6
Suggested Protocol for Handling Hospitalized Patients with Leptospirosis

- The cage should be appropriately labeled.
- Pregnant and immunocompromised staff should not handle the patient.
- The patient should be barrier-nursed from other dogs but housing in an isolation facility is not necessary.
- Appropriate PPE should be worn and should not leave the area: gloves, disposable impermeable barrier gown, boots, goggles/face shields.
- Supplies assigned to the patient should not be transferred to another patient.
- If possible, a urinary catheter should be placed to avoid the contamination of the environment. The urine should be collected in a biohazard bag which should be disposed of in the biohazard bin.
- Similarly, all material used for the patient (eg, cage pads, bandages) should be considered biohazardous material.
- If placing a urinary catheter is not possible the dog should be walked in an area that can be easily disinfected and is not frequented by other patients.
- If the patient has to be moved between different areas it should be carried (e.g, gurney).
- 10% bleach, iodine-based disinfectants, accelerated hydrogen peroxide, and quaternary ammonium solutions are effective.
- The urine is believed to be cleared of leptospires and no longer poses a risk after 3 days of antibiotic treatment at which stage the urinary catheter can be removed.

TABLE 10
Examples of Available Canine Vaccines Against *Leptospira* in Different Geographic Regions

Country	Currently Available Serovars and/or Serogroups Contained Within Vaccines
Globally	*L. interrogans* Serogroup **Canicola** serovar Portland-vere + *L. interrogans* Serogroup **Icterohemorrhagiae** serovar Copenhageni
Europe	*L. interrogans* Serogroup **Canicola** serovar Portland-vere + *L. interrogans* Serogroup **Icterohemorrhagiae** serovar Copenhageni + *L. kirschneri* Serogroup **Grippotyphosa** serovar Dadas +/– *L. interrogans* Serogroup **Australis** serovar Bratislava
North + South America	*L. interrogans* serovar **Canicola** + *L. interrogans* serovar **Icterohemorrhagiae** + *L. kirschneri* serovar **Grippotyphosa** + *L. interrogans* serovar **Pomona**
Australia	*L. interrogans* serovar **Copenhageni** *L. interrogans* serovar **Australis** (limited permit)
New Zealand	*L. interrogans* serovar **Icterohemoarrhagiae** *L. interrogans* Serogroup Icterohemorrhagiae serovar **Copenhageni**, *L. interrogans* serovar **Pomona**, *L. borgpetersenii* serovar **Hardjo** (genotype Hardjobovis) (licensed for use in cattle, has been used off label for dogs) [292]
Asia	*L. interrogans* serovar **Canicola** + *L. interrogans* serovar **Icterohemorrhagiae** *L. interrogans* serovar **Canicola** + *L. interrogans* serovar **Icterohemorrhagiae** + *L. interrogans* serovar **Pomona** + *L. kirschneri* serovar **Grippotyphosa**
Additionally in Japan	*L. interrogans* serovar **Copenhageni** + *L. interrogans* serovar **Canicola** + *L.interrogans* serovar **Hebdomanis**

Note that depending on the manufacturer and the importance of Serovars in the respective geographic region the description of the vaccine will be based on Serogroup or serovar contained (shown in bold).

Available vaccines can be used in puppies from the age of 6 weeks and maternally derived antibodies do not interfere with vaccine efficacy [168]. Two doses should be given 2 to 4 weeks apart. Yearly boosters are recommended. In dogs in which more than 15 months have elapsed since the last vaccination, two doses of vaccine should be given 2 to 4 weeks apart to re-establish immunity, followed by annual boosters [169].

Studies to test the efficacy of vaccines usually involve the experimental infection of vaccinated and control dogs through intraconjunctival and/or intraperitoneal inoculation with Serovars used in the vaccine. Dogs are usually challenged shortly after the primary vaccination course (onset of immunity) [168,170–172] and 6 to 12 months or even later (duration of immunity) [170–175]. Dogs are then monitored for clinical signs, clinicopathological abnormalities, antibody response,

leptospiraemia, and shedding (culture) and histopathological changes [175,176]. Clinical signs in vaccinated dogs are usually rare, mild, and transient after challenge. In studies, fatal leptospirosis has been prevented in all vaccinated dogs after the challenge with vaccine Serovars. None of the dogs developed a renal carrier state 4 to 5 weeks after primary vaccination (onset of immunity) [168,170–172]; however, some did after 6 to 12 months (duration of immunity). [170–175,177]. Protection was not only demonstrated against vaccine Serovars but also against Serovars of the same Serogroup [164].

While the efficacy of vaccines is generally high, fully vaccinated dogs can develop clinical leptospirosis [3,12,13,37,39,42,45,46,57,59,60,64,70,71,115,166,178,179]. Vaccination is thought to result in less severe disease in dogs developing leptospirosis [180]; however, case fatalities do occur [70]. The development of leptospirosis in fully vaccinated dogs could be due to the absence of the etiologic Serovar in the vaccine and limited cross-protection, host immune response, and virulence of the infecting strain.

Seroconversion after vaccination can differ considerably among individual dogs and among the vaccine Serogroups [181,182]. Antibody titers peaked 3 weeks after the first [173] and 2 to 6 weeks after the second injection in different studies [173,177,183] and then declined and became very low at 15 [177,182] to 16 weeks [184]. Most dogs are antibody negative 1 year after vaccination [182]. Importantly, MAT titers against nonvaccine Serovars could be induced by vaccination. In one study all vaccinated puppies developed antibody titers to Serovars Pomona and Autumnalis after vaccination with Serovars Pomona and Grippotyphosa; however, none developed antibodies against Serovar Grippotyphosa [184]. Therefore, studies evaluating seroconversion after vaccination for different vaccines are important to be able to correctly interpret antibody titers in vaccinated dogs with suspected leptospirosis. However, the measurement of antibody response after vaccination is not useful to evaluate the level of protection and vaccine efficacy.

There has been vaccination hesitancy among both veterinarians and dog owners due to the belief that the leptospirosis vaccine is associated with a heightened risk of adverse events, especially in small breed dogs [167]. The evidence for this is poor, and two studies indicated no greater risk from *Leptospira* bacterins [185,186]. In a study investigating side effects after vaccination with a quadrivalent vaccine, mild and transient clinical signs were found in 23% after the first and 10% within 5 days after the second vaccination; however, no changes in hematology, biochemistry, cTNI, and echocardiography results were observed [181]. Recommendations from veterinarians not to vaccinate against leptospirosis decreased vaccination rates and further studies are needed to investigate why some veterinarians recommend against vaccination [187,188].

Future Avenues for Investigation

The recent advances in molecular diagnostics are promising and allow more accurate characterization of pathogenic *Leptospira* species and Serovars in different geographic regions than the MAT. However, more studies are needed to develop a complete genomic database for different leptospiral Serovars. Commercially available genome sequencing would be an invaluable diagnostic tool for the investigation and characterization of leptospirosis worldwide.

Leptospiral General Secretory Protein D (GspD) is a secretin that elicits complement-independent bactericidal antibodies against diverse *Leptospira* species and Serovars. In a recent study, this protein was investigated as a potential antigen in a multi-valent subunit vaccine formulation [189]. A vaccine like this could protect against the vast majority of pathogenic *Leptospira* and would negate the need to determine causative Serovars in different geographic regions. Other antigens which could be potential candidates for vaccine development or could be useful to differentiate infected from vaccinated animals (DIVA) are proteins that are only present in pathogenic species of *Leptospira* such as LipL32 and immunoglobulin-like (Lig) proteins LigA and LigB [143,190].

SUMMARY

Canine leptospirosis affects dogs worldwide and can have a fatal outcome not only due to life-threatening complications such as severe AKI with oliguria/anuria or LPHS but also due to limited access to treatment facilities and the high cost of treatment. Causative Serovars vary between geographic regions. Generally, the causative Serovar is defined as the Serovar to which the highest MAT titer is detected. However, numerous studies have shown that the MAT is unreliable to determine the causative Serovar. Therefore, despite the abundance of literature regarding canine leptospirosis, there is still a lack of knowledge about the prevalence of infecting Serovars and new studies using molecular methods are needed to characterize these better. Monovalent to quadrivalent inactivated vaccines containing Serovars relevant to the respective geographic region are available. While they offer Serogroup-specific immunity, they only offer partial immunity to heterologous Serogroups and hence fully vaccinated dogs can develop fatal leptospirosis. Therefore, risk mitigation measures are of utmost importance. Overall, comparison between studies and therefore developing a global overview of canine leptospirosis is difficult due to differences in study design, criteria used to establish a diagnosis of leptospirosis and Serovars used in MAT.

CLINICS CARE POINTS

- In dogs with suspected leptospirosis rapid point-of-care tests are useful to aid in the early diagnosis and implementation of biosecurity measures; however, false-positive and false-negative results can occur.

- Confirmation of the diagnosis relies on further testing including PCR tests and convalescent MAT titers.
- A dog with suspected leptospirosis should be treated like a dog with confirmed leptospirosis.
- Antibiotics should never be withheld pending confirmatory results.
- Penicillin derivatives can be used initially; however, a 14-day course of doxycycline should be started as soon as oral medication can be given to clear the infection from the renal tubules.
- Hemodialysis is indicated in dogs with fluid overload, anuria/oliguria with adequate volume status and refractory to diuretics, azotemia not responding to adequate fluid therapy within 24 hours and hyperkalemia refractory to medical treatment.
- In dogs with LPHS treatment with glucocorticoids, desmopressin, theophylline, and frusemide are currently not recommended.

DISCLOSURE

The authors have nothing to disclose.

REFERENCES

[1] Reagan KL, Sykes JE. Diagnosis of canine leptospirosis. Vet Clin Small Anim Pract 2019;49(4):719–31.

[2] Schuller S, Francey T, Hartmann K, et al. European consensus statement on leptospirosis in dogs and cats. J Small Anim Pract 2015;56(3):159–79.

[3] Geisen V, Stengel C, Brem S, et al. Canine leptospirosis infections - clinical signs and outcome with different suspected Leptospira Serogroups (42 cases). J Small Anim Pract 2007;48(6):324–8.

[4] Miller MD, Annis KM, Lappin MR, et al. Variability in results of the microscopic agglutination test in dogs with clinical leptospirosis and dogs vaccinated against leptospirosis. J Vet Intern Med 2011;25(3):426–32.

[5] Lizer J, Velineni S, Weber A, et al. Evaluation of 3 serological tests for early detection of Leptospira-specific antibodies in experimentally infected dogs. J Vet Intern Med 2018;32(1):201–7.

[6] Goldstein RE, Lin RC, Langston CE, et al. Influence of infecting Serogroup on clinical features of leptospirosis in dogs. J Vet Intern Med 2006;20(3):489–94.

[7] Tangeman LE, Littman MP. Clinicopathologic and atypical features of naturally occurring leptospirosis in dogs: 51 cases (2000-2010). J Am Vet Med Assoc 2013;243(9):1316–22.

[8] Jimenez-Coello M, Vado-Solis I, Cárdenas-Marrufo MF, et al. Serological survey of canine leptospirosis in the tropics of Yucatan Mexico using two different tests. Acta tropica 2008;106(1):22–6.

[9] Suepaul S, Carrington C, Campbell M, et al. Seroepidemiology of leptospirosis in dogs and rats in Trinidad. Trop Biomed 2014;31(4):853–61.

[10] Adler B. Leptospira and leptospirosis, Vol. 387. Heidelberg: Springer Berlin; 2014.

[11] Vincent AT, Schiettekatte O, Goarant C, et al. Revisiting the taxonomy and evolution of pathogenicity of the genus Leptospira through the prism of genomics. PLoS Negl Trop Dis 2019;13(5):e0007270.

[12] Bertasio C, Boniotti MB, Lucchese L, et al. Detection of new leptospira genotypes infecting symptomatic dogs. is a new vaccine formulation needed? Pathogens 2020;9(6):484.

[13] Rahman SA, Khor KH, Khairani-Bejo S, et al. Detection and characterization of Leptospira spp. in dogs diagnosed with kidney and/or liver disease in Selangor, Malaysia. J Vet Diagn Invest 2021;33(5):834–43.

[14] Silva ÉF, Cerqueira GM, Seyffert N, et al. Leptospira noguchii and human and animal leptospirosis, Southern Brazil. Emerging Infect Dis 2009;15(4):621.

[15] Miotto BA, Moreno LZ, Guilloux AGA, et al. Molecular and serological characterization of the first Leptospira santarosai strain isolated from a dog. Acta tropica 2016;162:1–4.

[16] Ko AI, Goarant C, Picardeau M. Leptospira: the dawn of the molecular genetics era for an emerging zoonotic pathogen. Nat Rev Microbiol 2009;7(10):736–47.

[17] Klarenbeek A, Voet J. The dog as carrier of weil's disease. Nederlands Tijdschrift voor Geneeskunde 1933;77:398–400.

[18] Boey K, Shiokawa K, Rajeev S. Leptospira infection in rats: a literature review of global prevalence and distribution. PLoS Negl Trop Dis 2019;13(8):e0007499.

[19] Delaude A, Rodriguez-Campos S, Dreyfus A, et al. Canine leptospirosis in Switzerland—a prospective cross-sectional study examining seroprevalence, risk factors and urinary shedding of pathogenic leptospires. Prev Vet Med 2017;141:48–60.

[20] Taylor C, O'Neill DG, Catchpole B, et al. Incidence and demographic risk factors for leptospirosis in dogs in the UK. Vet Rec 2021;190(6):e512.

[21] Putz EJ, Nally JE. Investigating the immunological and biological equilibrium of reservoir hosts and pathogenic leptospira: balancing the solution to an acute problem? Front Microbiol 2020;11:2005.

[22] Dreyfus A, Wilson P, Benschop J, et al. Seroprevalence and herd-level risk factors for seroprevalence of Leptospira spp. in sheep, beef cattle and deer in New Zealand. New Zealand Vet J 2018;66(6):302–11.

[23] Jansen A, Luge E, Guerra B, et al. Leptospirosis in urban wild boars, Berlin, Germany. Emerging Infect Dis 2007;13(5):739.

[24] Straub MH, Church M, Glueckert E, et al. Raccoons (procyon lotor) and striped skunks (mephitis mephitis) as potential reservoirs of leptospira spp. in California. Vector-Borne Zoonotic Dis 2020;20(6):418–26.

[25] Richardson DJ, Gauthier JL. A serosurvey of leptospirosis in Connecticut peridomestic wildlife. Vector-Borne Zoonotic Dis 2003;3(4):187–93.

[26] Grimm K, Rivera NA, Fredebaugh-Siller S, et al. Evidence Of leptospira Serovars in wildlife and leptospiral DNA in water sources in a natural area in east-central Illinois, USA. J Wildl Dis 2020;56(2):316–27.

[27] Ayral F, Djelouadji Z, Raton V, et al. Hedgehogs and mustelid species: major carriers of pathogenic Leptospira, a survey in 28 animal species in France (20122015). PLoS One 2016;11(9):e0162549.

[28] Nau L, Obiegala A, Król N, et al. Survival time of Leptospira kirschneri Serovar Grippotyphosa under different environmental conditions. PLoS One 2020; 15(7):e0236007.

[29] Rossetti CA, Liem M, Samartino LE, et al. Buenos Aires, a new Leptospira Serovar of Serogroup Djasiman, isolated from an aborted dog fetus in Argentina. Vet Microbiol 2005;107(3–4):241–8.

[30] Kim S, Lee DS, Suzuki H, et al. Detection of Brucella canis and Leptospira interrogans in canine semen by multiplex nested PCR. J Vet Med Sci 2006;68(6):615–8.

[31] Sykes JE, Hartmann K, Lunn K, et al. 2010 ACVIM small animal consensus statement on leptospirosis: diagnosis, epidemiology, treatment, and prevention. J Vet Intern Med 2011;25(1):1–13.

[32] Medeiros Fda R, Spichler A, Athanazio DA. Leptospirosis-associated disturbances of blood vessels, lungs and hemostasis. Acta Trop 2010;115(1–2):155–62.

[33] Maissen-Villiger CA, Schweighauser A, van Dorland HA, et al. Expression profile of cytokines and enzymes mRNA in blood leukocytes of dogs with leptospirosis and its associated pulmonary hemorrhage syndrome. PLoS One 2016;11(1):e0148029.

[34] Schuller S, Callanan JJ, Worrall S, et al. Immunohistochemical detection of IgM and IgG in lung tissue of dogs with leptospiral pulmonary haemorrhage syndrome (LPHS). Comp Immunol Microbiol Infect Dis 2015;40:47–53.

[35] Sonderegger F, Nentwig A, Schweighauser A, et al. Association of markers of endothelial activation and dysfunction with occurrence and outcome of pulmonary hemorrhage in dogs with leptospirosis. J Vet Intern Med 2021;35(4):1789–99.

[36] Levett PN. Usefulness of serologic analysis as a predictor of the infecting Serovar in patients with severe leptospirosis. Clin Infect Dis 2003;36(4):447–52.

[37] Kohn B, Steinicke K, Arndt G, et al. Pulmonary abnormalities in dogs with leptospirosis. J Vet Intern Med 2010;24(6):1277–82.

[38] Mayer-Scholl A, Luge E, Draeger A, et al. Distribution of leptospira Serogroups in dogs from Berlin, Germany. Vector-Borne Zoonotic Dis 2013;13(3):200–2.

[39] Knopfler S, Mayer-Scholl A, Luge E, et al. Evaluation of clinical, laboratory, imaging findings and outcome in 99 dogs with leptospirosis. J Small Anim Pract 2017; 58(10):582–8.

[40] Gerlach T, Stephan I. Epidemiologische situation der kaninen leptospirose in norddeutschland in den Jahren 2003–2006. Tierärztliche Praxis Ausgabe K: Kleintiere/ Heimtiere 2007;35(06):421–9.

[41] Keller SP, Kovacevic A, Howard J, et al. Evidence of cardiac injury and arrhythmias in dogs with acute kidney injury. J Small Anim Pract 2016;57(8):402–8.

[42] Major A, Schweighauser A, Francey T. Increasing incidence of canine leptospirosis in Switzerland. Int J Environ Res Public Health 2014;11(7):7242–60.

[43] Francey T. Clinical features and epidemiology of presumptive canine leptospirosis in Western Switzerland, 2003–2005. J Vet Intern Med 2006;20:1530–1.

[44] Fraune CK, Schweighauser A, Francey T. Evaluation of the diagnostic value of serologic microagglutination testing and a polymerase chain reaction assay for diagnosis of acute leptospirosis in dogs in a referral center. J Am Vet Med Assoc 2013;242(10):1373–80.

[45] Magnin M, Barthélemy A, Sonet J, et al. Pulmonary dysfunction as a component of a multiple organ dysfunction syndrome in dogs with leptospirosis. Revue Vétérinaire Clinique. 2020;55(3):95–103.

[46] Barthélemy A, Magnin M, Pouzot-Nevoret C, et al. Hemorrhagic, hemostatic, and thromboelastometric disorders in 35 dogs with a clinical diagnosis of leptospirosis: a prospective study. J Vet Intern Med 2017; 31(1):69–80.

[47] Ayral FC, Bicout DJ, Pereira H, et al. Distribution of Leptospira Serogroups in cattle herds and dogs in France. Am J Trop Med Hyg 2014;91(4):756.

[48] Renaud C, Andrews S, Djelouadji Z, et al. Prevalence of the Leptospira Serovars bratislava, grippotyphosa, mozdok and pomona in French dogs. Vet J 2013;196(1): 126–7.

[49] Prescott JF, McEwen B, Taylor J, et al. Resurgence of leptospirosis in dogs in Ontario: recent findings. Can Vet J 2002;43(12):955–61.

[50] Alton GD, Berke O, Reid-Smith R, et al. Increase in seroprevalence of canine leptospirosis and its risk factors, Ontario 1998–2006. Can J Vet Res 2009;73(3):167.

[51] Gautam R, Wu C-C, Guptill LF, et al. Detection of antibodies against Leptospira Serovars via microscopic agglutination tests in dogs in the United States, 2000–2007. J Am Vet Med Assoc 2010;237(3):293–8.

[52] Moore GE, Guptill LF, Glickman NW, et al. Canine leptospirosis, United States, 2002–2004. Emerging Infect Dis 2006;12(3):501.

[53] Grayzel SE, DeBess EE. Characterization of leptospirosis among dogs in Oregon, 2007–2011. J Am Vet Med Assoc 2016;248(8):908–15.

[54] Davis M, Evermann J, Petersen C, et al. Serological survey for antibodies to Leptospira in dogs and raccoons in Washington State. Zoonoses and Public Health 2008; 55(8-10):436–42.

[55] Adin CA, Cowgill LD. Treatment and outcome of dogs with leptospirosis: 36 cases (1990–1998). J Am Vet Med Assoc 2000;216(3):371–5.

[56] Ghneim GS, Viers JH, Chomel BB, et al. Use of a case-control study and geographic information systems to determine environmental and demographic risk factors for canine leptospirosis. Vet Res 2007;38(1):37–50.

[57] Hennebelle JH, Sykes JE, Carpenter TE, et al. Spatial and temporal patterns of Leptospira infection in dogs from northern California: 67 cases (2001–2010). J Am Vet Med Assoc 2013;242(7):941–7.

[58] Sykes J., Bryan J., Armstrong P., Comparison of clinical findings associated with canine leptospirosis between two teaching hospitals, Paper presented at: Journal of Veterinary Internal Medicine, 21, 2007, 624.

[59] Rentko VT, Clark N, Ross LA, et al. Canine leptospirosis. A retrospective study of 17 cases. J Vet Intern Med 1992; 6(4):235–44.

[60] Birnbaum N, Barr SC, Center SA, et al. Naturally acquired leptospirosis in 36 dogs: serological and clinico-pathological features. J Small Anim Pract 1998;39(5): 231–6.

[61] Ward MP, Guptill LF, Prahl A, et al. Serovar-specific prevalence and risk factors for leptospirosis among dogs: 90 cases (1997–2002). J Am Vet Med Assoc 2004;224(12):1958–63.

[62] Ward MP, Guptill LF, Wu CC. Evaluation of environmental risk factors for leptospirosis in dogs: 36 cases (1997–2002). J Am Vet Med Assoc 2004;225(1):72–7.

[63] Lippi I, Puccinelli C, Perondi F, et al. Predictors of fatal pulmonary haemorrhage in dogs affected by leptospirosis approaching haemodialysis. Vet Sci 2021;8(2):25.

[64] Raj J, Campbell R, Tappin S. Clinical findings in dogs diagnosed with leptospirosis in England. Vet Rec 2021;189(7):e452.

[65] Juvet F, Schuller S, O'Neill E, et al. Urinary shedding of spirochaetes in a dog with acute leptospirosis despite treatment. Vet Record-English Edition 2011;168(21): 564.

[66] Weekes C, Everard C, Levett P. Seroepidemiology of canine leptospirosis on the island of Barbados. Vet Microbiol 1997;57(2–3):215–22.

[67] Paz LN, Dias CS, Almeida DS, et al. Multidisciplinary approach in the diagnosis of acute leptospirosis in dogs naturally infected by Leptospira interrogans Serogroup Icterohaemorrhagiae: a prospective study. Comp Immunol Microbiol Infect Dis 2021;77:101664.

[68] Penna B, Marassi CD, Libonati H, et al. Diagnostic accuracy of an in-house ELISA using the intermediate species Leptospira fainei as antigen for diagnosis of acute leptospirosis in dogs. Comp Immunol Microbiol Infect Dis 2017;50:13–5.

[69] Romero-Vivas CM, Cuello-Pérez M, Agudelo-Flórez P, et al. Cross-sectional study of Leptospira seroprevalence in humans, rats, mice, and dogs in a main tropical seaport city. Am J Trop Med Hyg 2013;88(1):178.

[70] Griebsch C, Kirkwood N, Ward MP, et al. Emerging leptospirosis in urban Sydney dogs: a case series (2017-2020). Aust Vet J 2022;100:190–200.

[71] Koizumi N, Muto MM, Akachi S, et al. Molecular and serological investigation of Leptospira and leptospirosis in dogs in Japan. J Med Microbiol 2013;62(4):630–6.

[72] Saeki J, Tanaka A. Canine Leptospirosis Outbreak in Japan. Front Vet Sci 2021;8.

[73] Zhang C, Xu J, Zhang T, et al. Genetic characteristics of pathogenic Leptospira in wild small animals and livestock in Jiangxi Province, China, 2002–2015. PLoS Negl Trop Dis 2019;13(6):e0007513.

[74] Sathiyamoorthy A, Selvaraju G, Palanivel K, et al. Seroprevalence of canine leptospirosis in namakkal, tamil nadu by microscopic agglutination test. J Cell Tissue Res 2017;17(1):5991–6.

[75] Kumar RS, Pillai R, Mukhopadhyay H, et al. Seroepidemiology of canine leptospirosis by iELISA and MAT. Vet World 2013;6(11):926.

[76] Ambily R, Mini M, Joseph S, et al. Canine leptospirosis-a seroprevalence study from Kerala, India. Vet World 2013;6(1):42–4.

[77] Sant'Anna da Costa R, N Di Azevedo MI, dos Santos Baptista Borges AL, et al. Persistent high leptospiral shedding by asymptomatic dogs in endemic areas triggers a serious public health concern. Animals 2021; 11(4):937.

[78] Ward MP. Seasonality of canine leptospirosis in the United States and Canada and its association with rainfall. Prev Vet Med 2002;56(3):203–13.

[79] Miller RI, Ross SP, Sullivan ND, et al. Clinical and epidemiological features of canine leptospirosis in North Queensland. Aust Vet J 2007;85(1–2):13–9.

[80] Kikuti M, Langoni H, Nobrega D, et al. Occurrence and risk factors associated with canine leptospirosis. J Venomous Anim Toxins including Trop Dis 2012; 18:124–7.

[81] Taylor C, Brodbelt D, Dobson B, et al. Spatio-temporal distribution and agroecological factors associated with canine leptospirosis in Great Britain. Prev Vet Med 2021;193:105407.

[82] Jorge S, Schuch RA, de Oliveira NR, et al. Human and animal leptospirosis in Southern Brazil: a five-year retrospective study. Trav Med Infect Dis 2017;18: 46–52.

[83] Smith AM, Arruda AG, Evason MD, et al. A cross-sectional study of environmental, dog, and human-related risk factors for positive canine leptospirosis PCR test results in the United States, 2009 to 2016. BMC Vet Res 2019;15(1):1–12.

[84] Lee H, Levine M, Guptill-Yoran C, et al. Regional and temporal variations of Leptospira seropositivity in dogs in the United States, 2000–2010. J Vet Intern Med 2014;28(3):779–88.

[85] Gautam R, Guptill LF, Wu CC, et al. Spatial and spatio-temporal clustering of overall and Serovar-specific Leptospira microscopic agglutination test (MAT) seropositivity among dogs in the United States from 2000 through 2007. Prev Vet Med 2010;96(1–2):122–31.

[86] Ward MP, Glickman LT, Guptill LF. Prevalence of and risk factors for leptospirosis among dogs in the United States and Canada: 677 cases (1970-1998). J Am Vet Med Assoc 2002;220(1):53–8.

[87] Ricardo T, Previtali MA, Signorini M. Meta-analysis of risk factors for canine leptospirosis. Prev Vet Med 2020;181:105037.

[88] Raghavan R, Brenner K, Higgins J, et al. Evaluations of land cover risk factors for canine leptospirosis: 94 cases (2002–2009). Prev Vet Med 2011;101(3–4):241–9.

[89] Raghavan RK, Brenner KM, Higgins JJ, et al. Neighborhood-level socioeconomic and urban land use risk factors of canine leptospirosis: 94 cases (2002–2009). Prev Vet Med 2012;106(3–4):324–31.

[90] Raghavan R, Brenner K, Higgins J, et al. Evaluations of hydrologic risk factors for canine leptospirosis: 94 cases (2002–2009). Prev Vet Med 2012;107(1–2):105–9.

[91] Iverson SA, Levy C, Yaglom HD, et al. Clinical, diagnostic, and epidemiological features of a community-wide outbreak of canine leptospirosis in a low-prevalence region (Maricopa County, Arizona). J Am Vet Med Assoc 2021;258(6):616–29.

[92] Boutilier P, Carr A, Schulman RL. Leptospirosis in dogs: a serologic survey and case series 1996 to 2001. Vet Ther 2003;4(4):387–96.

[93] Harkin KR, Roshto YM, Sullivan JT, et al. Comparison of polymerase chain reaction assay, bacteriologic culture, and serologic testing in assessment of prevalence of urinary shedding of leptospires in dogs. J Am Vet Med Assoc 2003;222(9):1230–3.

[94] Sant'Anna R, Vieira A, Oliveira J, et al. Asymptomatic leptospiral infection is associated with canine chronic kidney disease. Comp Immunol Microbiol Infect Dis 2019;62:64–7.

[95] Adamus C, Buggin-Daubie M, Izembart A, et al. Chronic hepatitis associated with leptospiral infection in vaccinated beagles. J Comp Pathol 1997;117(4):311–28.

[96] Bishop L, Strandberg J, Adams R, et al. Chronic active hepatitis in dogs associated with leptospires. Am J Vet Res 1979;40(6):839–44.

[97] McCallum KE, Constantino-Casas F, Cullen JM, et al. Hepatic leptospiral infections in dogs without obvious renal involvement. J Vet Intern Med 2019;33(1):141–50.

[98] Boomkens SY, Slump E, Egberink HF, et al. PCR screening for candidate etiological agents of canine hepatitis. Vet Microbiol 2005;108(1–2):49–55.

[99] Hutchins RG, Breitschwerdt EB, Cullen JM, et al. Limited yield of diagnoses of intrahepatic infectious causes of canine granulomatous hepatitis from archival liver tissue. J Vet Diagn Invest 2012;24(5):888–94.

[100] Habuš J, Poljak Z, Štritof Z, et al. Prognostic factors for survival of canine patients infected with Leptospira spp. Veterinarski arhiv 2020;90(2):111–28.

[101] Schweighauser A, Francey T. Pulmonary haemorrhage as an emerging complication of acute kidney injury due to canine leptospirosis.: abstract# 48. J Vet Intern Med 2008;22(6):1473–4.

[102] Schweighauser A, Burgener IA, Gaschen F, et al. Small intestinal intussusception in five dogs with acute renal failure and suspected leptospirosis (L. australis). J Vet Emerg Crit Care 2009;19(4):363–8.

[103] Greenlee JJ, Bolin CA, Alt DP, et al. Clinical and pathologic comparison of acute leptospirosis in dogs caused by two strains of Leptospira kirschneri Serovar grippotyphosa. Am J Vet Res 2004;65(8):1100–7.

[104] Mastrorilli C, Dondi F, Agnoli C, et al. Clinicopathologic features and outcome predictors of Leptospira interrogans Australis Serogroup infection in dogs: a retrospective study of 20 cases (2001-2004). J Vet Intern Med 2007;21(1):3–10.

[105] Loftis A, Castillo-Alcala F, Bogdanovic L, et al. Fatal canine leptospirosis on St. Kitts. Vet Sci 2014;1(3):150–8.

[106] Rissi DR, Brown CA. Diagnostic features in 10 naturally occurring cases of acute fatal canine leptospirosis. J Vet Diagn Invest 2014;26(6):799–804.

[107] Greenlee JJ, Alt DP, Bolin CA, et al. Experimental canine leptospirosis caused by Leptospira interrogans Serovars pomona and bratislava. Am J Vet Res 2005;66(10):1816–22.

[108] Townsend WM, Stiles J, Krohne SG. Leptospirosis and panuveitis in a dog. Vet Ophthalmol 2006;9(3):169–73.

[109] Gallagher A. Leptospirosis in a dog with uveitis and presumed cholecystitis. J Am Anim Hosp Assoc 2011;47(6):e162–7.

[110] Harkin KR, Roshto YM, Sullivan JT. Clinical application of a polymerase chain reaction assay for diagnosis of leptospirosis in dogs. J Am Vet Med Assoc 2003;222(9):1224–9.

[111] Paz LN, Dias CS, de Carvalho VMP, et al. Unusual case of polyarthritis and hepatorenal syndrome associated with Leptospira interrogans infection in a dog: a case report. Res Vet Sci 2021;134:186–90.

[112] Furlanello T, Reale I. First description of reactive arthritis secondary to leptospirosis in a dog. Iran J Vet Res 2020;21(2):146.

[113] Bovens C, Fews D, Cogan T. Leptospirosis and immune-mediated haemolytic anaemia in a dog. Vet Rec Case Rep 2014;2(1):e000065.

[114] Furlanello T., Reale I., Leptospirosis and immune-mediated hemolytic anemia: A lethal association, Paper presented at: Veterinary Research Forum, 10 (3), 2019, 261-265

[115] Barthélemy A, Violé A, Cambournac M, et al. Hematological and hemostatic alterations associated with a single extracorporeal renal replacement therapy in dogs with acute kidney injury associated leptospirosis: a pilot study. Top companion Anim Med 2020;38:100406.

[116] Davenport A, Rugman FP, Desmond MJ, et al. Is thrombocytopenia seen in patients with leptospirosis immunologically mediated? J Clin Pathol 1989;42(4):439–40.

[117] Lee SH, Kim KA, Park YG, et al. Identification and partial characterization of a novel hemolysin from Leptospira interrogans Serovar lai. Gene 2000;254(1–2):19–28.

[118] Zaragoza C, Barrera R, Centeno F, et al. Characterization of renal damage in canine leptospirosis by sodium dodecyl sulphate–polyacrylamide gel electrophoresis (SDS–PAGE) and Western Blotting of the urinary proteins. J Comp Pathol 2003;129(2–3):169–78.

[119] Dias C, Paz L, Solcà M, et al. Kidney Injury Molecule-1 in the detection of early kidney injury in dogs with leptospirosis. Comp Immunol Microbiol Infect Dis 2021;76:101637.

[120] Allen AE, Buckley GJ, Schaer M. Successful treatment of severe hypokalemia in a dog with acute kidney injury caused by leptospirosis. J Vet Emerg Crit Care 2016;26(6):837–43.

[121] Zamagni S, Troìa R, Zaccheroni F, et al. Comparison of clinicopathological patterns of renal tubular damage in dogs with acute kidney injury caused by leptospirosis and other aetiologies. Vet J 2020;266:105573.

[122] Gendron K, Christe A, Walter S, et al. Serial CT features of pulmonary leptospirosis in 10 dogs. Vet Rec 2014;174(7):169.

[123] Miotto BA, Tozzi BF, Penteado MS, et al. Diagnosis of acute canine leptospirosis using multiple laboratory tests and characterization of the isolated strains. BMC Vet Res 2018;14(1):222.

[124] Stoddard RA, Gee JE, Wilkins PP, et al. Detection of pathogenic leptospira spp. through TaqMan polymerase chain reaction targeting the LipL32 gene. Diagn Microbiol Infect Dis 2009;64(3):247–55.

[125] Miotto BA, Hora ASd, Taniwaki SA, et al. Development and validation of a modified TaqMan based real-time PCR assay targeting the lipl32 gene for detection of pathogenic Leptospira in canine urine samples. Braz J Microbiol 2018;49:584–90.

[126] Rojas P, Monahan A, Schuller S, et al. Detection and quantification of leptospires in urine of dogs: a maintenance host for the zoonotic disease leptospirosis. Eur J Clin Microbiol Infect Dis 2010;29(10):1305–9.

[127] Xu C, Loftis A, Ahluwalia SK, et al. Diagnosis of canine leptospirosis by a highly sensitive FRET-PCR targeting the lig genes. PLoS One 2014;9(2):e89507.

[128] Miotto BA, Guilloux AGA, Tozzi BF, et al. Prospective study of canine leptospirosis in shelter and stray dog populations: Identification of chronic carriers and different Leptospira species infecting dogs. PLoS One 2018;13(7):e0200384.

[129] Llewellyn J-R, Krupka-Dyachenko I, Rettinger AL, et al. Urinary shedding of leptospires and presence of Leptospira antibodies in healthy dogs from Upper Bavaria. Berliner und Munchener Tierarztliche Wochenschrift 2016;129(5–6):251–7.

[130] Khorami N, Malmasi A, Zakeri S, et al. Screening urinalysis in dogs with urinary shedding of leptospires. Comp Clin Pathol 2010;19(3):271–4.

[131] Gay N, Soupé-Gilbert M-E, Goarant C. Though not reservoirs, dogs might transmit Leptospira in New Caledonia. Int J Environ Res Public Health 2014;11(4):4316–25.

[132] Fink JM, Moore GE, Landau R, et al. Evaluation of three 5′ exonuclease–based real-time polymerase chain reaction assays for detection of pathogenic Leptospira species in canine urine. J Vet Diagn Invest 2015;27(2):159–66.

[133] Gentilini F, Zanoni RG, Zambon E, et al. A comparison of two real-time polymerase chain reaction assays using hybridization probes targeting either 16S ribosomal RNA or a subsurface lipoprotein gene for detecting leptospires in canine urine. J Vet Diagn Invest 2015;27(6):696–703.

[134] Midence JN, Leutenegger CM, Chandler AM, et al. Effects of recent Leptospira vaccination on whole blood real-time PCR testing in healthy client-owned dogs. J Vet Intern Med 2012;26(1):149–52.

[135] Orr B, Westman ME, Malik R, et al. Leptospirosis is an emerging infectious disease of pig-hunting dogs and humans in north Queensland. PLOS Negl Trop Dis 2022;16(1):e0010100.

[136] Boon R. Some observations on cystitis, nephritis and leptospirosis in small animals. Aust Vet J 1952;28(3):81–4.

[137] Troìa R, Balboni A, Zamagni S, et al. Prospective evaluation of rapid point-of-care tests for the diagnosis of acute leptospirosis in dogs. Vet J 2018;237:37–42.

[138] Ribotta MJ, Higgins R, Gottschalk M, et al. Development of an indirect enzyme-linked immunosorbent assay for the detection of leptospiral antibodies in dogs. Can J Vet Res 2000;64(1):32.

[139] Sathiyamoorthy A, Selvaraju G, Palanivel K, et al. Development of indirect enzyme-linked immunosorbent assay for diagnosis of canine leptospirosis. Vet World 2017;10(5):530.

[140] Subathra M, Senthilkumar T, Ramadass P. Recombinant OmpL1 protein as a diagnostic antigen for the detection of canine leptospirosis. Appl Biochem Biotechnol 2013;169(2):431–7.

[141] La-Ard A, Amavisit P, Sukpuaram T, et al. Evaluation of recombinant Lig antigen-based ELISA for detection of leptospiral antibodies in canine sera. Southeast Asian J Trop Med Public Health 2011;42(1):128.

[142] Ye C, Yan W, Xiang H, et al. Recombinant antigens rLipL21, rLoa22, rLipL32 and rLigACon4-8 for serological diagnosis of leptospirosis by enzyme-linked immunosorbent assays in dogs. PLoS One 2014;9(12):e111367.

[143] Behera S, Sabarinath T, Deneke Y, et al. Evaluation of the diagnostic potential and DIVA capability of recombinant LigBCon1-5 protein of Leptospira interrogans Serovar Pomona in canine leptospirosis. Iran J Vet Res 2021;22(2):120.

[144] Palaniappan RU, Chang Y-F, Hassan F, et al. Expression of leptospiral immunoglobulin-like protein by

Leptospira interrogans and evaluation of its diagnostic potential in a kinetic ELISA. J Med Microbiol 2004; 53(10):975–84.

[145] Andre-Fontaine G, Aviat F, Marie J-L, et al. Undiagnosed leptospirosis cases in naïve and vaccinated dogs: properties of a serological test based on a synthetic peptide derived from Hap1/LipL32 (residues 154–178). Comp Immunol Microbiol Infect Dis 2015;39:1–8.

[146] Dey S, Mohan CM, Kumar TS, et al. Recombinant LipL32 antigen-based single serum dilution ELISA for detection of canine leptospirosis. Vet Microbiol 2004; 103(1–2):99–106.

[147] Subathra M, Senthilkumar T, Ramadass P, et al. Development of rapid flow-through-based dot-immunoassay for serodiagnosis of leptospirosis in dogs. Comp Immunol Microbiol Infect Dis 2011;34(1):17–22.

[148] Subathra M, Senthilkumar T, Ramadass P, et al. Evaluation of the cocktail recombinant antigens, LipL32 and LipL41 for serodiagnosis of canine leptospirosis. World J Microbiol Biotechnol 2011;27(5):1077–82.

[149] Altheimer K, Jongwattanapisan P, Luengyosluechakul S, et al. Leptospira infection and shedding in dogs in Thailand. BMC Vet Res 2020;16(1):1–13.

[150] Adeniyi Okewole E, Oluremi Ayoola M. Seroprevalence of leptospiral Serovars other than Canicola and Icterohaemorrhagiae in dogs in the Southwestern Nigeria. Veterinarski arhiv 2009;79(1):87–96.

[151] Klopfleisch R, Kohn B, Plog S, et al. An emerging pulmonary haemorrhagic syndrome in dogs: similar to the human leptospiral pulmonary haemorrhagic syndrome? Vet Med Int 2010;2010:928541.

[152] Cole LP, Jepson R, Dawson C, et al. Hypertension, retinopathy, and acute kidney injury in dogs: a prospective study. J Vet Intern Med 2020;34(5):1940–7.

[153] Schweighauser A, Francey T. Treatment of pulmonary haemorrhage in canine leptospirosis with desmopressin and dexamethasone.: abstract# 49. J Vet Intern Med 2008;22(6):1456–83.

[154] Barmettler R, Schweighauser A, Bigler S, et al. Assessment of exposure to Leptospira Serovars in veterinary staff and dog owners in contact with infected dogs. J Am Vet Med Assoc 2011;238(2):183–8.

[155] Guagliardo SAJ, Iverson SA, Reynolds L, et al. Despite high-risk exposures, no evidence of zoonotic transmission during a canine outbreak of leptospirosis. Zoonoses and Public Health 2019;66(2):223–31.

[156] Whitney EAS, Ailes E, Myers LM, et al. Prevalence of and risk factors for serum antibodies against Leptospira Serovars in US veterinarians. J Am Vet Med Assoc 2009; 234(7):938–44.

[157] Mauro T, Harkin K. Persistent leptospiruria in five dogs despite antimicrobial treatment (2000–2017). J Am Anim Hosp Assoc 2019;55(1):42–7.

[158] Mansur FAF, Mohamed NA, Omar MR, et al. Canine-sourced leptospirosis. Int Med J 2020;27(5):602–3.

[159] Goh SH, Ismail R, Lau SF, et al. Risk factors and prediction of leptospiral seropositivity among dogs and dog handlers in Malaysia. Int J Environ Res Public Health 2019;16(9):1499.

[160] Trevejo RT, Rigau-Pérez JG, Ashford DA, et al. Epidemic leptospirosis associated with pulmonary hemorrhage—Nicaragua, 1995. J Infect Dis 1998;178(5):1457–63.

[161] Muñoz-Zanzi C, Mason MR, Encina C, et al. Leptospira contamination in household and environmental water in rural communities in southern Chile. Int J Environ Res Public Health 2014;11(7):6666–80.

[162] Tromp S. Report on leptospirosis between cardwell and babinda. Far North Queensland; 2006.

[163] Buser F, Schweighauser A, im Hof-Gut M, et al. Evaluation of C-reactive protein and its kinetics as a prognostic indicator in canine leptospirosis. J Small Anim Pract 2019;60(8):477–85.

[164] Bouvet J, Lemaitre L, Cariou C, et al. A canine vaccine against Leptospira Serovars Icterohaemorrhagiae, Canicola and Grippotyphosa provides cross protection against Leptospira Serovar Copenhageni. Vet Immunol immunopathology 2020;219:109985.

[165] Klaasen HLE, Adler B. Recent advances in canine leptospirosis: focus on vaccine development. Vet Med Res Rep 2015;6:245.

[166] Claus A, Van de Maele I, Pasmans F, et al. Leptospirosis in dogs: a retrospective study of seven clinical cases in Belgium. Vlaams Diergeneeskundig Tijdschrift 2008; 77(4):259–64.

[167] Day MJ, Horzinek M, Schultz R, et al. WSAVA guidelines for the vaccination of dogs and cats. J small Anim Pract 2016;57(1):E1.

[168] Klaasen H, Van Der Veen M, Molkenboer M, et al. A novel tetravalent Leptospira bacterin protects against infection and shedding following challenge in dogs. Vet Rec 2013;172(7):181.

[169] Day M, Crawford C, Marcondes M, et al. Recommendations on vaccination for Latin American small animal practitioners: a report of the WSAVA Vaccination Guidelines Group. J Small Anim Pract 2020;61(6):E1–35.

[170] Minke JM, Bey R, Tronel JP, et al. Onset and duration of protective immunity against clinical disease and renal carriage in dogs provided by a bi-valent inactivated leptospirosis vaccine. Vet Microbiol 2009;137(1–2):137–45.

[171] Bouvet J, Cariou C, Valfort W, et al. Efficacy of a multivalent DAPPi-Lmulti canine vaccine against mortality, clinical signs, infection, bacterial excretion, renal carriage and renal lesions caused by Leptospira experimental challenges. Vaccin Rep 2016;6:23–8.

[172] Klaasen HL, Molkenboer MJ, Vrijenhoek MP, et al. Duration of immunity in dogs vaccinated against leptospirosis with a bivalent inactivated vaccine. Vet Microbiol 2003;95(1–2):121–32.

[173] Wilson S, Stirling C, Thomas A, et al. Duration of immunity of a multivalent (DHPPi/L4R) canine vaccine against four Leptospira Serovars. Vaccine 2013;31(31): 3126–30.

[174] Grosenbaugh DA, Pardo MC. Fifteen-month duration of immunity for the Serovar Grippotyphosa fraction

of a tetravalent canine leptospirosis vaccine. Vet Rec 2018;182(23):665.

[175] Klaasen HL, van der Veen M, Sutton D, et al. A new tetravalent canine leptospirosis vaccine provides at least 12 months immunity against infection. Vet Immunol Immunopathol 2014;158(1–2):26–9.

[176] Schreiber P, Martin V, Najbar W, et al. Prevention of renal infection and urinary shedding in dogs by a Leptospira vaccination. Vet Microbiol 2005;108(1–2):113–8.

[177] Schreiber P, Martin V, Grousson D, et al. One-year duration of immunity in dogs for Leptospira interrogans Serovar icterohaemorrhagiae after vaccination. Int J Appl Res Vet Med 2012;10:305–10.

[178] Scanziani E, Calcaterra S, Tagliabue S, et al. Serological findings in cases of acute leptospirosis in the dog. J Small Anim Pract 1994;35(5):257–60.

[179] Andre-Fontaine G. Diagnosis algorithm for leptospirosis in dogs: disease and vaccination effects on the serological results. Vet Rec 2013;172(19):502.

[180] Andre-Fontaine G, Triger L. MAT cross-reactions or vaccine cross-protection: retrospective study of 863 leptospirosis canine cases. Heliyon 2018;4(11):e00869.

[181] Spiri AM, Rodriguez-Campos S, Matos JM, et al. Clinical, serological and echocardiographic examination of healthy field dogs before and after vaccination with a commercial tetravalent leptospirosis vaccine. BMC Vet Res 2017;13(1):138.

[182] Martin LE, Wiggans KT, Wennogle SA, et al. Vaccine-associated Leptospira antibodies in client-owned dogs. J Vet Intern Med 2014;28(3):789–92.

[183] Curtis K, Foster P, Smith P, et al. Performance of a recombinant LipL32 based rapid in-clinic ELISA (SNAP® Lepto) for the detection of antibodies against Leptospira in dogs. Int J Appl Res Vet Med 2015;13(3):182–9.

[184] Barr SC, McDonough PL, Scipioni-Ball RL, et al. Serologic responses of dogs given a commercial vaccine against Leptospira interrogans Serovar pomona and Leptospira kirschneri Serovar grippotyphosa. Am J Vet Res 2005;66(10):1780–4.

[185] Yao PJ, Stephenson N, Foley JE, et al. Incidence rates and risk factors for owner-reported adverse events following vaccination of dogs that did or did not receive a Leptospira vaccine. J Am Vet Med Assoc 2015;247(10):1139–45.

[186] Moore GE, Guptill LF, Ward MP, et al. Adverse events diagnosed within three days of vaccine administration in dogs. J Am Vet Med Assoc 2005;227(7):1102–8.

[187] Eschle S, Hartmann K, Rieger A, et al. Canine vaccination in Germany: A survey of owner attitudes and compliance. PloS one 2020;15(8):e0238371.

[188] Public Chemical Registration Information System Search. https://portal.apvma.gov.au. Accessed January 19, 2021.

[189] Schuler E, Marconi R. The Leptospiral General Secretory Protein D (GspD), a secretin, elicits complement-independent bactericidal antibody against diverse Leptospira species and Serovars. Vaccin X. 2021;7:100089.

[190] Thomé S, Lessa-Aquino C, Ko AI, et al. Identification of immunodominant antigens in canine leptospirosis by Multi-Antigen Print ImmunoAssay (MAPIA). BMC Vet Res 2014;10(1):1–9.

[191] Krawczyk M. Serological evidence of leptospirosis in animals in northern Poland. Vet Rec 2005;156(3):88–9.

[192] Llewellyn J, Krupka-Dyachenko I, Rettinger A, et al. Prevalenced of leptospira urinary shedding in healthy dogs from Southern Germany; ISCAID-O4. J Vet Intern Med 2014;28(2):711–44.

[193] Houwers DJ, Goris MG, Abdoel T, et al. Agglutinating antibodies against pathogenic Leptospira in healthy dogs and horses indicate common exposure and regular occurrence of subclinical infections. Vet Microbiol 2011;148(2–4):449–51.

[194] Arent Z, Andrews S, Adamama-Moraitou K, et al. Emergence of novel Leptospira Serovars: a need for adjusting vaccination policies for dogs? Epidemiol Infect 2013; 141(6):1148–53.

[195] Burriel A, Dalley C, Woodward MJ. Prevalence of Leptospira species among farmed and domestic animals in Greece. Vet Rec 2003;153(5):146–8.

[196] Piredda I, Ponti MN, Piras A, et al. New insights on leptospira infections in a canine population from North Sardinia, Italy: a sero-epidemiological study. Biology 2021;10(6):507.

[197] Bertelloni F, Cilia G, Turchi B, et al. Epidemiology of leptospirosis in North-Central Italy: fifteen years of serological data (2002–2016). Comp Immunol Microbiol Infect Dis 2019;65:14–22.

[198] Tagliabue S, Figarolli BM, D'Incau M, et al. Serological surveillance of Leptospirosis in Italy: two-year national data (2010–2011). Vet Ital 2016;52:129–38.

[199] Scanziani E, Origgi F, Giusti A, et al. Serological survey of leptospiral infection in kennelled dogs in Italy. J Small Anim Pract 2002;43(4):154–7.

[200] López MC, Vila A, Rodón J, et al. Leptospira seroprevalence in owned dogs from Spain. Heliyon 2019;5(8): e02373.

[201] Millán J, Candela MG, López-Bao JV, et al. Leptospirosis in wild and domestic carnivores in natural areas in Andalusia, Spain. Vector-borne zoonotic Dis 2009;9(5): 549–54.

[202] Hernández MB, Vicente J, Díaz P, et al. COMPARISON OF THE PREVALENCE OF THE INFECTION BY Leptospira spp, Leishmania infantum AND Ehrlichia canis IN DOGS IN THE COMUNIDAD VALENCIANA (SPAIN). Epidemiol et sante anim 2005;45:83–6.

[203] Schuller S, Arent Z, Gilmore C, et al. Prevalence of anti-leptospiral serum antibodies in dogs in Ireland. Vet Rec 2015;177(5):126.

[204] Van den Broek A, Thrusfield M, Dobbiet G, et al. A serological and bacteriological survey of leptospiral infection in dogs in Edinburgh and Glasgow. J Small Anim Pract 1991;32(3):118–24.

[205] Spangler D, Kish D, Beigel B, et al. Leptospiral shedding and seropositivity in shelter dogs in the Cumberland

Gap Region of Southeastern Appalachia. Plos one 2020; 15(1):e0228038.

[206] Stokes JE, Kaneene JB, Schall WD, et al. Prevalence of serum antibodies against six Leptospira Serovars in healthy dogs. J Am Vet Med Assoc 2007;230(11): 1657–64.

[207] Cardenas-Marrufo MF, Vado-Solis I, Perez-Osorio CE, et al. Seropositivity to leptospirosis in domestic reservoirs and detection of Leptospira spp. from water sources, in farms of Yucatan, Mexico. Trop Subtropical Agroecosystems 2011;14(1):185–9.

[208] Domínguez SdCB, Dzib MYC, Velázquez MGM, et al. Detection of reactive canines to Leptospira in Campeche City, Mexico. Revista argentina de microbiología 2013;45(1):34–8.

[209] Hernández-Ramírez C, Gaxiola-Camacho S, Enriquéz-Verdugo I, et al. Leptospira Serovars and of contagion risks in humans and dogs from Culiacan City, in Sinaloa, Mexico. Abanico Veterinario 2020;10:1–16.

[210] Jimenez-Coello M, Ortega-Pacheco A, Guzman-Marin E, et al. Stray dogs as reservoirs of the zoonotic agents Leptospira interrogans, Trypanosoma cruzi, and Aspergillus spp. in an urban area of Chiapas in southern Mexico. Vector-Borne Zoonotic Dis 2010;10(2): 135–41.

[211] Ortega-Pacheco A, Colin-Flores R, Gutiérrez-Blanco E, et al. Frequency and type of renal lesions in dogs naturally infected with Leptospira species. Ann N Y Acad Sci 2008;1149(1):270–4.

[212] Abdoel TH, Houwers DJ, van Dongen AM, et al. Rapid test for the serodiagnosis of acute canine leptospirosis. Vet Microbiol 2011;150(1–2):211–3.

[213] Pratt N, Conan A, Rajeev S. Leptospira seroprevalence in domestic dogs and cats on the Caribbean Island of Saint Kitts. Vet Med Int 2017;2017.

[214] Adesiyun A, Hull-Jackson C, Mootoo N, et al. Seroepidemiology of canine leptospirosis in Trinidad: Serovars, implications for vaccination and public health. J Vet Med Ser B. 2006;53(2):91–9.

[215] da Rocha Albuquerque M, dos Reis TA, de Souza Rocha K, et al. Evidence of exposure to Leptospira spp. in dogs at a zoonosis control center in Brazil. Rev Acad Ciênc Anim 2020;18:e18301.

[216] Bernardino MG, Costa DF, Nogueira DB, et al. Cross-sectional survey for canine leptospirosis in an Atlantic Rainforest area of the semiarid of Paraíba state, Northeastern Brazil. Pesquisa Veterinária Brasileira 2021; 41(3):1–8.

[217] do Nascimento Benitez A, Monica TC, Miura AC, et al. Spatial and simultaneous seroprevalence of anti-Leptospira antibodies in owners and their domiciled dogs in a major city of Southern Brazil. Front Vet Sci 2020;7.

[218] Ornellas R.O., Albuquerque D.D.Ad, Cordeiros J.L.P., et al. Seroprevalence of leishmaniasis, toxoplasmosis, and leptospirosis in the domestic fauna of an anthropized environment of the atlantic forest in the city of Rio de Janeiro, Archives of Veterinary Science 2020, 25 (2), 13-20.

[219] Sevá AP, Brandão APD, Godoy SN, et al. Seroprevalence and incidence of Leptospira spp. in domestic dogs in the Southeast region of São Paulo State, Brazil. Pesquisa Veterinária Brasileira 2020;40:399–407.

[220] de Abreu JAP, da Silva Krawczak F, Guedes IB, et al. Frequency of anti-Leptospira spp. antibodies in dogs and wild small mammals from rural properties and conservation units in southern Brazil. One health 2019;8: 100104.

[221] de Lima Brasil AW, da Costa DF, Pimenta CLRM, et al. Prevalence and risk factors to Leptospira sp. infection in dogs attended at veterinary clinics in João Pessoa, Paraíba State, Northeastern Brazil. Braz J Vet Res Anim Sci 2018;55(3):e144154.

[222] Hafemann DCM, Merlini LS, Gonçalves DD, et al. Detection of anti-Leptospira spp., anti-Brucella spp., and antiToxoplasma gondii antibodies in stray dogs. Semina: Ciências Agrárias 2018;39(1):167–76.

[223] Latosinski GS, Fornazari F, Babboni SD, et al. Serological and molecular detection of Leptospira spp in dogs. Revista da Sociedade Brasileira de Medicina Trop 2018;51:364–7.

[224] SanT'Anna R, Vieira A, Grapiglia J, et al. High number of asymptomatic dogs as leptospiral carriers in an endemic area indicates a serious public health concern. Epidemiol Infect 2017;145(9):1852–4.

[225] de Freitas Siqueira ERD, Castro V, das Graças Prianti M, et al. Occurrence of antibodies against Leptospira spp in dogs from Teresina, Piauí, Brazil. Braz J Vet Res Anim Sci 2017;54(1):88–91.

[226] Paz GSd, Rocha KdS, Lima MdS, et al. Seroprevalence for brucellosis and leptospirosis in dogs from Belém and Castanhal, State of Pará, Brazil. Acta Amazonica 2015;45:265–70.

[227] de Oliveira LA, Zaniolo MM, Dias EH, et al. Leptospirosis and brucellosis seroepidemiology in sheep and dogs from non-mechanized rural properties in the northwestern region in the state of Paraná. Semina: Ciências Agrárias 2016;37(5):3147–58.

[228] Dreer MKdP, Gonçalves DD, Caetano ICdS, et al. Toxoplasmosis, leptospirosis and brucellosis in stray dogs housed at the shelter in Umuarama municipality, Paraná, Brazil. J Venomous Anim Toxins including Trop Dis 2013;19:1–5.

[229] Fonzar UJV, Langoni H. Geographic analysis on the occurrence of human and canine leptospirosis in the city of Maringá, state of Paraná, Brazil. Revista da Sociedade Brasileira de Medicina Trop 2012;45:100–5.

[230] Lavinsky MO, Abou Said R, Strenzel GMR, et al. Seroprevalence of anti-Leptospira spp. antibodies in dogs in Bahia, Brazil. Prev Vet Med 2012;106(1):79–84.

[231] Azócar-Aedo L, Monti G, Jara R. Serological conversion for anti-leptospira antibodies among domestic dogs from southern chile, a prospective study. J Vet Med Res 2018;5(8):1154.

[232] Lelu M, Muñoz-Zanzi C, Higgins B, et al. Seroepidemiology of leptospirosis in dogs from rural and slum communities of Los Rios Region, Chile. BMC Vet Res 2015; 11(1):1–9.

[233] Myers D. Leptospiral antibodies in stray dogs of Moreno, Province of Buenos Aires, Argentina. Revista Argentina de Microbiologia 1980;12(1):18–22.

[234] Murcia CA, Astudillo M, Romero MH. Prevalence of leptospirosis in vaccinated working dogs and humans with occupational risk. Biomédica 2020;40:62–75.

[235] Cárdenas NC, Infante GP, Pacheco DAR, et al. Seroprevalence of Leptospira spp infection and its risk factors among domestic dogs in Bogotá, Colombia. Vet Anim Sci 2018;6:64–8.

[236] Calderón A, Rodríguez V, Máttar S, et al. Leptospirosis in pigs, dogs, rodents, humans, and water in an area of the Colombian tropics. Trop Anim Health Prod 2014;46(2):427–32.

[237] Roqueplo C, Davoust B, Marié J-L, et al. Serological study of leptospirosis in dogs from French Guiana. Int J Infect Dis 2019;79:121–2.

[238] Zwijnenberg R, Smythe L, Symonds M, et al. Cross-sectional study of canine leptospirosis in animal shelter populations in mainland Australia. Aust Vet J 2008; 86(8):317–23.

[239] O'Keefe J, Jenner J, Sandifer N, et al. A serosurvey for antibodies to Leptospira in dogs in the lower North Island of New Zealand. New Zealand Vet J 2002;50(1):23–5.

[240] Collings D. Leptospira interrogans infection in domestic and wild animals in Fiji. New Zealand Vet J 1984; 32(3):21–4.

[241] Senthil N, Palanivel K, Rishikesavan R. Seroprevalence of leptospiral antibodies in canine population in and around Namakkal. J Vet Med 2013;2013.

[242] Jittapalapong S, Sittisan P, Sakpuaram T, et al. Coinfection of leptospira spp and toxoplasma gondii among stray dogs in Bangkok, Thailand. Southeast Asian J Trop Med Public Health 2009;40(2):247.

[243] Meeyam T, Tablerk P, Petchanok B, et al. Seroprevalence and risk factors associated with leptospirosis in dogs. Southeast Asian J Trop Med Public Health 2006; 37(1):148.

[244] Niwetpathomwat A, Assarasakorn S. Preliminary investigation of canine leptospirosis in a rural area of Thailand. Med Weter 2007;63(1):59–61.

[245] Pumipuntu N, Suwannarong K. Seroprevalence of Leptospira spp. in cattle and dogs in Mahasarakham Province, Thailand. J Health Res 2016;30(3):223–6.

[246] Goh SH, Khor KH, Radzi R, et al. Shedding and genetic diversity of leptospira spp. from urban stray dogs in Klang Valley, Malaysia. Top Companion Anim Med 2021;100562.

[247] Rani MA, Goh SH, Rahman MSA, et al. Serological Detection of Anti-Leptospira Antibodies among Animal Caretakers, Dogs and Cats Housed in Animal Shelters in Peninsular Malaysia. Sains Malaysiana 2020;49(5): 1121–8.

[248] Hua KK, Xian TW, Fong LS, et al. Seroprevalence and molecular detection of leptospirosis from a dog shelter. Trop Biomed 2016;33(2):276–84.

[249] Lau S, Wong J, Khor K, et al. Seroprevalence of leptospirosis in working dogs. Top companion Anim Med 2017;32(4):121–5.

[250] Lau S, Low K, Khor K, et al. Prevalence of leptospirosis in healthy dogs and dogs with kidney disease in Klang Valley, Malaysia. Trop Biomed 2016;33(3):469–75.

[251] Phumoonna T, Mutalib A, Bahaman A, et al. Leptospiral infection in stray dogs in malaysia. J Vet Malaysia 2009;21:23–7.

[252] Iwamoto E, Wada Y, Fujisaki Y, et al. Nationwide survey of Leptospira antibodies in dogs in Japan: results from microscopic agglutination test and enzyme-linked immunosorbent assay. J Vet Med Sci 2009;71(9): 1191–9.

[253] Aslantaş Ö, Özdemir V, Kiliç S, et al. Seroepidemiology of leptospirosis, toxoplasmosis, and leishmaniosis among dogs in Ankara, Turkey. Vet Parasitol 2005; 129(3–4):187–91.

[254] Avizeh R, Ghorbanpoor M, Hatami S, et al. Seroepidemiology of canine leptospirosis in Ahvaz, Iran. Iranian J Vet Med 2009;2(2):75–9.

[255] Roqueplo C, Marié J-L, André-Fontaine G, et al. Serological survey of canine leptospirosis in three countries of tropical Africa: Sudan, Gabon and Ivory Coast. Comp Immunol Microbiol Infect Dis 2015;38:57–61.

[256] Roach J, Van Vuuren M, Picard J. A serological survey of antibodies to Leptospira species in dogs in South Africa. J South Afr Vet Assoc 2010;81(3):156–9.

[257] Millán J, Chirife AD, Kalema-Zikusoka G, et al. Serosurvey of dogs for human, livestock, and wildlife pathogens, Uganda. Emerging Infect Dis 2013;19(4):680.

[258] Samir A, Soliman R, El-Hariri M, et al. Leptospirosis in animals and human contacts in Egypt: broad range surveillance. Revista da Sociedade Brasileira de Medicina Trop 2015;48:272–7.

[259] Habus J, Persic Z, Spicic S, et al. New trends in human and animal leptospirosis in Croatia, 2009–2014. Acta tropica 2017;168:1–8.

[260] Štritof Majetić Z, Habuš J, Milas Z, et al. A serological survey of canine leptospirosis in Croatia-the changing epizootiology of the disease. Veterinarski arhiv 2012; 82(2):183–91.

[261] Geisen V, Stengel C, Hartmann K. Epidemiologische Situation der Leptospirose beim Hund in Süddeutschland. Tierärztliche Praxis Ausgabe K: Kleintiere/Heimtiere. 2008;36(05):329–36.

[262] Brem S, Kopp H, Meyer P. Leptospira antibody detection in dog serum in the years 1985 to 1988. Berliner und Munchener Tierarztliche Wochenschrift 1990; 103(1):6–8.

[263] Prescott JF, Ferrier RL, Nicholson VM, et al. Is canine leptospirosis underdiagnosed in southern Ontario? A case report and serological survey. Can Vet J 1991; 32(8):481.

[264] Hrinivich K, Prescott JF. Leptospirosis in 2 unrelated dogs. Can Vet J 1997;38(8):509.

[265] Kalin M, Devaux C, DiFruscia R, et al. Three cases of canine leptospirosis in Quebec. Can Vet J 1999;40(3): 187.

[266] Ribotta M, Fortin M, Higgins R, et al. Canine leptospirosis: serology. Can Vet J 2000;41(6):494.

[267] Harkin KR, Gartrell CL. Canine leptospirosis in New Jersey and Michigan: 17 cases (1990-1995). J Am Anim Hosp Assoc 1996;32(6):495–501.

[268] Larson CR, Dennis M, Nair RV, et al. Isolation and characterization of Leptospira interrogans Serovar Copenhageni from a dog from Saint Kitts. JMM case Rep 2017; 4(10).

[269] Santos CM, Dias GCDRS, Saldanha AVP, et al. Molecular and serological characterization of pathogenic Leptospira spp. isolated from symptomatic dogs in a highly endemic area, Brazil. BMC Vet Res 2021;17(1): 1–11.

[270] Romero-Vivas CM, Thiry D, Rodríguez V, et al. Molecular Serovar characterization of Leptospira isolates from animals and water in Colombia. Biomédica 2013;33:179–84.

[271] Harland A, Cave N, Jones B, et al. A serological survey of leptospiral antibodies in dogs in New Zealand. New Zealand Vet J 2013;61(2):98–106.

[272] Patil D, Dahake R, Roy S, et al. Prevalence of leptospirosis among dogs and rodents and their possible role in human leptospirosis from Mumbai, India. Indian J Med Microbiol 2014;32(1):64–7.

[273] Paungpin W, Chaiwattanarungruengpaisan S, Mongkolphan C, et al. Genotyping of the causative Leptospira in symptomatic dogs in Thailand. Korean J Vet Res 2020;60(1):1–7.

[274] Llewellyn J, Krupka-Dyachenko I, Rettinger A, et al. Prevalence ofleptospirarinary shedding in healthy dogs from southern germany: iscaid-O-4. J Vet Intern Med 2014;28(2):711–44.

[275] Rühl-Fehlert C, Brem S, Feller W, et al. Clinical, microbiological and pathological observations in laboratory beagle dogs infected with leptospires of the Serogroup Sejroe. Exp toxicologic Pathol official J Gesellschaft Toxikologische Pathologie 2000;52(3):201–7.

[276] Vicari D, Percipalle M, Concetta LM, et al. Evidence of canine leptospirosis in kennels in Sicily, by PCR method. Rev Cubana Med Trop 2007;59(1):61–2.

[277] da Cunha CEP, Felix SR, Neto ACPS, et al. Infection with Leptospira kirschneri Serovar Mozdok: first report from the southern hemisphere. Am J Trop Med Hyg 2016;94(3):519.

[278] Rohilla P, Khurana R, Kumar A, et al. Detection of Leptospira in urine of apparently healthy dogs by quantitative polymerase chain reaction in Haryana, India. Vet World 2020;13(11):2411.

[279] Dash BR, Dhaygude VS, Gadhave PD, et al. Molecular detection of Leptospira spp. from canine kidney tissues and its association with renal lesions. Vet World 2018; 11(4):530.

[280] Kurilung A, Chanchaithong P, Lugsomya K, et al. Molecular detection and isolation of pathogenic Leptospira from asymptomatic humans, domestic animals and water sources in Nan province, a rural area of Thailand. Res Vet Sci 2017;115:146–54.

[281] Benacer D, Thong KL, Ooi P, et al. Serological and molecular identification of Leptospira spp. in swine and stray dogs from Malaysia. Trop Biomed 2017;34(1): 89–97.

[282] Zaidi S, Bouam A, Bessas A, et al. Urinary shedding of pathogenic Leptospira in stray dogs and cats, Algiers: A prospective study. PLoS One 2018;13(5):e0197068.

[283] Bergstrom BE, Stiles J, Townsend WM. Canine panuveitis: a retrospective evaluation of 55 cases (2000–2015). Vet Ophthalmol 2017;20(5):390–7.

[284] Munday JS, Bergen DJ, Roe WD. Generalized calcinosis cutis associated with probable leptospirosis in a dog. Vet Dermatol 2005;16(6):401–6.

[285] Berrocal A., Zuñiga F., Pérez M., FOCAL AND GENERALIZED CALCINOSIS CUTIS ASSOCIATED WITH LEPTOSPIROSIS IN TWO BEAGLES, presented at: ACVP/ASVCP Annual Meeting, December 5-9, 2009, Monterey California, USA (poster presentation).

[286] Avaiable at: http://www.iris-kidney.com. Accessed January 20, 2021.

[287] Bateman SW, Mathews KA, Abrams-Ogg AC, et al. Diagnosis of disseminated intravascular coagulation in dogs admitted to an intensive care unit. J Am Vet Med Assoc 1999;215(6):798–804.

[288] Forrest LJ, O'Brien RT, Tremelling MS, et al. Sonographic renal findings in 20 dogs with leptospirosis. Vet Radiol Ultrasound 1998;39(4):337–40.

[289] Blanchard S, Cariou C, Bouvet J, et al. Quantitative real-time PCR assays for the detection of pathogenic Leptospira species in urine, and blood samples in canine vaccine clinical studies: a rapid alternative to classical culture methods. J Clin Microbiol 2021;59(7): 03006–20.

[290] Pérez LJ, Lanka S, DeShambo VJ, et al. A Validated multiplex real-time PCR assay for the diagnosis of infectious leptospira spp.: a novel assay for the detection and differentiation of strains from both pathogenic groups I and II. Front Microbiol 2020;11:457.

[291] Ferreira AS, Costa P, Rocha T, et al. Direct detection and differentiation of pathogenic Leptospira species using a multi-gene targeted real time PCR approach. PLoS One 2014;9(11):e112312.

[292] Cave NJ, Harland AL, Allott SK. The serological response of working farm dogs to a vaccine containing Leptospira interrogans Serovars Copenhageni and Pomona, and L. borgpetersenii Serovar Hardjo. N Z Vet J 2014;62(2):87–90.

[293] Notomi T, Okayama H, Masubuchi H, et al. Loop-mediated isothermal amplification of DNA. Nucleic Acids Res 2000;28(12):e63.

[294] Gunasegar S, Neela VK. Evaluation of diagnostic accuracy of loop-mediated isothermal amplification

method (LAMP) compared with polymerase chain reaction (PCR) for Leptospira spp. in clinical samples: a systematic review and meta-analysis. Diagn Microbiol Infect Dis 2021;100(3):115369.

[295] Gentilini F, Zanoni RG, Zambon E, et al. A comparison of the reliability of two gene targets in loop-mediated isothermal amplification assays for detecting leptospiral DNA in canine urine. J Vet Diagn Invest 2017;29(1): 100–4.

[296] Grune Loffler S, Leiva CL, Scialfa EA, et al. Detection of pathogenic leptospiral DNA traces in canine sera serum samples by loop mediated isothermal amplification. LAMP; 2016.

[297] Thiel BE LL, Okwumabua O, Schultz SR. Comparison of a novel point-of-care diagnostic, PCRun, with real time Leptospira PCR for detection of Leptospira antigen in canine samples. Paper presented at: Conference of research workers in animal diseases.; December 7–9, 2014, 2014; Chicago.

[298] Weiss S, Menezes A, Woods K, et al. An extended multi-locus sequence typing (MLST) scheme for rapid direct typing of Leptospira from clinical samples. PLoS Negl Trop Dis 2016;10(9):e0004996.

[299] Balboni A, Zamagni S, Bertasio C, et al. Identification of Serogroups australis and icterohaemorrhagiae in two dogs with a severe form of acute leptospirosis in Italy. Pathogens 2020;9(5):351.

[300] Le Guyader M, Fontana C, Simon-Dufay N, et al. Successful Leptospira genotyping strategy on DNA extracted from canine biological samples. J Microbiol Methods 2020;176:106007.

[301] Harkin KR, Hays MP. Variable-number tandem-repeat analysis of leptospiral DNA isolated from canine urine samples molecularly confirmed to contain pathogenic leptospires. J Am Vet Med Assoc 2016;249(4): 399–405.

[302] Loffler SG, Passaro D, Samartino L, et al. Genotypes of Leptospira spp. strains isolated from dogs in Buenos Aires, Argentina. Revista Argentina de microbiologia 2014;46(3):201–4.

[303] Koizumi N, Muto MM, Izumiya H, et al. Multiple-locus variable-number tandem repeat analysis and clinical characterization of Leptospira interrogans canine isolates. J Med Microbiol 2015;64(3):288–94.

[304] Nickolyn-Martin JE. Optimizing main spectrum profiles for use in real-time MALDI-TOF mass spectrometry identification of Leptospira Serovars, Thesis, 2020. http://hdl.handle.net/2142/108114.

[305] Boonsilp S, Thaipadungpanit J, Amornchai P, et al. A single multilocus sequence typing (MLST) scheme for seven pathogenic Leptospira species. PLoS Negl Trop Dis 2013;7(1):e1954.

[306] Salaun L, Mérien F, Gurianova S, et al. Application of multilocus variable-number tandem-repeat analysis for molecular typing of the agent of leptospirosis. J Clin Microbiol 2006;44(11):3954–62.

[307] Balamurugan V, Thirumalesh SR, Alamuri A, et al. Evaluation of the diagnostic potential of recombinant leptospiral OMP A-like protein (Loa22) and transmembrane (OmpL37) protein in latex agglutination test for serodiagnosis of leptospirosis in animals. Lett Appl Microbiol 2021;72(6):730–40.

[308] Dey S, Mohan CM, Ramadass P, et al. Recombinant antigen-based latex agglutination test for rapid serodiagnosis of leptospirosis. Vet Res Commun 2007; 31(1):9–15.

[309] Winzelberg S, Tasse S, Goldstein R, et al. Evaluation of SNAP® Lepto in the Diagnosis of Leptospirosis Infections in dogs: Twenty two Clinical Cases. Int J Appl Res Vet Med 2015;13(3):193–8.

[310] Kodjo A, Calleja C, Loenser M, et al. A rapid in-clinic test detects acute leptospirosis in dogs with high sensitivity and specificity. Biomed Research International 2016;2016.

[311] Lizer J, Grahlmann M, Hapke H, et al. Evaluation of a rapid IgM detection test for diagnosis of acute leptospirosis in dogs. Vet Rec 2017;180(21):517.

[312] Gloor CI, Schweighauser A, Francey T, et al. Diagnostic value of two commercial chromatographic "patient-side" tests in the diagnosis of acute canine leptospirosis. J Small Anim Pract 2017;58(3):154–61.

SECTION V: NUTRITION

Advances in Small Animal Care 3 (2022) 221–227

ADVANCES IN SMALL ANIMAL CARE

Nutritional Management of Acute Pancreatitis

Daniel L. Chan, DVM, DACVECC, DECVECC, DACVIM(Nutrition)

Section of Emergency and Critical Care, Department of Clinical Science and Services, The Royal Veterinary College, Hawkshead Lane, North Mymms, Hertfordshire AL97TA, United Kingdom

KEYWORDS
- Enteral nutrition   • Parenteral nutrition   • Acute pancreatitis   • Feeding tubes   • Nasoesophageal feeding
- Esophagostomy feeding tube

KEY POINTS
- Nutritional support is considered a key part of management of patients with acute pancreatitis.
- Feeding should be attempted in all patients if cardiovascularly stable, and parenteral nutrition should not be considered unless enteral feeding is not tolerated.
- Placement of feeding tubes should be considered as the standard for providing nutritional support in hyporexic patients with acute pancreatitis.
- Parenteral nutrition still has a place in the management of patients with acute pancreatitis, but it is to be reserved for patients who fail to tolerate enteral nutrition.

INTRODUCTION

Acute pancreatitis (AP) is commonly encountered in both companion animals, particularly dogs. Although most cases are mild and self-limiting, some cases develop systemic complications that can result in death. Establishing a definitive diagnosis is sometimes difficult, especially in cats, and the successful management may depend on several factors. Experimental and clinical data strongly support that nutritional management plays an important therapeutic role in both veterinary and human patients suffering from AP [1–6]. Although the optimal nutritional management of AP in dogs and cats remains unclear and warrants further research, consensus is growing that enteral nutrition (EN) should be implemented in most cases, and earlier than previously thought [7]. Parenteral nutritional (PN) support, although no longer considered necessary, may be required in cases when EN is not tolerated.

SIGNIFICANCE

The underlying pathophysiology of AP is incompletely understood [7–9] but is thought to involve 2 key events:
- Colocalization of lysosomes and zymogen granules within acinar cells and
- Abnormal intra-acinar activation of digestive enzymes such as trypsinogen

The result of these events leads to interactions between inert pancreatic zymogens and lysosomal proteases within the acinar cells. Trypsin is then activated and leads to activation of the other pancreatic zymogens to active enzymes. Activated pancreatic enzymes are then released in the pancreatic tissue, and inflammation ensues. The initiating trigger for these events is currently unknown in dogs and cats, with the vast majority of cases classified as idiopathic.

E-mail address: dchan@rvc.ac.uk

https://doi.org/10.1016/j.yasa.2022.05.006

NUTRITIONAL MANAGEMENT STRATEGIES

The traditional nutritional approach to AP centered on the premise that withholding food ("pancreatic rest") would reduce pancreatic autodigestion by decreasing pancreatic stimulation and enzyme release [4,10,11]. However, it is now clear that the initiating events in the development of AP involve intracellular premature activation of proteolytic enzymes rather than pancreatic stimulation. Avoidance of feeding as a means to decrease pancreatic stimulation may be unwarranted because this could not only lead to malnutrition but also complicate the disease by potentially impairing gastrointestinal barrier function [12–14]. For these reasons, there should be particular consideration for implementing EN support in patients with AP unless contraindicated.

ENTERAL NUTRITION DURING ACUTE PANCREATITIS

Nutritional support during AP has been well documented to play a central role in the management of this condition in people. PN had been the standard therapy for many years, based on the theory that EN stimulated pancreatic secretion, potentially exacerbating the inflammatory response and delaying recovery. However, recent data suggest that EN in people is not only well tolerated but also safer and associated with fewer complications than with PN and is even associated with improved survival in some studies [3,6,15,16]. In recent years EN has become the new gold standard of nutritional therapy in managing AP in people [3,6,15–18].

The current consensus is also that EN should be initiated as early as possible (ideally within the first 48 hours of diagnosis) [12,18]. Although studies prospectively evaluating tolerance of EN in dogs and cats with AP are limited, there is growing evidence supporting this approach in dogs and cats with AP. Experimental studies in dogs with induced AP have compared the effects of early intrajejunal feedings and PN and showed no effect on serum concentrations of amylase and lysosomal enzyme activities relative to the PN group [2,19]. In addition, circulating plasma endotoxin activity and bacterial translocation was reduced significantly in the intrajejunal-fed group versus the PN group [2,19]. The intrajejunal-fed group also displayed improved gut barrier when assessed histopathologically by enteral villi height, and thickness of mucosa and bowel wall in the ileum and transverse colon.

In veterinary medicine there is a single small pilot study evaluating the tolerability of prepyloric EN in dogs with AP, which showed promising results with no exacerbation of pain or vomiting in the enterally fed group when compared with the parenterally fed group [1]. The frequency of vomiting or regurgitations episodes was higher in the group of dogs receiving PN, and it was hypothesized that EN may improve gut health and thereby reduces ileus and vomiting. In addition, no evidence of exacerbation of abdominal pain was found in the enterally fed group. However, due to the study's very small sample size (ie, 5 dogs in each group) further studies are warranted to confirm these findings.

Nasogastric tube feeding has been assessed retrospectively in 55 cats with AP. Administration of bolus feeding or continuous rate infusion were compared in addition to whether or not the cats had received an amino acid-dextrose solution [20]. In the study, nasogastric feeding was well tolerated and there was no significant difference between groups with respect to the clinical variables assessed before or after feeding (including frequency of vomiting, incidence of diarrhea, and hypersalivation) [20]. Complications were considered mild, and overall rate of complications was considered low. Based on broad evidence in human studies and the preliminary results of experimental and clinical studies in animals, EN, when possible, should be considered as the mode of choice for feeding patients with AP.

FEEDING TUBES AND ROUTES

Given the importance of EN in the management of patients with AP and the poor reliability of appetite stimulants or simply offering enticing food to animals suffering from AP, more effective means of nutritional support are often required. Although the use of capromorelin (a ghrelin receptor agonist) has been demonstrated to increase appetite in dogs, this study only evaluated dogs that did not require hospitalization or intravenous fluids [21]. Therefore it is unknown whether capromorelin would be an effective appetite stimulant in dogs with AP who typically require hospitalization and fluid therapy among other therapies. Feeding tubes have been demonstrated to be effective means of facilitating nutritional support in animals with AP, and several options are available [1,20,22,23]. Nasoesophageal feeding tubes (Fig. 1) are easily placed with a local anesthetic and do not require general anesthesia. These tubes are therefore an appropriate choice for short-term nutritional

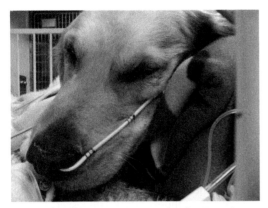

support of the severely debilitated patient, where a general anesthetic is contraindicated. The major disadvantage is their small diameter, which limits feeding to liquid enteral diets, and that these may clog more frequently. Moreover, currently available liquid veterinary diets have a relative high fat content (eg, 45% of total calorie content) to increase calorie density, which may not be ideal for dogs with hyperlipidemia-associated pancreatitis. Dogs with hyperlipidemia are at increased risk of developing pancreatitis, although the exact mechanism remains unclear [24]. Both fats and amino acids stimulate CCK release and induce pancreatic stimulation in normal dogs; however, the relationship between pancreatic stimulation and naturally occurring AP in dogs has not been proven. In a study evaluating experimentally induced AP in dogs, enteral feeding increased serum CCK concentrations but did not seem to stimulate pancreatic secretion, bringing into question the role of CCK in AP in dogs [2]. Fat content is not a typical concern in cats with AP. Although human liquid diets with a lower fat content are available, they should not be considered nutritionally complete with respect to amino acid composition and are therefore inappropriate for use in veterinary patients, especially cats, unless supplemented with various amino acids (eg, arginine).

Esophagostomy tubes (Fig. 2) require a short general anesthetic for placement, but are an excellent option for cats and dogs of most sizes and have the advantage that a liquidized complete diet can be fed, permitting better individualized diet selection (eg, lower fat content). There is a single small study demonstrating good results

when dogs with AP were fed a commercial low-fat diet via esophagostomy tubes [1]. In cases when surgery is required (eg, pancreatic abscess), placement of gastrostomy or jejunostomy feeding tubes ensures access for enteral feeding. Two retrospective veterinary studies described the application of jejunostomy tubes in dogs and cats with AP undergoing surgical management for pancreatitis [22,23]. These studies evaluated complications and potential prognostic factors but did not describe in detail the complications encountered in relation to jejunostomy tubes.

Minimally invasive techniques for placement of nasojejunal tubes using fluoroscopy or endoscopy in dogs has been described, but has not yet been widely adopted [25,26]. Feeding tubes were successfully placed in the jejunum in 74% to 78% of cases; however, in one study the success rate increased over time to 100%, indicating that technical proficiency improves with experience. The major complication was oral tube migration (less than a third of cases). AP was the primary diagnosis of dogs undergoing fluoroscopic wire-guided placement of nasojejunal tubes in one study [26]. Slow constant-rate infusion of a liquid diet ("trickle feeding") is recommended, and jejunostomy tubes are therefore only suitable for hospitalized patients.

Parenteral Nutrition

In patients with severe AP and intractable vomiting who do not tolerate EN, PN can be a valuable treatment modality to prevent malnutrition. Although compounding PN solutions requires specialized expertise and is limited to referral centers, readymade amino acid/glucose solutions for PN can be used in practice as interim solutions until the animal can tolerate either placement of a feeding tube or is voluntarily eating [27,28]. The sole use of PN in experimental animal models of AP has been associated with a high risk of infection and gut atrophy, with subsequent increased risk of bacterial translocation and sepsis [29]. However, there are no studies on PN in dogs or cats that indicate a high risk for infection or sepsis, and in the single veterinary study that specifically evaluated PN support in dogs with AP, no septic complications were identified [30]. Although most patients fed parenterally had to have demonstrated intolerance to enteral feeding initially, many may tolerate provision of trickle feeding and gradual weaning onto EN, which may help to maintain intestinal integrity and function. This introduction of enteral feeding should start as soon as possible and maybe within 24 hours of initiating parental nutrition. This approach is supported by the fact that early enteral feeding has been associated with

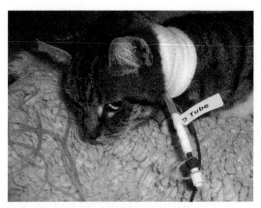

FIG. 2 Esophagostomy tubes (shown here in a cat) are particularly useful in managing patients requiring longer-term nutritional support, and their wider diameter allows the use of blenderized canned diets so that a greater variety of diets can be used.

earlier return of gastrointestinal motility and cessation of vomiting [31]. The time for initiation of PN is controversial in light of recent findings that initiation of PN in critically ill human patients in first 7 days of intensive care unit hospitalization could be harmful [32]. The effect of time to PN initiation or combination of PN with concurrent EN in veterinary patients has not been performed, so it is uncertain, but in most studies detailing PN in veterinary patients, the time to initiation is usually in the first 3 days of hospitalization [27,28,33].

Selection or formulation of an appropriate nutritional solution is critical when using PN, and it necessitates consideration of the caloric requirement of the patient and comorbidities present. Commercially available readymade parenteral solutions for people are not designed to meet the needs of animals, and may not provide adequate nutritional support [34]. Although a great proportion of energy in 3-in-1 PN solutions is derived from fat, there is currently no evidence to suggest that the lipid content in PN solutions is detrimental in the management of canine or feline pancreatitis. High-lipid formulations seem to be well-tolerated in nonhyperlipidemic AP [34]. The optimal solution for dogs with AP and hypertriglyceridemia is not known.

DIETARY CONSIDERATIONS

When implementing enteral feeding, an appropriate diet should be selected. Although there is a paucity of veterinary studies evaluating the influence of diet type on disease course, a highly digestible diet designed for patients with gastrointestinal disease is generally

recommended. Avoidance of a diet high in fat has been the general recommendation for years, although in naturally occurring disease, the link between a high dietary fat content and pancreatitis is not very clear. The presence of hypertriglyceridemia in certain dog breeds has been shown to act as a predisposing factor, and fat-restricted diets will therefore serve a benefit in the management of pancreatitis in these cases [35,36]. Although fat restriction is considered an important component of the management of chronic pancreatitis in dogs, the role in nonhypertriglyceridemic AP is not well understood.

Cats have specialized dietary requirements that differ considerably from those of dogs with respect to dietary fat and protein requirements, and may be more prone to carbohydrate intolerance. The high dietary protein requirement makes cats more susceptible to protein-energy malnutrition and lean muscle loss during stressed starvation. Cats have the ability to digest and use high levels of dietary fat, and there is no current evidence supporting restricting fat in the diet of cats with pancreatitis. In a retrospective study evaluating nasogastric tube feeding in cats with AP, feeding of a liquid enteral high-lipid diet (45% of total calories fed) was well tolerated [20].

FUTURE AVENUES TO INVESTIGATE
Emerging Role of Immunonutrition
In human medicine there is increasing evidence supporting the idea that certain nutrients such as glutamine, arginine, and fatty acids play a significant role in metabolic, inflammatory, and immune processes in AP. The use of these specific nutrients in the care of critically ill human patients, including those with AP, is becoming more common, with increasing evidence of their benefits with minimal risk of complications [37,38]. In relation to immunonutrition and AP, glutamine supplementation has particular applications to the management of AP, and a brief discussion is warranted.

Glutamine is the most abundant amino acid both in the plasma and in the muscle pool of amino acids and is essential for a wide variety of physiologic processes. The pancreas has a high protein turnover, and glutamine supplementation in animals has resulted in the prevention of atrophy of pancreatic acinar cells, improvement in pancreatic exocrine function, and improved outcomes following critical illness [39–42]. Glutamine has also been demonstrated to support gut barrier function, reduce intestinal permeability, and restore antioxidant defenses [5]. Human patients with severe AP treated with glutamine-enriched PN solutions demonstrated significant improvement in C-reactive protein concentrations and anti-inflammatory cytokines (IL-10), improved nitrogen balance as well as decreased dependence on PN, reduced infectious complications, and reduced length of hospitalization [38,43]. Glutamine-supplemented PN is challenged by the fact that glutamine is relatively unstable in solution and generally has to be provided as dipeptides to maintain stability [44]. Glutamine is currently not supplemented routinely to PN formulations in veterinary medicine, and no clinical trials evaluating its use in pancreatitis have been published. As many meta-analyses of the use of immune-enhancing diets in critically ill patients have shown a reduction of hospital stay and infection rate, but no adverse effect on mortality rate, this was deemed a safe therapeutic option [45].

SUMMARY

There is increasing evidence supporting the important role of early EN (within 48 hours of diagnosis of pancreatitis) in positively impacting outcome beyond simply proving energy and nutrients in AP. Nutritional support is now considered an integral and key aspect of the successful management of AP. Although not as extensively studied in veterinary medicine, limited clinical data do suggest enteral feeding to be considered to be safe, effective, and well tolerated in severe AP. Use of feeding tubes have been shown to be effective and safe in dogs and cats and should be used unless specific contraindications are identified. The exact composition of the diet has not been identified, but diets commonly used for convalescent dogs and cats or diets used for gastrointestinal disorders have been used successfully. Avoidance of high fat content does not seem to be necessary in most patients. Despite the growing evidence that EN can be used effectively in the management patients with AP, there may still be patients requiring some form of PN until EN can be tolerated.

CLINICS CARE POINTS

- The standard of care for treating AP in hospitalized companion animals now includes the incorporation of nutritional support, which should be implemented within 48 to 72 hours of admission

- The preferred modality of nutritional support for patients with AP is EN, which often involves the placement of feeding tubes
- Short-term (<3 days) EN support may be achieved with nasogastric or nasoesophageal feeding tubes, which can be placed with local anesthesia rather than general anesthesia. These small tubes often only accommodate completely liquid diets
- Animals requiring more extended periods of nutritional support are best managed with esophagostomy tubes, which require a brief general anesthetic
- Diets most commonly used for managing patients with pancreatitis include convalescence and gastrointestinal diets
- A small subset of patients with AP that do not tolerate EN can be supported with short periods of PN

DISCLOSURE OF COMMERCIAL OR FINANCIAL CONFLICTS OF INTERESTS

The author declares no conflict of interest in relation to this article.

REFERENCES

[1] Mansfield CS, James FE, Steiner JM, et al. A pilot study to assess tolerability of early enteral nutrition via esophagostomy tube feeding in dogs with severe acute pancreatitis. J Vet Intern Med 2011;25:419–25.

[2] Qin HL, Su ZD, Hu LG, et al. Effect of parenteral and early intrajejunal nutrition on pancreatic digestive enzyme synthesis, storage and discharge in dog models of acute pancreatitis. World J Gastroenterol 2007;13: 1123–8.

[3] Petrov M, Kukosh M, Emelyanov N. A Randomized controlled trial of enteral versus parenteral feeding in patients with predicted severe acute pancreatitis shows a significant reduction in mortality and in infected pancreatic complications with total enteral nutrition. Dig Surg 2006;23:336–45.

[4] Petrov MS. Gastric feeding and "gut rousing" in acute pancreatitis. Nutr Clin Pract 2014;29(3):287–90.

[5] Pan L, Li J, Shamoon M, et al. Recent advances on nutrition in treatment of acute pancreatitis. Front Immunol 2017;8:762.

[6] Ramanathan M, Aadam AA. Nutrition management in acute pancreatitis. Nutr Clin Pract 2019;34(Suppl 1): S7–12.

[7] Forman MA, Steiner JM, Armstrong PJ, et al. ACVIM consensus statement on pancreatitis in cats. J Vet Intern Med 2021;35:703–23.

[8] Gukovskaya AS, Gukovsky I. Autophagy and pancreatitis. Am J Physiol Gastrointest Liver Physiol 2012;303: 993–1003.

[9] Gukovsky I, Pandol SJ, Gukovskaya AS. Organellar dysfunction in the pathogenesis of pancreatitis. Antioxidant Redox Signal 2011;15:2699–710.

[10] Simpson K, Lamb C. Acute Pancreatitis. Practice 1995;17: 328–37.

[11] Williams DA. Diagnosis and management of pancreatitis. J Small Anim Pract 1994 1995;35:445–54.

[12] Nathens AB, Curtis JR, Beale RL, et al. Management of the critically ill patient with severe acute pancreatitis. Crit Care Med 2004;32:2524–36.

[13] Ioannidis O, Lavrentieva A, Botsios D. Nutrition support in acute pancreatitis. J Pancreas 2008;9:375–90.

[14] Curtis CS, Judsk KA. Nutrition Support in Pancreatitis. Surg Clin North America 2007;87:1403–15.

[15] Spanier BWM, Bruno MJ, Mathus-Vliegen EMH. Enteral nutrition and acute pancreatitis: a review. Gastroenterol Res Pract 2011;9:10–2.

[16] Guptaa R, Patela K, Calderb PC, et al. A randomised clinical trial to assess the effect of total enteral and total parenteral nutritional support on metabolic, inflammatory and oxidative markers in patients with predicted severe acute pancreatitis (APACHE II $\geq$6). Pancreatology 2003;3:406–13.

[17] McClave SA. Defining the new gold standard for nutritional support in acute pancreatitis. Nutr Clin Pract 2004;19:1–4.

[18] Gianotti L, Meier R, Lobo DN, et al. ESPEN Guidelines on Parenteral Nutrition: Pancreas. Clin Nutr 2009;28: 428–35.

[19] Qin HL, Su ZD, Hu LG, et al. Parenteral versus early intrajejunal nutrition: effect on pancreatitic natural course, entero-hormones release and its efficacy on dogs with acute pancreatitis. World J Gastroenterol 2003;9:2270–3.

[20] Klaus J, Rudloff E, Kirby R. Nasogastric tube feeding in cats with suspected acute pancreatitis: 55 cases (2001-2006). J Vet Emerg Crit Care 2009;19:337–46.

[21] Zollers B, Wofford JA, Heinen E, et al. A Prospective, Randomized, Masked, Placebo-Controlled Clinical Study of Capromorelin in Dogs with Reduced Appetite. J Vet Intern Med 2016;30(6):1851–7.

[22] Son TT, Thompson L, Serrano S, et al. Surgical intervention in the management of severe acute pancreatitis in cats: 8 cases (2003-2007). J Vet Emerg Crit Care 2010; 20:426–35.

[23] Thompson LJ, Seshadri R, Raffe MR. Characteristics and outcomes in surgical management of severe acute pancreatitis: 37 dogs (2001-2007). J Vet Emerg Crit Care 2009;19:165–73.

[24] Xenoulis PG, Steiner JM. Canine hyperlipidaemia. J Small Anim Pract 2015;56:595–605.

[25] Pápa K, Psáder R, Sterczer A, et al. Endoscopically guided nasojejunal tube placement in dogs for short-term post-duodenal feeding. J Vet Emerg Crit Care 2009;19: 554–63.

[26] Beal MW, Brown AJ. Clinical experience utilizing a novel fluoroscopic technique for wire-guided nasojejunal tube placement in the dog: 26 cases (2006-2010). J Vet Emerg Crit Care 2011;21:151–7.

[27] Gajanayake I, Wylie CE, Chan DL. Clinical experience with a lipid-free, ready-made parenteral nutrition solution in dogs: 70 cases (2006-2012). J Vet Emerg Crit Care 2013;23.

[28] Olan NV, Prittie J. Retrospective evaluation of Procal-Amine administration in a population of hospitalized ICU dogs: 36 cases (2010-2013). J Vet Emerg Crit Care 2015;25(3):405–12.

[29] Alverdy J, Ayos E, Moss G. Total parenteral nutrition promotes bacterial translocation from the gut. Surgery 1988; 104:185–90.

[30] Freeman L, Labato M, Rush J, et al. Nutritional support in pancreatitis: a retrospective study. J Vet Emerg Crit Care 1995;5:32–41.

[31] Wernerman J. Guidelines for nutritional support in intensive care unit patients: a critical analysis. Curr Opin Clin Nutr Metab Care 2005;8:171–5.

[32] Casaer MP, Mesotten D, Hermans G, et al. Early versus Late Parenteral Nutrition in Critically Ill Adults. New Engl J Med 2011;365:506–17.

[33] Chan DL, Freeman LM, Labato M, et al. Retrospective evaluation of partial parenteral nutrition in dogs and cats. J Vet Intern Med 2002;16:440–5.

[34] Campbell SJ, Karriker MJ, Fascetti AJ. Central and peripheral parenteral nutrition. Waltham Focus 2006;16: 22–30.

[35] Verkest K, Fleeman L, Rand J, et al. Subclinical pancreatitis is more common in overweight and obese dogs if peak postprandial triglyceridemia is >445 mg/dL (Abstr). J Vet Intern Med 2008;22:820.

[36] Fleeman LM. Is hyperlipidemia clinically important in dogs? Vet J 2010;183:10.

[37] Cetinbas F, Yelken B, Gulbas Z. Role of glutamine administration on cellular immunity after total parenteral nutrition enriched with glutamine in patients with systemic inflammatory response syndrome. J Crit Care 2010;25:61.e1-6.

[38] Ockenga J, Borchert K, Rifai K, et al. Effect of glutamine-enriched total parenteral nutrition in patients with acute pancreatitis. Clin Nutr 2002;21:409–16.

[39] Fan B, Salehi A, Sternby B, et al. Total parenteral nutrition influences both endocrine and exocrine function of rat pancreas. Pancreas 1997;15:147–53.

[40] Helton W, Jacobs D, Bonner-Weir S, et al. Effects of glutamine-enriched parenteral nutrition on the exocrine pancreas. J Parenteral Enteral Nutr 1990; 14:344–52.

[41] Zou X, Chen M, Wei W, et al. Effects of enteral immunonutrition on the maintenance of gut barrier function and immune function in pigs with severe acute pancreatitis. J Parenter Enteral Nutr 2010;34:554–66.

[42] Belmonte L, Coëffier M, Le Pessot F, et al. Effects of glutamine supplementation on gut barrier, glutathione content and acute phase response in malnourished rats

during inflammatory shock. World J Gastroenterol 2007; 13:2833–40.

[43] Fuentes-Orozco C, Cervantes-guevara G, Mucino-Hernandez I, et al. L-alanul-L-glutamine-supplemented parenteral nutrition decreases infectious morbidity rates in patients with severe acute pancreatitis. JPEN J Parenter Enteral Nutr 2008;32:403–11.

[44] Khan K, Hardy G, McElroy B, et al. The stability of L-glutamine in total parenteral nutrition solutions. Clin Nutr 1991;10:193–8.

[45] Galbán C, Montejo J, Mesejo A, et al. An immune-enhancing enteral diet reduces mortality rate and episodes of bacteremia in septic intensive care unit patients. Critial Care Med 2003;28:643–8.

Advances in Small Animal Care 3 (2022) 229–238

ADVANCES IN SMALL ANIMAL CARE

Creating a Weight Loss Plan with Owner Engagement

Camille Torres, DVM, DABVP, DACVIM (Nutrition)[a,*], Jonathan Stockman, DVM, DACVIM (Nutrition)[b]

[a]Colorado State University, James L. Voss Veterinary Teaching Hospital, 300 W Drake, Fort Collins, CO 80523, USA; [b]Long Island University, 720 Northern Boulevard, Greenvale, NY 11548, USA

KEYWORDS

• Obesity • Weight loss • Diet • Physical activity • Hurdles

KEY POINTS

- Pet obesity has a substantial impact on the quality of life, risk of concurrent disease, and longevity.
- Although any dog and cat can become overweight or obese, it is important to recognize those who are at increased risk and prevent weight gain.
- Many owners may not recognize their pet as overweight and may not understand the implications.
- The weight loss process requires participation of all members of the household that interact with the pet and provide food.
- The veterinarian should be aware of the possible hurdles for successful weight loss and how to mitigate them as needed.

INTRODUCTION—WHY IS WEIGHT LOSS IMPORTANT?

Pet obesity is a highly common yet complex problem with many contributing factors. It has considerable implications on the pet's health and quality of life. Despite increased awareness by veterinarians of the harmful implications of excess bodyweight, the prevalence of obesity in dogs and cats appears to be increasing in the western world. It is currently estimated that more than 50% of companion dogs and cats are overweight or obese [1–3]. Many owners are unaware of the consequences of excess bodyweight or may not recognize their own pet as being overweight or obese [4].

Owner perception of their own pet's body condition may also be influenced by the fact that show dogs and cats that are supposedly ideal examples of their respective breeds are often overweight or obese [5,6]. Changing an owner's perception regarding excess bodyweight is imperative because this is associated with several concurrent diseases that may affect the quality of life and reduce longevity. Some examples of obesity-related diseases include diabetes mellitus, osteoarthritis, cardiovascular disease, dermatological disease, increased risk for pancreatitis, and hyperlipidemia. Diabetes mellitus is an endocrine disease that is defined by the relative or absolute lack of insulin. In cats, insulin sensitivity is known to decrease with obesity [7]. The same occurs in dogs, although obese dogs may be able to compensate better than cats by increasing insulin secretion [8]. Diabetes mellitus in dogs and cats may have life-threatening complications, such as diabetes ketoacidosis, as well as an ongoing impact on the pet's quality of life and care required by the owner, including insulin injections and blood glucose monitoring, which further leads to additional financial expense.

Osteoarthritis is a common disease in dogs and cats with increased prevalence in older animals. This is a complex degenerative process, which may involve a shift in the normal cartilage production and degradation. Surveys have identified radiographic evidence of osteoarthritis in up to 61% of cats aged older than

---

*Corresponding author, *E-mail address:* c.torres-henderson@colostate.edu

https://doi.org/10.1016/j.yasa.2022.06.002
2666-450X/22/

6 years [9]. The prevalence of clinical disease due to osteoarthritis may be harder to assess, especially when clinical signs are subtle; but according to medical record surveys clinical osteoarthritis in dogs may reach 20% [10]. The pathophysiology of this disease is not entirely known; however, it is hypothesized that repeated joint loading in obese individuals could cause osteoarthritis in some cases [11]. Obesity can exacerbate signs associated with osteoarthritis. Even more importantly, weight loss may result in significant improvement in clinical signs of osteoarthritis [12].

Obese dogs have also been found to be at higher risk of cardiovascular disease [13]. Although dogs and cats do not suffer from atherosclerosis as humans and other species do, obesity can complicate clinical management of cardiovascular disease and has a negative impact on the quality of life. Exercise intolerance in obese dogs with cardiovascular disease may be exacerbated; these may become more dyspneic than dogs with a healthy bodyweight. Additional evidence indicates that energy restriction can increase longevity in dogs. It was shown that labrador dogs that had been restricted in their food intake lived significantly longer than their paired littermates and had a later onset of age-related disease [14].

Risk Factors for Obesity

Although the imbalance between energy intake and energy expenditure is ultimately the cause of weight gain, not all dogs and cats are at the same risk of becoming overweight or obese. For example, some dog breeds such as labrador retrievers are known to be at higher risk for obesity [10]. This increased risk of obesity in labradors is related to a genetic mutation involving a 14 bp deletion in the pro-opiomelanocortin gene, which results in the disruption of the melanocyte-stimulating hormone and β-endorphin genes and leads to increased body weight, increased adiposity, and increased food-seeking behavior [15]. Although the hereditary or genetic component is not known in other dogs, there are additional breeds at high risk for obesity including pug, beagle, rottweiler, Shetland sheepdog, border terrier, cocker spaniel, English springer spaniel, dachshund, and dalmatian [16–18].

Conflicting reports exist regarding the prevalence of obesity in various cat breeds. Previous reports found that purebred cats were less likely to be overweight or obese compared with domestic shorthair cats [19]. Of the purebred cats, a previous report indicated that Norwegian Forest cats are at higher risk of obesity compared with other breeds such as Siamese [20]; however, this is in contrast to another report of show cats that did not find a breed association with obesity although this

might have resulted from a low number of surveyed cats [6].

Neuter status may also impact risk for obesity, which is an important consideration as the vast majority of companion animals in North America are spayed and neutered [21,22]. It is generally accepted that energy requirements are reduced in both male and female dogs and cats once castrated; therefore, without adjustments in food intake after castration, these animals are at an increased risk for weight gain and obesity [23–27]. Some published findings indicate weight gain is associated with castration in males but not in females [28].

An additional risk factor is aging, which generally results in a decreased metabolic rate that may increase the risk of weight gain, although this is a complex process and several parallel changes may occur with contrasting results pertaining to weight gain and weight loss. Another age-related factor is age at onset of obesity because young animals that become overweight are at higher risk of obesity later in life. Obesity in growing animals is also associated with other disease conditions related to skeletal deformities because growth may be accelerated [29].

Principles of Clinical Management of Weight Loss

Identifying pets in need of weight loss relies on accurately assessing and documenting body condition score [30,31]. There are multiple scales for body condition score, and these are useful to determine if there is excess adiposity and to quantify it. These scales are also a useful tool to qualitatively monitor the weight loss progress in addition to monitoring bodyweight trends.

Weight loss is achieved by altering the balance between caloric intake and expenditure to achieve a net negative energy balance, thereby inducing catabolism. The weight loss process should begin with an initial caloric intake restriction selected as a starting point. This can be further modified according to the weight trends of the patient. A thorough diet history is incredibly helpful in starting off the weight loss process successfully because it accounts for all caloric intake in a typical day including the main meal, treats, and supplements (such as fish oil). If possible, discussion of diet amounts should be done in weight units (gram, kilogram, pound) rather than volume for accuracy because volume amounts may be subjective and highly variable [32].

Typically, a 20% reduction from the current intake is an acceptable starting point; however, this may depend on the individual animal, concurrent diseases, and current diet. When energy intake is unknown the calculated resting energy requirement (RER, kilocalories per day) of the pet at its current weight or its approximated ideal bodyweight can be used as a starting point in dogs, and $0.8 \times$ RER is often used in cats. RER can be calculated in either of the following equations [33,34]:

1. $RER = 70 \times BW_{(kg)}^{0.75}$
2. $RER = 30 \times BW_{(kg)} + 70$

The second equation is not accurate in very large or very small animals such as those weighing less than 2 kg or greater than 45 kg; therefore, the first equation is often preferred. Whichever approach is used to determine new caloric intake, it should only be considered a starting point, and frequent reassessment is necessary. Follow-up appointments provide an opportunity to adjust intake as needed to achieve the desired weight loss rate. It is generally recommended that weight loss should be maintained between a rate of 1% and 2% of the total bodyweight per week in healthy dogs [35]. Some owners may find the food restriction and the frequent follow-up appointments daunting, so it is important to prepare them in advance. It is also important to prepare owners for the possible duration of the process because it may take several weeks to months. To determine the estimated time until ideal weight is achieved, the veterinarian should calculate the patient's ideal weight, and the difference between the current weight and ideal weight is determined. This assessment may use the clinician's assessment of the pet's body condition score because each point on the body condition score scale above 5 (using the 9 point scale) represents a 10% to 15% deviation from the ideal body condition score [30,31]. For example, if a dog weighing 50 lbs has a body condition score of 7 out of 9, the patient is estimated to be 20% overweight, and the ideal bodyweight would be estimated as approximately 40 lbs.

The risk associated with the necessary restriction of food for weight loss purposes is that this may result in nutritional deficiencies, including protein malnutrition, which may be highly consequential during weight loss because it exacerbates muscle catabolism and a decline in lean body mass during weight loss. The rate of weight loss may need to be attenuated in some patients where a fast weight loss rate or food restriction may be of concern. For example, in patients with renal disease that require a protein-restricted diet, food restriction may result in protein malnutrition that may be avoided by a more modest energy restriction.

Daily protein recommended allowance in adult dogs and cats is expressed by the following equations [36]:

Daily protein recommended allowance for an adult dog at maintenance (g/day): $3.28 \text{ g}/BW_{(kg)}^{0.75}$

Daily protein recommended allowance for an adult cat at maintenance (g/day): $4.96 \text{ g}/BW_{(kg)}^{0.67}$

The amount of protein in the diet can be calculated using the label; however, the percent of crude protein reflects the number of grams of protein in 100 g of food. Therefore, to determine how much protein is provided by the diet every day, the percent crude protein is divided by the caloric density of the food (kcal/kg) and then multiplied by 1000, which will provide the grams of protein per 100 kcal (a value which is sometimes provided by the manufacturer). This is then multiplied by the patient's caloric intake divided by 100 to determine the daily protein intake (Box 1).

Diet selection for the duration of the weight loss period is imperative. Although some owners may be reluctant to transition their pet from the current over-the-counter (OTC) diet; these are many times inadequate for weight loss. Although OTC diets are designed to meet the nutritional requirements of healthy animals, these diets often do not provide sufficient amounts of essential nutrients when food intake is restricted [37]. Veterinary therapeutic diets are formulated to help with weight loss in several ways, including improved satiety by higher protein and fiber content, enhancing water intake by adding sodium, and decreased caloric density. Importantly, these diets are nutrient dense so that caloric restriction is less likely to result in nutritional deficiencies. OTC diets designated as "light" or "lite" are not equivalent to therapeutic veterinary diets. Lite or light diets typically do not have the same nutrient density found in veterinary weight loss diets, although per definition lite dry dog food cannot contain more than 3100 kcal/kg, and lite dry cat food cannot contain more than 3250 kcal/kg [38]. Light diets are mostly recommended for animals at risk of becoming overweight or obese, or those animals close enough to an ideal body condition score that only require minimal weight loss. It has been shown that caloric restriction with the use of light diets did achieve weight loss with energy allowances of 80% and 70% of the maintenance energy intake in dogs and cats, respectively, although this did result in several deficiencies of essential nutrients including selenium, choline, potassium, and riboflavin in some animals [39].

Pet related hurdles

Many dog and cat owners struggle adhering to a weight reduction plan for their pets because of unwanted pet behavior that often increases due to reduced food intake. Increased begging behavior may raise concerns regarding the pet's well-being. In addition, dogs and

---

BOX 1
Example of determining if a daily diet provides enough protein to meet the recommended allowance [36]

Example: A 20 kg dog is fed a diet that has minimum 26% crude protein and 4050 kcal/kg

Step 1: Calculate the dog's daily protein requirement

(20 kg $^{0.75}$) × 3.28 = 31 g of protein per day required to meet NRC recommended allowance

Step 2: Determine daily caloric intake if feeding RER

(20 kg^0.75) × 70 = 662 kcal per day

Step 3: Determine amount of protein in diet on an energy basis:

(26/4050) × 1000 = 6.4 g of protein/100 kcal

Determine how much protein how much protein the dog will receive from the diet if fed current RER:

662/100 = 6.62

6.62 × 6.4 = 42.3 g of protein per day

Conclusion: This diet would meet this dog's daily recommended allowance for protein (31 g of protein required, the diet would provide 42.3 g of protein if the dog was fed RER).

This will need to be recalculated as the patient's caloric intake is adjusted.

---

cats may seek out food, leading to destructive behavior such as chewing through barriers, or may begin to eat unwanted objects such as feces, plants, or sticks, which may lead to medical complications such as a gastrointestinal foreign body obstruction. Additionally, attention-seeking behavior such as vocalizing or pacing may be exhibited, or in some cases, pets may demonstrate signs of hunger-related aggression. One of the authors (C.T.) had managed a feline patient with specific aggressive behavior toward the owner when food was reduced to facilitate weight loss. The cat would bite the back of the owner's leg until food was added to the food bowl. These types of behaviors can affect the human–animal bond and can lead to a decline in owner compliance to the diet plan, and this behavior may be further reinforced if the pet receives food or treats as a result. In a survey of pet owners from Brazil, China, Russia, United Kingdom, and United States, 54% of pet owners often or always gave their dog or cat food if they begged, and 22% of pet owners overfed their pet as a result of this behavior [40].

Owner-related hurdles

Several surveys found an association between owner's age or owners that are less physically active with an increased likelihood to have overweight dogs [1,41]. Food and feeding are often adhered to the emotional bond between owner and pet in addition to food intake being viewed often as a measure of health and well-being. The enthusiasm some dogs and cats demonstrate during mealtime creates a positive experience for the owner, and food is also used for important activities

such as training and socialization. These interactions may be disrupted during the planned weight loss unless the veterinarian and the owner take steps to maintain them while avoiding excess energy intake. It may be important to assess the pet owner's readiness to make daily routine changes that may affect their interaction with their pet, as well as explore factors that may prevent the owner from being able to follow through with the diet plan. In some cases, there are multiple people in the family that may participate in pet feeding, and all should be included in the conversation regarding weight loss.

Multipet households create a unique set of challenges for the owner, especially when one pet has unique medical needs such as obesity. For example, there may be a scenario where there is an overweight pet and an underweight pet in the same house. The owner may wish to have food left out throughout the day to encourage intake for the underweight pet; however, this may directly interfere with weight loss goals for the overweight pet. Automated pet feeders equipped with a sensor can be helpful to mitigate the challenges in the weight loss process specifically in multipet household. Although dry food tends to be more practical for automatic feeders, there are also feeders that have ice packs to keep canned food fresh for several hours. Alternative solutions can include building a feeding station or using baby gates to create separate feeding stations. To allow the underweight pet to feed separately, a hole may be cut in a ventilated container and a pet door flap may inserted. The hole may be cut so that it is too narrow for the overweight pet, or by the use of programmable doors that respond to the pet's microchip.

Excess treats and human food may contribute to obesity. Treats do not provide a balanced nutrition, and there is a risk for malnutrition when treats exceed 10% of the total daily caloric intake. Treats can be included in the daily diet in a variety of ways, which may not always be easily identified. For example, some owners may provide medications with cheese or peanut butter, not realizing the contribution those provide to the daily calories. This emphasizes the importance of obtaining a complete diet history including assessment of treats, human food and supplements that are being given to the dog or cat.

These challenges may only be mitigated by creating a partnership between the veterinary care team and the owner and their family. This requires an understanding of potential barriers for a successful weight loss plan and finding solutions that are effective and acceptable to all.

Veterinarian-related hurdles

One of the challenges many veterinarians face is how to deliver optimal care to a large number of diverse patients within stringent time limitations. Some veterinarians may be concerned that the appointment will take more time if clients are asked too many open-ended questions and may opt for targeted closed-ended questions with an intention to improve efficiency [42]; however, this has the potential to lead to an abbreviated or inaccurate assessment of the patient history. Owner compliance can be directly influenced by the of communication between the veterinarian and the pet owner, and this in turn can influence the outcomes of a weight loss plan [43–45]. Veterinarians are often viewed as being approachable, sensitive, sympathetic, and understanding, which helps build a trusting relationship with pet owners [46]. However, this relationship can be tested when the veterinary recommendations do not align with the client's perception. Some veterinarians avoid discussing topics that may be contentious. Addressing weight loss in pets may also be more difficult if the owners themselves are overweight or if they refuse to recognize obesity in their pet. However, veterinarians may also need to recognize of weight bias that may affect their treatment and owner communication [47].

Important components of a weight loss program

Several components can contribute to the success of a weight loss plan. These include understanding the client's motivation and commitment to the weight loss plan, individualization of the diet plan and follow-up and reassessment [48]. Determining the client's perception regarding their pets' weight as well as determining the readiness to change are important steps in the multifactorial approach to creating an effective weight loss plan [48,49]. The body condition scoring (BCS) system is ubiquitous and well-established method for the assessment of adiposity in pets [50]; however, it can be difficult for a pet owner to understand the meaning behind it [51]. Some pet owners may find percentage of body fat a more tangible concept as body mass index, which is correlated with body fat and is commonly used in human health care. To address this, the percentage of body fat can be estimated using the body condition score where a BCS of 4 on a 9-point scale would correspond with 15% to 19% body fat, and a BCS of 9 on a 9-point scale would be greater than 40% body fat [52].

The veterinary team can use strategies to modify owners' behavior, such as goal setting, defining a specific outcome, education, and feedback because this may increase the chances of successful weight loss. Further research is needed to establish which strategies are most beneficial for a successful weight loss plan [53].

Overcoming pet-related and owner-related hurdles

The owners provide positive reinforcement when "giving in" and providing food in response to begging, and this can jeopardize the success of the weight loss plan. The owner can redirect their response to begging behavior by engaging in a different activity, such as taking their pet for a walk, playing fetch, brushing, and so forth. It may also be effective to disassociate the owner from being a source of food by using a sensor-activated feeder or food timer. Additional approaches to consider:

- Avoid feeding the dog or cat at the table
- Keep the pets away from the area where the family eats meals
  - Use baby gates to block off the area
  - Have the dog stay in his or her kennel during meals
- Teach obedience commands to reduce unwanted behavior
- Ignore begging behavior
- Reward positive behavior

For some pet owners, the concerns regarding their pet acting hungry may be alleviated knowing that their diet is providing all the nutrients required to maintain health while achieving a caloric deficit for weight loss. Conveying the mechanism behind satiety and hunger in simplified terms owners can understand improves adherence to a weight loss plan. Satiety and hunger involve complex mechanisms, which are regulated by a variety of anorexigenic and orexigenic signals. Anorexigenic hormones such as leptin, insulin, peptide YY and glucagon-like peptide signal satiety, whereas orexigenic hormones, such as ghrelin, signal for increased feeding behavior [36]. Leptin is released from adipose tissue and is an important anorexigenic hormone that signals satiety and increases the metabolic rate, and while leptin release is increased with increased adipose tissue, the response to it decreases in obese individuals [54]. Begging behavior is often triggered by increased orexigenic signals and is further exacerbated by decreased satiety due to decreased response to leptin an anorexigenic signal. As the patient loses weight and the amount of adipose tissue decreases, the response to leptin improves [55]. If the owners remain committed to the weight loss plan long enough to have a reduction in adipose tissue, the begging behavior may improve coinciding with a reduction in leptin in circulation.

Increased food-seeking behavior is often reported at the initial visit in the beginning of the weight loss process; however, this behavior usually improves over the subsequent visits [56].

As discussed above, a veterinary therapeutic weight loss by a reputable manufacturer is highly recommended during caloric restriction. Feeding a diet that is of low caloric density but high in nutrient density allows the owner to feed more food while reducing the calories being fed and with reduced risk of malnutrition. In addition, these diets are often higher in fiber and protein to promote satiety [57]. Increasing the moisture in the diet by adding water or feeding canned food may also help promote satiety and reduce begging behavior. Some dogs and cats will not eat their food after water has been added. To improve their acceptance of added moisture only a small amount of water should be added intially. This amount can be gradually increased over several days to weeks. If there is food left behind, it should be discarded after 30 minutes to reduce the risk of bacterial contamination [34].

Using lower calorie treat options such as vegetables or fruits provide a solution to preserve the interaction while at the same time reducing calories. Activities where food is used as a reward, such as training or behavior modification, may also be an important factor for some families when considering creating a diet plan. Finding high reward, but low-calorie treats can be a solution. Some commercial cat treats are 1 to 2 kcal per treat and are often highly palatable to both dogs and cats. Giving guidance on the precise number of calories that can come from treats and including favorite treats whenever possible can improve compliance. Calories coming from treats should not exceed 10% of the total daily caloric intake.

Durable food timers may help prevent destructive behavior aimed at obtaining food and food puzzles or toys can increase mental stimulation and positive foraging behavior [58]. Food puzzles have also been shown to encourage weight loss, slow the rate of food intake, as well as provide enrichment in companion animals [59,60]. It is important to try several different types of food puzzles to determine what the pet is most interested in as well has discussing expectations with the pet owner. For example, if a mobile food puzzle is used, dry food may end up throughout the house. If this is not acceptable from the owner's standpoint, then a stationary food puzzle may be more appropriate. It is also possible that over time the cat or dog will lose interest in the puzzle; therefore, it may be helpful to consider using different types of puzzles, moving the puzzle to a new location, or introduce a puzzle that is more difficult to get food from [61].

Overcoming veterinary related hurdles

Time limitations may reduce the thoroughness of the diet history. One solution is to have owners fill out a diet history before they arrive or while they are waiting. There are several resources that provide a template for this purpose; one example is World Small Animal Veterinary Association short diet history form that may help the practitioner standardize the history-taking process and saving time during the appointment [https://wsava.org/wp-content/uploads/2020/01/Diet-History-Form.pdf].

It may be that weight loss discussions would need to be postponed if the pet is healthy or if the owner is not yet ready for this. Weight loss discussions and follow-up can also be delegated to other members of the veterinary team that may be trained to monitor patients undergoing weight loss to help decrease the time commitment by the veterinarian. The weight management team can be responsible for questions, weigh-ins, and arranging a follow-up plan. However, if the weight loss is not occurring as expected, the veterinarian should be consulted for diet adjustment recommendations.

Most veterinarians do not care for difficult conversations with clients. However, most owners ultimately appreciate a candid and factual discussion done

compassionately. Creating a partnership and utilizing valuable communication skills can help:
Eliciting the client's perspective:
"How do you feel about Fluffy's weight?"
Asking permission:
"I am concerned about Fluffy's weight, is that something you would be willing to discuss today?"

From the 2 questions above, the veterinarian can receive valuable insight on the clients understanding of their pet's weight as well as if they are willing to address it. If the client does not feel their dog or cat is overweight, most of the conversation may be directed toward helping the client understand the physical examination findings that indicate there is excess body fat. If the client is aware their pet is overweight but they do not feel ready to address it, then more effort may be invested in understanding why. Understanding the obstacles the owner is facing can help the veterinary care team to provide the necessary support.
"What concerns do you have about a weight loss plan for Fluffy?"
"I understand you do not feel a weight loss plan will work for Fluffy, can you tell me more about your concerns?"

Physical activity and weight loss plan

Physical activity promotes health in people by increasing energy expenditure and supporting lean body mass anabolism, which are important particularly during weight loss [62]. Furthermore, exercise may help improve metabolic abnormalities that are associated with obesity, even without changes in percentage of body fat [63]. This suggests that even if an ideal body condition is not achieved, exercise could lead to an improvement in the pet's quality of life and overall health. It has been shown that as the time dedicated to exercise increases per week, there is a decreased risk of obesity in dogs, therefore discussing exercise during young dog and young cat wellness visits could have a benefit [64]. One study that looked at dietary energy intake and physical activity in dogs determined that increased activity was associated with increased energy intake but the dogs were still able to maintain weight loss goals [65]. In a prospective study looking at dogs undergoing a weight loss program, lean body mass was preserved in the group of dogs that participated in an exercise plan along with caloric restriction, whereas the group with caloric restriction alone lost lean body mass [66]. However, exercise without caloric restriction is usually inadequate for successful weight loss [67]. For example, in a study looking at exercise and weight loss in 5 healthy men, 80% reduction in

fat mass while maintaining lean body mass was achieved by exercising 6 days a week, twice a day at 55% of their VO_2 max [68]. Studies looking at the effects of exercise on weight loss in dogs are limited; however, evidence suggests that a formal exercise plan in combination with client education may improve the rate of weight loss [67].

Veterinarians play an important role in the connection among human, animal, and environmental health, also known as One Health [46]. Because lack of physical inactivity in people has been identified as a risk factor for overall morbidity and mortality and is considered a leading threat to human health globally, dog ownership is associated with increased physical activity [69,70]. Several studies indicate that encouraging physical activity with a dog may help promote physical activity and wellness for the owner [71–73].

It is vital to consider the dog owner's medical conditions if any, as well as their fitness level. Certainly, any medical conditions the dog or cat may have will also affect their ability to perform physical activities such as walking, playing, swimming, and physical therapy.

SUMMARY

A successful weight loss plan requires a multifaceted approach considering the environmental factors as well as the pet's medical history. Early understanding of pet, owner, and veterinarian-related limiting factors can help increase the chances of success. This can be achieved with a thorough diet history and by eliciting the client's perspective, which may help the veterinary care team to gain valuable insights into obstacles to weight loss.

An individualized diet plan designed to meet the unique needs of the pet as well as the owner and their household should include specific feeding guidelines, as well as a follow-up plan to ensure a successful outcome. It is important to acknowledge that weight loss is challenging but a challenge nonetheless that must be faced head-on to improve the quality of life of the pet and prevent concurrent disease.

CLINICS CARE POINTS

1. When discussing pet obesity with pet owners, veterinarians should consider the individual circumstances of the owner and their household in order to identify possible hurdles to weight loss.

2. Reinforcing unwanted begging behaviors can jeopardize the success of the weight loss plan.
3. A therapeutic weight loss diet is highly recommended to minimize the risk of nutritional deficiencies that may occur when food amount is restricted.
4. Follow-up and caloric intake adjustments are paramount to help pets reach their target bodyweight.

DISCLOSURE

J. Stockman is a consultant for Petco Health and Wellness Company, Inc. and for Mars PetCare. He has received research grants from Royal Canin and from Hill's Pet Nutrition Inc. C. Torres is a consultant for Healthy Pet Advisory Council and Mars Petcare and a board member of Pet Nutrition Alliance. She has recieved research grants from Nestle Purina Pet Care

REFERENCES

[1] Courcier E, Thomson R, Mellor D, et al. An epidemiological study of environmental factors associated with canine obesity. J Small Anim Pract 2010;51:362–7.
[2] Courcier EA, O'Higgins R, Mellor DJ, et al. Prevalence and risk factors for feline obesity in a first opinion practice in Glasgow, Scotland. J Feline Med Surg 2010;12:746–53.
[3] Cave N, Allan F, Schokkenbroek S, et al. A cross-sectional study to compare changes in the prevalence and risk factors for feline obesity between 1993 and 2007 in New Zealand. Prev Vet Med 2012;107:121–33.
[4] Kluess HA, Jones RL, Lee-Fowler T. Perceptions of body condition, diet and exercise by sports dog owners and pet dog owners. Animals 2021;11:1752.
[5] Corbee RJ. Obesity in show dogs. J Anim Physiol N 2013;97:904–10.
[6] Corbee RJ. Obesity in show cats. J Anim Physiol N 2014;98:1075–80.
[7] Appleton D, Rand J, Sunvold G. Insulin sensitivity decreases with obesity, and lean cats with low insulin sensitivity are at greatest risk of glucose intolerance with weight gain. J Feline Med Surg 2001;3:211–28.
[8] Verkest K, Fleeman L, Morton J, et al. Compensation for obesity-induced insulin resistance in dogs: assessment of the effects of leptin, adiponectin, and glucagon-like peptide-1 using path analysis. Domest Anim Endocrinol 2011;41:24–34.
[9] Slingerland L, Hazewinkel H, Meij B, et al. Cross-sectional study of the prevalence and clinical features of osteoarthritis in 100 cats. Vet J 2011;187:304–9.
[10] O'Neill DG, Church DB, McGreevy PD, et al. Prevalence of disorders recorded in dogs attending primary-care veterinary practices in England. PLoS One 2014;9:e90501.
[11] Marshall W, Bockstahler B, Hulse D, et al. A review of osteoarthritis and obesity: current understanding of the relationship and benefit of obesity treatment and prevention in the dog. Vet Comp Orthopaedics Traumatol 2009;22:339–45.
[12] Impellizeri JA, Tetrick MA, Muir P. Effect of weight reduction on clinical signs of lameness in dogs with hip osteoarthritis. J Am Vet Med Assoc 2000;216:1089–91.
[13] Thengchaisri N, Theerapun W, Kaewmokul S, et al. Abdominal obesity is associated with heart disease in dogs. BMC Vet Res 2014;10:1–7.
[14] Kealy R, Lawler D, Ballam J, et al. Effects of diet restriction on life span and age-related changes in dogs. J Am Vet Med Assoc 2002;220:1315–20.
[15] Raffan E, Dennis Rowena J, O'Donovan Conor J, et al. A deletion in the canine POMC gene is associated with weight and appetite in obesity-prone labrador retriever dogs. Cell Metab 2016;23:893–900.
[16] Kronfeld DS, Donoghue S, Glickman LT. Body condition and energy intakes of dogs in a referral teaching hospital. J Nutr 1991;121:S157–8.
[17] Lund EM, Armstrong P, Kirk CA, et al. Prevalence and risk factors for obesity in adult cats from private US veterinary practices. Intern J Appl Res Vet Med 2005;3:88–96.
[18] Pegram C, Raffan E, White E, et al. Frequency, breed predisposition and demographic risk factors for overweight status in dogs in the UK. J Small Anim Pract 2021;62(7):521–30.
[19] Colliard L, Paragon B-M, Lemuet B, et al. Prevalence and risk factors of obesity in an urban population of healthy cats. J Feline Med Surg 2009;11(2):135–40.
[20] Kienzle E, Moik K. A pilot study of the body weight of pure-bred client-owned adult cats. Br J Nutr 2011;106:S113–5.
[21] Chu K, Anderson WM, Rieser MY. Population characteristics and neuter status of cats living in households in the United States. J Am Vet Med Assoc 2009;234:1023–30.
[22] Trevejo R, Yang M, Lund EM. Epidemiology of surgical castration of dogs and cats in the United States. J Am Vet Med Assoc 2011;238:898–904.
[23] Jeusette I, Detilleux J, Cuvelier C, et al. Ad libitum feeding following ovariectomy in female Beagle dogs: effect on maintenance energy requirement and on blood metabolites. J Anim Physiol N 2004;88:117–21.
[24] Flynn M, Hardie E, Armstrong P. Effect of ovariohysterectomy on maintenance energy requirement in cats. J Am Vet Med Assoc 1996;209:1572–81.
[25] Pedrinelli V, Porsani MYH, Lima DM, et al. Predictive equations of maintenance energy requirement for healthy and chronically ill adult dogs. J Anim Physiol N 2019;105(S2):63–9.
[26] Bermingham EN, Thomas DG, Cave NJ, et al. Energy requirements of adult dogs: a meta-analysis. PLoS One 2014;9:e109681.
[27] Wei A, Fascetti AJ, Kim K, et al. Early effects of neutering on energy expenditure in adult male cats. PLoS One 2014;9:e89557.

[28] Bjørnvad C, Gloor S, Johansen S, et al. Neutering increases the risk of obesity in male dogs but not in bitches—A cross-sectional study of dog-and owner-related risk factors for obesity in Danish companion dogs. Prev Vet Med 2019;170:104730.

[29] Salt C, Morris PJ, Butterwick RF, et al. Comparison of growth patterns in healthy dogs and dogs in abnormal body condition using growth standards. PLoS One 2020;15:e0238521.

[30] Laflamme D. Development and validation of a body condition score system for cats: a clinical tool. (Santa Barbara, Calif: 1990)(USA): Feline practice; 1997.

[31] Laflamme D. Development and validation of a body condition score system for dogs. Canine Pract 1997; 22(4):10–5.

[32] Coe JB, Rankovic A, Edwards TR, et al. Dog owner's accuracy measuring different volumes of dry dog food using three different measuring devices. Vet Rec 2019;185:599.

[33] Kleiber M. The Fire of Life: an Introduction to Animal Energetics. New York: Wiley; 1961.

[34] Thatcher C, Hand MS, Thatcher CD, et al. Small animal clinical nutrition: an iterative process Small Animal Clinical Nutrition. 4th. Topeka, KS: Mark Morris Institute; 2000. p. 1–19.

[35] Diez M, Nguyen P, Jeusette I, et al. Weight loss in obese dogs: evaluation of a high-protein, low-carbohydrate diet. J Nutr 2002;132:1685S–7S.

[36] National Research Council (NRC). Nutrient requirements of dogs and cats. Washington, DC: National Academies Press; 2006.

[37] Linder DE, Freeman LM, Morris P, et al. Theoretical evaluation of risk for nutritional deficiency with caloric restriction in dogs. Vet Quart 2012;32:123–9.

[38] Model regulations for pet food and spefty pet food under the model bill. Association of American Feed Control Officials: In: 2019 Official Publication, 2019.

[39] Keller E, Sagols E, Flanagan J, et al. Use of reduced-energy content maintenance diets for modest weight reduction in overweight cats and dogs. Res Vet Sci 2020;131: 194–205.

[40] Mars Petcare, 2018. Survey weighs up potential reasons behind the pet obesity crisis. [Online] Available at: https://www.waltham.com/news-events/nutrition/survey-reasons-pet-obesity [Accessed 6 2 2022].

[41] German AJ, Blackwell E, Evans M, et al. Overweight dogs exercise less frequently and for shorter periods: results of a large online survey of dog owners from the UK. J Nutr Sci 2017;6:e11.

[42] Coe J. A focus group study of veterinarians' and pet owners' perceptions of veterinarian-client communication in companion animal practice. J Am Vet Med 2008;233:1072–80.

[43] Dysart L. Analysis of solicitation of client concerns in companion animal practice. J Amer Vet Med 2011;238: 1609–15.

[44] Kanji N. Effect of veterinarian-client-patient interactions on client adherence to dentistry and surgery recommendations in companion-animal practice. J Am Vet Med Assoc 2012;240:427–36.

[45] Janke N. Pet owners' and veterinarians' perceptions of information exchange and clinical decision-making in companion animal practice. PLoS One 2021;16:e0245632.

[46] Kedrowicz A. A comparison of public perceptions of physicians and veterinarians in the United States. Vet Sci 2020;7:50.

[47] Pearl RL, Wadden TA, Bach C, et al. Who's a good boy? Effects of dog and owner body weight on veterinarian perceptions and treatment recommendations. Int J Obes 2020;44:2455–64.

[48] Churchill, J., 2010. Vetlearn.com. [Online] Available at: https://scholar.google.com/scholar_lookup?title=Increase%20the%20success%20of%20weight%20loss%20programs%20by%20creating%20an%20environment%20for%20change&publication_year=2010&author=J.%20Churchill. Accessed 2 February 2022.

[49] Linder D. Pet obesity management: beyond nutrition. Vet Clin North Am Small Anim Pract 2014;44(4): 789–806.

[50] Santarossa A, Parr JM, Verbrugghe A. Assessment of canine and feline body composition by veterinary health care teams in Ontario, Canada. Can Vet J 2018;59: 1280–6.

[51] White G. Canine obesity: is there a difference between veterinarian and owner perception? J Small Anim Pract 2011;52:622–6.

[52] Cline M. 2021 AAHA Nutrition and Weight Management. J Am Anim Hosp Assoc 2021;57:153–78.

[53] Krasuska M. How effective are interventions designed to help owners to change their behaviour so as to manage the weight of their companion dogs? A systematic review and meta-analysis. Prev Vet Med 2018;159: 40–50.

[54] Houseknecht K. The biology of leptin: a review. J Anim Sci 1998;76:1405–20.

[55] Kil D. Endocrinology of obesity. Vet Clin Small Anim 2010;40:205–19.

[56] Flanagan J. Success of a weight loss plan for overweight. PLoS One 2017. https://doi.org/10.1371/journal.pone.0184199.

[57] Butterwick R. Advances in dietary management of obesity in dogs and cats. J Nutr 1998;128:2771S–5S.

[58] Schipper L. The effect of feeding enrichment toys on the behaviour of kennelled dogs (Canis familiaris). Appl Anim Behav Sci 2008;114:182–95.

[59] German. Cohort Study of the Success of Controlled Weight Loss Programs for Obese Dogs. J Vet Intern Med 2015;29(6):1547–55.

[60] Clarke D. Using environmental and feeding enrichment to facilitate feline weight loss 2005.

[61] Dantas L. Food puzzles for cats: feeding for physical and emotional wellbeing. J Feline Med Surg 2016;18:723–32.

[62] JM Jakicic AO. Physical activity considerations for the treatment and prevention of obesity. Am J Clin Nutr 2005;82:226–9.

[63] P Roudebush WS, Delaney SJ. An evidence-based review of the use of therapeutic foods, owner education, exercise, and drugs for the management of obese and overweight pets. J Am Vet Med Assoc 2008;233:717–25.

[64] Robertson I. The association of exercise, diet and other factors with owner-perceived obesity in privately owned dogs from metropolitan Perth, WA. Prev Vet Med 2003; 58:75–83.

[65] Wakshlag J. Evaluation of dietary energy intake and physical activity in dogs undergoing a controlled weight-loss program. J Am Vet Med Assoc 2012;240:413–9.

[66] Vitger A. Integration of a physical training program in a weight loss plan for overweight pet dogs. J Am Vet Med Assoc 2016;248:174–82.

[67] Chauvet A. Incorporation of exercise, using an underwater treadmill, and active client education into a weight management program for obese dogs. Can Vet J 2011; 52:491–6.

[68] Bouchard C. Long-term exercise training with constant energy intake. 1: Effect on body composition and selected metabolic variables. Int J Obes 1990;14:57–73.

[69] Christian H. Dog ownership and physical activity: a review of the evidence. J Phys Act Health 2013;10:750–9.

[70] Thornton J. Physical activity prescription: a critical opportunity to address a modifiable risk factor for the prevention and management of chronic disease: a position statement by the Canadian Academy of Sport and Exercise Medicine. Br J Sports Med 2016;26(4):259–65.

[71] Johnson R. Dog-walking: motivation for adherence to a walking program. Clin Nurs Res 2012;19:387–402.

[72] Ham SA, Epping J. Dog walking and physical activity in the United States. Prev Chronic Dis 2006;3(2):A47.

[73] Westgarth C. Dog owners are more likely to meet physical activity guidelines than people without a dog: an investigation of the association between dog ownership and physical activity levels in a UK community. Sci Rep 2019;9(1):5704.

Moving?

Make sure your subscription moves with you!

To notify us of your new address, find your **Clinics Account Number** (located on your mailing label above your name), and contact customer service at:

Email: journalscustomerservice-usa@elsevier.com

800-654-2452 (subscribers in the U.S. & Canada)
314-447-8871 (subscribers outside of the U.S. & Canada)

Fax number: 314-447-8029

Elsevier Health Sciences Division
Subscription Customer Service
3251 Riverport Lane
Maryland Heights, MO 63043

*To ensure uninterrupted delivery of your subscription, please notify us at least 4 weeks in advance of move.

Printed and bound by CPI Group (UK) Ltd, Croydon, CR0 4YY

08/05/2025

01864713-0007